Reading:

A selection of papers edited
and with introd
Jessie F. Re

Ward Lock Educational

ISBN 0 7062 3344 1 hardbound
ISBN 0 7062 3122 8 paperback

This collection © Ward Lock Educational 1972.

Set in 10 on 11 point Monotype Baskerville
by Richard Clay (The Chaucer Press), Ltd.,
Bungay, Suffolk
for Ward Lock Educational
116 Baker Street, London w1m 2bb
Made in England

Contents

Contents

4

Acknowledgments

The publishers would like to thank the following for permission to reproduce copyright material:
Advisory Centre for Education and John E. Merritt for 'What is reading readiness?' from *Where?* (1970) 49; American Academy of Cerebral Palsy and T. T. S. Ingram, A. W. Mason and I. Blackburn for 'A retrospective study of 82 children with reading disability' from *Developmental Medicine and Child Neurology* (1970) 12, 3; Appleton-Century-Crofts and G. L. Bond and M. A. Tinker for 'Basic principles of remedial instruction' from *Reading Difficulties: Their Diagnosis and Correction* (1957); 'Learning in the disadvantaged' by Cynthia P. Deutsch, from *The Disadvantaged Child*, edited by Martin Deutsch and Associates. © by Martin Deutsch, Basic Books Inc. Publishers, New York; Vernon, M. D. *Reading and its Difficulties* © 1971, Cambridge University Press; Centre for Research in Educational Sciences, University of Edinburgh for 'Children's comprehension of syntactic features found in some extension readers' (1972); the Controller of Her Majesty's Stationery Office for 'Children with specific reading difficulties', paras 2–10 from the *Tizard Report* (1972); Educational and Psychological Measurement and Selma G. Sapir and Bernice Wilson for 'A developmental scale to assist in the prevention of learning disability' from *Educational and Psychological Measurement* (1967) 27; International Reading Association and Charlotte Sonenberg and Gerald Glass for 'Reading and speech: an incidence and treatment study' from *The Reading Teacher* (1965), December; Invalid Children's Aid Association and Gill Cotterell for 'Teaching procedures' from A. W. Franklin and S. Naidoo (eds) *Assessment and Teaching of Dyslexic Children* (1970); S. Karger AG and H. Lytton for 'Some psychological and sociological characteristics of "good" and "poor" achievers (boys) in remedial reading groups: clinical case studies' from *Human Development* (1968) 11; S. Karger AG and M. L. Kellmer Pringle and V. Bossio 'A study of deprived children, part 2: Language development and reading attainment' from *Vita Humana* (1958) 1; Longman and M. Rutter and W. Yule for 'Reading retardation and antisocial behaviour—the nature of the association' and M. Rutter, J. Tizard and K. Whitmore for 'Implications for services: a postscript to the surveys' from *Education, Health and Behaviour* (1970); Longman and D. Mackay, B. Thompson and P. Shaub for 'Breakthrough to Literacy in the remedial situation' a revised version of chapter 9 from *Breakthrough to Literacy Teacher's Manual* (1970); Davenport Plumer and Markham Publishing Company, *Language and Poverty* by F. Williams, selection by D. Plumer; National Foundation for Educational

Acknowledgments

Research for 'Dyslexia: a problem of communication' from *Educational Research* (1969) 10, 2; John Downing 'ita and slow learners: a reappraisal' from *Educational Research* (1969) 11, 3; D. Lawrence 'The effects of counselling on retarded readers' from *Educational Research* (1971) 13, 2; Asher Cashdan and P. D. Pumfrey 'Some effects of the remedial teaching of reading' from *Educational Research* (1969) 11, 2; N. J. Georgiades for 'An experiment with ita in remedial reading' from *New Education* (1967) September; A. E. G. Pilliner for 'The definition and measurement of reading problems'; Professional Press and K. Wedell for 'Diagnosing learning difficulties: a sequential strategy' from *Journal of Learning Disabilities* (1970) 3, 6; Routledge and Kegan Paul and Geoffrey R. Roberts for 'A method to meet the needs of backward readers' from *Reading in Primary Schools* (1969); Routledge and Kegan Paul and A. E. Tansley for 'Reading failure: its causes and prevention' from *Reading and Remedial Reading* (1967); Scottish Academic Press and Sandhya Naidoo for 'Specific developmental dyslexia' from the *British Journal of Educational Psychology* (1971) 31; Tavistock Publications Limited and Margaret Donaldson for 'The prediction of ability' from *A Study of Children's Thinking* (1963); United Kingdom Reading Association and the following authors: M. L. Kellmer Pringle for 'Language development and reading attainment of deprived children', Geoffrey R. Roberts for 'Implications of recent research for teaching techniques' both from *Reading: Influences on Progress* (1969); Asher Cashdan for 'Backward readers—research on auditory-visual integration' from *Reading Skills: Theory and Practice* (1970); Gilbert R. Gredler for 'Severe reading disability—some important correlates', David Mackay for 'The materials' reprinted from 'Breakthrough to Literacy' both from *Reading and the Curriculum* (1971); Alan Little, Christine Mabey and Jennifer Russell for 'Class size, pupil characteristics and reading attainment', John E. Merritt for 'Reading failure: a reexamination', David V. Moseley for 'The English Colour Code programmed reading course' all from *Literacy at all levels* (1972); University of Chicago Press and Helen Robinson for 'Emotional and personality problems of severely retarded readers' from *Why Pupils Fail in Reading* (1946) © Helen Robinson 1946.

Foreword

Efforts to simplify the learning of reading go back several hundred years. The consciousness that reading problems can exist is therefore in that sense not a new phenomenon. However, reading difficulties have been given fresh importance within this century because of changes in society. Some of these changes have been social and political. For instance, the introduction of universal primary education in 1870 in England, and 1872 in Scotland, exposed the entire population of five and six year olds to the task of learning to read and write in a way that had never been done before. This innovation represented a change in society's view of equality of opportunity, but a change which brought its own problems. The most recent manifestations of this kind of social concern have been the findings of the Plowden Committee and the designating of Educational Priority Areas, and more recently still the decision by the Secretary of State for Education and Science to set up a nationwide inquiry into reading attainment. A second type of change has consisted in an increase in the need for literacy arising from the demands of bureaucratic government. Many of these demands are of course the result of better social services, but they are demands which the less than literate adult is often unable to meet. Yet another kind of change is that which results from a shorter working week and increased leisure. People are becoming conscious that those who cannot turn to books to fill part of their extra amount of spare time will sometimes turn to pursuits which are not very desirable.

Another source of fresh importance has been the growing study of human ability. We now know a great deal more than we did seventy or eighty years ago about the ways in which human intelligence develops and functions and about the range of individual differences to be found when different intellectual capacities are measured. Techniques of measurement have also multiplied and diversified, though with the result that there is perhaps more scepticism about the measurement of intelligence now than there was seventy years ago.

There have been changes too in educational practice. The use which is made of literacy in the school has changed very much in the last century in that pupils are now much more likely to be given the task of finding something out for themselves from books than they are to be told it in a manner which simply requires them to be passive listeners. In addition, the rise of the school psychological services and of the medical disciplines of developmental neurology and child psychiatry has given a new impetus to the study of individual cases of severe reading difficulty.

This book of readings is intended as an overview of the main parts of this large field of social, professional and political concern. It begins with a section in which reading problems are defined and the most recent evidence as to their scope surveyed. Then follow two sections on correlates and causes. The first of these deals with correlates of social and emotional origin and the second with the difficult and controversial topic of developmental reading disability. The next section looks at some current views of diagnosis, assessment and treatment, and the final section at some of the fields which seem to offer the best hope for effective prevention. Within each section an attempt has been made to put the papers in an order which follows some sort of logical sequence, but they can obviously be studied in any order a reader may choose.

Because of limitations of space there is no separate section devoted to writing problems. The intimate connection between the receptive and expressive sides of literacy has however been recognized in many of the papers, and there is certainly no suggestion that reading should be regarded as an isolated function.

E. B. Huey called the evolution of literacy 'the most remarkable, specific performance that civilization has learned in all its history'. It is hoped that this collection of papers will help to throw some light on those many performers who for one reason or another have failed to learn their parts.

REFERENCES AND FURTHER READING

Throughout this volume references have been printed at the end of individual papers. Works which it is felt would be of particular benefit for further reading have been marked with an asterisk in these reference lists. In addition it will of course be appropriate for the reader to consult the books from which extracts have been taken. A further brief bibliography of recommended books not mentioned elsewhere in the text appears at the end of the volume.

1 Definition and scope of the problem of reading failure

Introduction

In studying any problem it is important to begin by asking the following questions:

1   What are we talking about?
2   What concepts are we operating with?
3   What terminology has been and is in use to talk about these concepts?
4   Given that we have defined the phenomena in which we are interested, what is the extent and severity of the problem they represent?

The first set of papers in this volume is concerned with these questions.

The conception of 'a reading problem' as a discrepancy between performance and potential is the basis for the whole enterprise of remedial and preventive work in literacy. It is appropriate therefore that the first paper should be one which deals with some aspects of the concept of potential and its nonrealization. The paper is not specifically about attainment in reading, but this is irrelevant. It is about those underlying assumptions concerning attainment of any kind without which none of the studies of diagnosis, treatment and prevention of reading problems would make any sense.

The second paper, which is in two sections, follows on from the discussion by Donaldson by looking first at the terminology in most common use in the field of reading, and at the conceptual distinctions which the terms have been used to make—distinctions which indicate how some other writers have viewed the intelligence/attainment relationship. Some of the main sources of confusion are pointed out, but no glossary, however exhaustive, can be a substitute for a careful scrutiny of the context in which any term is used in a particular instance. The second part of the paper deals with problems of measurement, especially as they relate to the conceptual problems already discussed.

The third paper is a collation of information from recent surveys and studies of reading. It presents the main facts and figures in terms of which action—remedial and preventive—is seen to be necessary.

1.1 The prediction of ability

MARGARET DONALDSON

Department of Psychology, University of Edinburgh

Reprinted from Margaret Donaldson (1963) *A Study of Children's Thinking*
Tavistock Publications, pp. 1–9

We are all constantly making predictions. We predict that there will soon be snow; or that we shall not reach home before we run out of petrol; or that the government will be defeated at the next election. Also, however, we make predictions of a slightly different kind. We say, for instance: 'Listen to that noise! There must be a mouse gnawing at the wood.' This last example is different from the others in that we are here not really foretelling the future, except in so far as we are predicting what we should find if we were to look to see; and it would be possible to argue that this should not be called prediction at all. But it is important to realize that many of the predictions of science are of this latter kind. The laws of science often do not tell us about sequences of events following one another in time, so that knowledge of earlier ones enables us to predict later ones, but rather about interrelated happenings, so that knowledge of one enables us to know about others that are occurring at the same moment.

An analogy may help to make this point clearer. In recent years people have begun to study seriously what is now called 'extrasensory perception' —that is, awareness of things which have not been directly perceived by the senses—and it is claimed that there are two cases to be distinguished. One of these is 'precognition' or knowledge of events which have not yet happened. This is the counterpart of what many people think of as the only type of scientific prediction. But there is also 'clairvoyance' which is claimed to consist in a knowledge of events or states of affairs that are contemporary but inaccessible to the normal organs of sense-perception. And this has its scientific counterpart as well.

It may seem a little fanciful to speak of science as an instrument of extrasensory perception—and yet this, in a way, is what it is. It enables us to know about things and events which we have not perceived directly. And it has its 'clairvoyant' as well as its 'precognitive' side. In the former case, what is predicted is that if you look to see you will observe that some specified event is occurring or has occurred or that some specified relationships hold. It is then only the looking to see which is in the future.

In the scientific study of human behaviour we are concerned, as in all science, with prediction. Here, as elsewhere, attention has tended to concentrate in the past on precognitive prediction. It may be that in this study the clairvoyant types of prediction will prove to be of particular importance. Perhaps some of the greatest practical consequences will rest in the end on increases in our ability to make inferences about a present state of affairs from rather limited evidence.

Within the class of precognitive predictions, there is a distinction to be made that deserves attention. This is the distinction which Karl Popper (1957) has drawn between what he calls the 'prophetic' and the 'technological' or 'conditional' predictions. The prophetic predictions are the foretellings of things which it is beyond our power to prevent or control, such as the coming of a typhoon. The technological predictions, by contrast, tell us by what means a given event can be brought about: they tell us what we must do if we want to achieve something. Popper's own example of a conditional or technological prediction is the statement that if we want to build a shelter to withstand the force of a typhoon we must build it in a certain way.

When Popper makes this distinction he is discussing and criticizing notions of history as a process of inevitable unfolding about which only prophetic predictions can be made. However, not only the history of mankind but also the individual history of each one of us has been held by some people to be, in certain respects at least, an inevitable unfolding. And there is nothing of which this has been claimed more forcibly than the development of intelligence.

The great early advocate of this view was Francis Galton. In 1869 he published his book *Hereditary Genius*, the main argument of which was that intelligence is largely independent of environmental variation and that in each one of us its development is governed by hereditary constitution.

But, of course, if the *whole* of our intellectual development were inevitably determined from the start, much of education as we know it would be superfluous. If, then, a prophetic view of intelligence is to be reconciled with the retention of schools, a distinction has to be drawn between what can be prophesied and what cannot; and this has commonly been done by means of the distinction between intelligence and attainment. Galton himself did not make much of this distinction, and indeed he came near at times to expressing the opinion that education *was* superfluous, at least for the most able; but those who have come after him and who have agreed with him in his conception of intelligence have for the most part seen attainment as subject to a limited measure of conditional prediction, the limitation being imposed by intelligence. Intelligence is then regarded as the 'innate potential', that which makes attainment possible. Education has only to make it actual—and can, indeed, do no more.

This view is much less widely held than it used to be and many educationists and psychologists seriously mistrust it; but it still underlies much educational thinking in Britain and in the United States. It is a curious fact that the country which is at present most influenced by a conception of history as an inevitable unfolding—namely, the Soviet Union—is much less influenced than Western countries by a similar conception of the development of the individual.

We might ask what is the evidence one way or the other? And this question has been asked repeatedly. It may be more illuminating, however, to begin by asking not what evidence we possess but what evidence we would be justified in accepting as conclusive proof of inevitability; for the answer to this question may perhaps determine how efforts to get evidence ought to be directed.

For this purpose, let us suppose first of all that arguments about how to test intelligence were settled, so that no difficulties of measurement would be complicating the issue. What sort of evidence would we then require?

It turns out that this question is hard to answer. It would not be enough for our purpose to have evidence that one set of environmental variations had not affected the issue—not enough, for instance, to know that a pair of identical twins, reared in different environments from infancy and tested in adulthood, had proved in the end to be of very similar intelligence. It would not even be enough to know that a very considerable number of different sets of variations had not caused intelligence to vary. (This is not in any way intended as a summary of the results of actual inquiries of this kind. We are considering here not what evidence is available but what evidence would be necessary.) For the claim we are considering is that *nothing* in the way of environmental variation (given, of course, an environment sufficiently favourable to sustain life) can cause intelligence to vary—and this is a very big claim. J. B. S. Haldane (1955) has remarked that if we make a claim of this kind we are behaving rather like the physicists of a century ago who called certain gases 'permanent', meaning by this that they could not be liquefied. It turned out in the event that these gases were no more 'permanent' than any others: it was merely that the physicists who so described them did not know how to liquefy them. When they said the gases could not be liquefied they were describing their own incapacity.

Environmental variations that might conceivably affect intelligence are of so many different kinds that the task of testing their effects, even by very limited sampling, would present enormous problems and has certainly never been attempted. But even if it were done—and this is the point which most needs to be stressed—no evidence that development was unaffected by fortuitous environmental variation could ever establish the impossibility of affecting it by deliberate action in the light of real understanding. The history of the physicists and the gases is again relevant. The discovery of impermanence did not come in the end through a random sampling of all the innumerable possible conditions that might affect gases: it came as all discoveries come (though sometimes chance helps them) through careful research and the gradual growth of knowledge. In the same way we shall discover, if we ever do discover, how to affect the development of intelligence. But meantime, there is no justification at all, and it is hard to see how there ever could be justification, for a claim that its development is inevitably predetermined and entirely beyond our control. (This is not at all the same as saying that heredity contributes nothing or only a little to the development.)

It is worth noting that this argument amounts to a rejection of any absolute and final distinction between things which can be conditionally predicted and those which can be prophesied, given that the criterion of a prophecy is our inability to affect the issue. This is because we can never be sure that our inability is final, and consequently anything which at one time admits only of prophetic prediction may come, with advance in our understanding, into some possibility of control. Popper would presumably accept this, because it is part of his own argument that the progress of our knowledge is itself something we can never predict. Thus it cannot be maintained that there is anything which we can never come to know —except for this one limit: that we cannot know what we shall know.

If the above arguments are sound, we must cease to claim that intelligence is innately determined—if by this we mean that environment cannot affect the issue. (There are, of course, very few people who would want to make this extreme claim. Our concern is not so much to refute this claim, as to show what are the implications of accepting it as untenable.) In this case, though, what becomes of the distinction between intelligence and attainment? Clearly, the old basis for distinguishing the two has gone. On the view that intelligence was 'innate potential', its relation to attainment was that of 'rendering possible'. But if we are not prepared to assert that the whole development of intelligence is innately determined, can we still hold to the view that intelligence is in some sense 'potential', or must we abandon that conception also? Can we give up trying to distinguish between what is 'innate' and what is 'acquired', yet still keep the distinction between 'intelligence' and 'attainment' and the notion that the one 'makes possible' the other?

There are two circumstances which would lead many people to give a negative answer to this question. In the first place, there is the old habitual association of the words 'innate' and 'potential'. These two have been used together so regularly and for so long now that their inseparability is liable to be taken for granted. When words come to be linked in this way, it grows easy after a while to slip into the unreflecting assumption that the one notion implies the other, so that the possibility of retaining one and rejecting the other is not even considered.

But there is a second reason why the idea of intelligence as potential is in danger of rejection. There is a current tendency to have misgivings about the whole concept of potential ability and its value for any scientific study. This appears to arise from the idea that whatever is potential is quite unobservable, an idea which is seriously, and curiously, mistaken. We are constantly observing potential. When we say of someone, 'He could be a strong swimmer, if he knew how', we are making a judgment of potential that is based on direct observation of physical characteristics such as well-developed muscles.

It is of more than incidental interest to notice that the distinction between potential and realized ability is more likely to be overlooked by an English speaker because of the fact that in his language the one word 'could' is used in both senses: 'He could be a strong swimmer, if he could swim', we might say, though we would tend to avoid this awkward juxta-position wherever possible. In the French language, however, the distinction is very neatly provided for by the words *pouvoir* and *savoir*. The English 'he cannot swim' is quite ambiguous. But the French clearly distinguish *il ne peut pas nager* (because of lack of potential, a radical incapacity) from *il ne sait pas nager* (because he has never learned, never realized his perfectly adequate potential for the achievement of this skill).

Now the question of whether the strength of a man's muscles is innately determined raises just the same difficulties as does the similar question about the development of his intelligence, and these we have already considered. What must now be observed is that our inability to prove the complete innateness of his muscle strength in no way prevents us from regarding that strength as potential. And we can regard it in this way without necessarily being in a position to say exactly what influences have been exerted on this development by the food he has eaten or the ways in which he has exercised his body. Our ignorance on these matters does not alter the fact that, in relation to the specific attainment of swimming, his muscles represent a potential of unrealized ability.

In a similar way, the concept of intelligence as potential ability is not necessarily bound to the concept of intelligence as innate, and we can perfectly well give up the latter without having to deny the notion that intelligence makes attainment possible.

There is, however, a difficulty still to be considered. In so far as intelli-gence is not an inevitable unfolding, it may very justly be claimed that it is itself a form of attainment. And if intelligence is allowed to be attain-ment, what becomes then of the distinction between the two?

This difficulty is not so great as it at first seems. The fact that man is an animal does not mean that we cannot distinguish him from other animals or that we may not sometimes be justified in using the word 'animal' in a way which contrasts with, instead of including, 'man'. Similarly, then, there may be certain sorts of attainment which, because of some dis-tinguishing features, can reasonably and usefully be given a special name: the name 'intelligence'. And it would be in keeping with traditional usage if this name were reserved for attainments which can be shown to be of special value for the clairvoyant and precognitive prediction of other attainments. But Ferguson (1954) expresses an important truth when he says: 'The concept of intelligence . . . is no longer a useful scientific concept except as subsuming some defined set of clearly distinguishable abilities.'

It has been argued so far that we cannot prove that the development of intelligence is a process of inevitable unfolding. At the same time, it has been pointed out that this is by no means equivalent to an assertion that heredity does not affect the issue or affects it only a little. A sensible suggestion by Hebb (1949), which has been fairly widely adopted and has done a great deal to clear up confusion, is that we assume the existence of a certain genetic complement which is relevant to the development of intellectual power. This we call Intelligence A. We acknowledge, however, from the beginning, that we cannot directly test Intelligence A—that is, innate capacity in the strict sense. What we can hope to measure with some success is Intelligence B—the individual's effective developed intelligence.

Now the practical implications of giving up all claim to be able to test Intelligence A are worthy of consideration. So long as we speak or think as if we aim to find out about innate capacity we shall be tempted to try to use our test results for long-term prediction—to forecast, for instance, when a child is eleven or younger how he will perform in an examination that is five or six years away; or to forecast when a student enters a university how he will do in his final examinations. This is because innate capacity is something which lends itself to prophetic prediction, and prophetic predictions tend to be (though, as Popper points out, they need not be) long-term ones. Obviously enough, if we think we are dealing with an inevitable unfolding, we shall feel justified in making predictions about the fairly remote future. But if, on the other hand, we conceive ourselves to be dealing with a potential ability which develops and increases in the measure in which it is realized, we shall not be so likely to proceed in this way, for we shall understand that the child's abilities five years from now may depend not only on his present state but on what happens to him—and on what he does—in the interval. Consequently, we shall realize that where there is any proposal to select a child for one kind of education rather than another, our prediction will affect its own fulfilment, for what the child's abilities will be five years from now may depend in some measure on what education we decide he is to have.

This sort of circumstance is one which all students of human behaviour have to be prepared to encounter, as Karl Popper points out. In the social sciences, he says, a prediction 'may in an extreme case even *cause* the happening it predicts: the happening might not have occurred at all if it had not been predicted'.

How, then, would it be reasonable to make use of tests of intelligence if it is allowed that the development of ability may not be wholly predetermined, and unaffected by our decisions or actions? The implication would seem to be that they should be used not so much for long-term as for very immediate prediction. It would be reasonable to use them to tell us what a child is ready to go on to *now*, to indicate whether we can expect him, in his present stage of development, to start successfully on this or that new attempt at learning. The importance of the tests would not be reduced by this way of regarding them, because an unsuccessful learning attempt can be very damaging, and we want to see that children are not asked to tackle something for which they are not fit. But it is important to notice that this way of looking at the tests would have the effect of emphasizing the notion of 'readiness' and suggesting that, although the child is not ready now, this need not be final: perhaps he could be ready in a year—or less—and perhaps, if we understood more of his difficulties, we could even help him towards that readiness. However, before we can hope to help him as effectively as possible, we must understand better than we do at present, and in much greater detail, how his powers of thinking develop.

References

FERGUSON, G. A. (1954) On learning and human ability *Canadian Journal of Psychology* 8

GALTON, F. (1869) *Hereditary Genius: An Inquiry into its Laws and Consequences* London: Macmillan; Collins Fontana 1962

HALDANE, J. B. S. (1955) A logical basis for genetics *British Journal for the Philosophy of Science* 6

HEBB, D. O. (1949) *The Organization of Behaviour* London: Chapman and Hall

POPPER, K. (1957) *The Poverty of Historicism* London: Routledge and Kegan Paul

1.2 The definition and measurement of reading problems

A. E. G. PILLINER and JESSIE F. REID

Centre for Research in Educational Sciences,
University of Edinburgh

First publication

One of the main aims in any field of study claiming to be scientific has always been to achieve a language which will be more precise and therefore more intelligible for scientific purposes than everyday language. It is very difficult, however, to create a technical language which will be both clear and consistent, and it is an ironic truth that in many instances communication has been hindered rather than assisted by the proliferation of terms which are either imperfectly defined or inconsistently used.

The field of reading is no exception. A certain amount of clarification is however possible. The first part of this paper sets forth the principal terms likely to be encountered in current literature on reading problems, together with some account of the ways in which the terms have chiefly been used. Many of the terms are of course concerned with questions of measurement, and for this reason the second section of the paper deals with problems in this area, and particularly with their relevance to the definition of certain key concepts.

Terminology

The terminological difficulties in the discussion of reading problems are of several kinds. One kind arises from the sheer diversity of terms used to talk about the problems. The other arises from the variety of ways in which certain of the terms have been defined, and this means, in many cases, ways in which the variables referred to are measured. The techniques used for this measurement assume that the attainment or 'learned behaviour' being measured forms a *continuum*—an unbroken gradation from zero to some unspecified upper limit. When we talk about this concept, the language we use has certain characteristics which sometimes cause confusion in communication. Take, for example, the continuum of extension in space in one dimension—what we call 'length' or 'width' if the extension is horizontal, 'height' if it is vertical upwards, and 'depth' if it is vertical downwards. These nouns, and the adjectives with which they are cognate, behave in a curious way. Each adjective is one of a *pair* of adjectives which we use to indicate extremes—short *long*; narrow *wide*; low *high*; shallow *deep*. But when asking the question 'how much?', we most commonly use the italicized one. We say 'How long is it?' 'How high is it?' and so on. In this case, the adjective becomes as it were neutral or 'nonpolar', in the same way as the nouns are 'nonpolar' in sentences like 'The *length* of the tiny fish is one centimetre.' The tiny fish is, relative to fishes in general, very *short*, but we do not say 'The shortness of the tiny fish is one centimetre.' We use the noun as the name of a dimension. And in this use it has no opposite.

The words we use to talk about the continuous dimensions in educational measurement behave in much the same way. We use the word 'intelligent' to indicate one pole of a continuum, and 'stupid' or 'unintelligent' to indicate the other. Yet we talk of measuring 'intelligence' and not 'stupidity' even when we are assessing a feeble-minded person, who would be described as 'of very low intelligence', not 'of very high stupidity'. We talk of an 'able reader' and a 'disabled reader' but we measure 'reading ability' or 'reading competence'. We talk of an 'illiterate man' and a 'literate man', but we assess 'literacy'. In these cases, the nouns 'intelligence', 'ability', 'competence', 'literacy', are names for the dimensions, not for one extreme, and have no opposites. But it is also possible to say: 'It needs intelligence to be a teacher.' 'He is a man of ability.' 'I admire her competence.' 'Literacy is an essential in our society.' In these cases, the nouns are names for one part of the dimension—that lying towards the upper end. It is therefore possible to talk of someone's 'stupidity', 'disability' (or 'inability'), 'incompetence' and 'illiteracy' (though it should be noted that 'disability' and 'inability' are not synonyms, and that they always refer to *specific areas* of deficit).

A further note about the word 'intelligent': psychologists commonly talk of 'intelligent behaviour' when they intend to contrast it, not with *unintelligent* behaviour, but with behaviour that is not mediated by any kind of thinking, or planning, or understanding at all. Donaldson (1963) makes this point:

> There are, of course, activities of kinds which cannot be performed either intelligently or stupidly, such as sneezing or digesting one's dinner. . . .

The use of the word 'intelligent' in this sense (contrasted with, say, 'automatic') is necessitated by the lack of a separate neutral adjective. In an earlier work Donaldson (1956) proposed the use of the term 'intelligential' to make this contrast.

In many cases, the reader's sense of the context will prevent misunderstanding. But it is as well to be on the alert for the subtle shifts of meaning which have been illustrated here because an unnoticed shift can lead to notable errors in argument (see Donaldson 1963, pp. 15–16).

The notion of literacy

Let us turn now to a more detailed examination of some specific terminology, beginning with the set of terms centring on the notion of *literacy*—the word literacy itself, and the cognate terms 'literate', 'semiliterate', and 'illiterate'.

Those adjectives represent a spectrum of attainment, of which it might be thought that one end (the 'negative' end) is more clearly defined than the other. In the past this was almost certainly true. An illiterate person used to be (and still is, in some contexts) one who, *at an age where he would be expected to have done so*, has not learned to read and write. (The italicized clause is important: we do not call a five year old illiterate. The term is used mostly to describe children over the age of twelve, and adults.) Sometimes the reference is more to writing than to reading. For instance, in World War II the Army Personnel Selection staff defined as 'illiterate', 'those recruits who could not produce legible answers to the questionnaire or qualification form filled up on entry to the service' (Ministry of Education 1950). But a search through the literature reveals that the term illiterate is sometimes used in a very different way, for instance, to describe university examination scripts which contain a lot of spelling mistakes, or are in untidy handwriting, or display an incomplete grasp of syntax. What has happened when these, or their producers, are described as illiterate is that the norm has been moved up the scale of performance; in other words the term has become relative. This shift in meaning is commented on in the Ministry of Education (1950) document referred to above:

The definition of illiteracy
The word illiterate, which originally meant unlettered, has, over several hundred years, acquired so many shades of meaning that it has ceased to be immediately usable for exact thought. The purposes for which written or printed words are used are so varied that it is quite easy to be fully competent in one situation and not in another. Thus it has been said that 'It is common knowledge that our professional students and candidates for the PH.D are illiterate.' No doubt these students and candidates may sometimes have difficulty in presenting an account of a complicated piece of research, but they would certainly be able to make out a washing list for the laundry. Or, again, the *Encylopedia Britannica* states that 'In the more restricted and technical sense of the term an illiterate is one who is unable to read and write his own language. The tests of this ability vary greatly, but all are so simple that a person could easily pass them and yet be illiterate in the wider sense.' But even 'to read and write one's own

language' is not a clear definition—to read an erudite work of literary criticism is quite a different occupation from reading an account of a football match. In truth most definitions of illiteracy amount to this —'that he is illiterate who is not as literate as someone else thinks he ought to be'.

The contrasted term 'literate' has suffered a similar fate. Literate means in some contexts, as it used to do, 'able to read and write for practical purposes of daily life' (Ministry of Education 1950). W. S. Gray (1956) coined the term 'functional literacy' to describe this level of competence. But we also now use literate as a term of approbation, just as we use illiterate as a term of censure, to mean 'capable of handling written language with skill and elegance', or sometimes 'very well versed in literature'. There are, in short, various degrees and kinds of literacy.

The term 'semiliterate', however, has retained rather more of the earlier meaning of literate and is used much more technically than the two other terms, with, usually, an 'operational' definition. That is to say, it is defined in terms of some explicit action or operation (like the application of a particular test or other objective criterion). To quote the Ministry of Education document again, semiliterate is defined there as 'having a reading age of seven years or greater, but less than nine years'. This of course is only one quantitative definition of the term and is put in here for illustration. But all definitions of semiliterate would be likely to make some reference to explicit standards of achievement, in adults or older children, which fall somewhere between complete illiteracy in the earlier sense, and a degree of competence which matches the average performance found in the later years of primary school.

Backwardness

Adults or school-leavers who are not functionally literate fall into the category of the 'backward', in the sense that they perform at a level well below the *average for their age*. This term, however, is used much less of adults than of children still at school. The term backward probably became part of the educational vocabulary through the work of Burt and Schonell. *The Backward Child* and *Backwardness in the Basic Subjects*, were pioneer works and standard references, not only because of their detailed examination of correlates of failure, but because of their treatment of the question of measurement.

The point to note about the term backward is that it means 'falling short of an age criterion by some specified amount'. A backward child is below the average for his age. The whole problem of measurement is dealt with in the second section of this paper, but it ought to be stressed at once that in any group or population with a spread of ability, roughly half will be 'below average', regardless of the absolute standards reached. There are therefore serious logical difficulties in any notion of 'bringing backward children up to the average of their group'. The average will retreat, like the carrot in front of the donkey's nose, because it is 'fixed to the cart'. Yet the 'conditional prediction' (see Donaldson 1963, p. 2) on which remedial work is based, is that backward readers can, given suitable help, be 'brought up' in some sense to a higher level of attainment. In one important recent instance, namely the Ministry of Education Pamphlet already referred to, the term 'backward' was used in conjunction with the terms 'illiterate' and 'semiliterate', to designate three categories of poor achievement in reading. The writers define the categories thus:

Backward readers are those whose reading ages are more than 20 per cent below their chronological ages; in the case of children, those whose reading quotients are below 80. In the case of adults, the expected average reading age may be taken as 15.0 years, hence backward readers are those with reading ages below 12.0 years.
Illiterate readers are those whose reading age (regardless of chronological age) is less than 7.0 years. (This figure differs from Burt's $6\frac{1}{2}$ years merely because the reading test . . . did not readily measure the $6\frac{1}{2}$ year level.)
Semiliterate readers are those whose reading age is 7.0 or greater, but less than 9.0 years. (1938 norms Ed.)

They comment that 'since backwardness is a matter of degree, the proportions of backward or illiterate individuals will naturally depend on just where the dividing lines are drawn. Hence an attempt has been made in this, and later, sections to adhere to a few uniform divisions.' (p. 34)

Retardation

Burt, Schonell and many others have made a further distinction—that between the child of limited ability and the child of normal or good ability who, in the well-known words of countless school reports, 'could do better'. That is, they distinguished 'capacity' or 'potential' from 'attainment'. By the 1950s, a new term—the word 'retarded'—had been adopted to designate those children who fell short of their capacity.

This distinction is clearly brought out in an article by Kellmer Pringle (1956). In this article, however, she not only distinguishes backwardness from retardation, but states that (a) some backwardness is not remediable, while retardation is, and (b) retardation, being relative to mental age and not to chronological age, may exist in a child who is not backward in relation to his age-group. Concerning backwardness, she wrote:

Comparing a child's attainment with that of his contemporaries implies that potentially every pupil can reach a level of educational achievement commensurate with his chronological age. But this is not the case. Since about 10 per cent of children are intellectually dull, they cannot by definition achieve the same standards as the majority of their contemporaries.

By contrast, retardation was described as 'underfunctioning' and Kellmer Pringle went on to say:

> The scholastic attainments of a retarded pupil fall seriously below the level of his capacity. . . . Thus, while in backwardness a child's attainments are compared with those of his contemporaries, in retardation one considers a pupil's achievements in relation to his mental capacity.

She noted further that some children are both backward and retarded— i.e. both behind their age norm and their own mental capacity.

This view of the relationship between capacity and achievement has been seriously challenged by P. E. Vernon (1956, 1960). His arguments are based on the nature of educational measurement. His conclusions amount to a calling in question of the whole 'up to capacity' notion, though *not* of the notion that a given child who happens to be towards the lower end of his age-group in attainment 'could do better': indeed he is prepared rather to make this hopeful forecast of all children, and not just of those whose IQs were promisingly high:

> It is definitely untrue that all dull children are inevitably backward, or that a low IQ absolves us from the need to do our best to explore the underlying causes—to see whether a changed environment, medical attention, or a new approach to teaching might not help such children.

Throughout the literature, unfortunately, the two terms have not consistently been used to make the distinction made by Kellmer Pringle, and the confusion has been made worse by the use of the phrase 'mentally retarded' in a different context, to indicate a condition that (a) refers to capacity itself and (b) has little or no connotation of remediability. The only recourse a reader has is to ensure that he is as clear as possible about how any particular term is being used in any given context. Various other terms relating to backwardness and retardation are also found. The term 'slow learner' has come to be a euphemism for a child who is generally backward. The term 'reluctant reader' is sometimes used to denote a child who lacks motivation or who has for some reason developed an aversion to reading.

Reading disability

The group of terms which have perhaps caused most trouble, however, consist of those coined and used throughout the discussions of 'reading disability'. This term itself is used in two senses. One of these is almost synonymous with 'reading retardation'. The other has a more precise meaning, that of a deficit of some kind, predisposing to, or resulting in, very severe difficulty in learning to read and write. Sometimes the word 'difficulty' is used instead of 'disability', and in recent years the second sense, as defined above, has been distinguished from the first by the addition of the word 'specific' (see Reid (1968) in this volume). It is notable that the Tizard Report (HMSO 1972) has adopted this term and is actually called *Children with Specific Reading Difficulties*. (See this volume, pages 127–129.)

The task of discussing the topic without proliferating terms seems almost impossible. Here is Money (1966) writing in *The Disabled Reader*:

> The *disabled* reader is one whose condition is that of being unable to thrive pedagogically, unable to profit from standard methods of instruction, and unable to learn to read. The resultant *illiteracy*, or *defective literacy* is to be distinguished from that which results simply from educational neglect or inadequate instruction. Characteristically, the *disabled* reader is arrested at the beginner or near-beginner level, making the typical beginner's mistakes. Thus, reading *disability* can be suspected and recognized in the first and second grades. In the higher grades, it is a rule of thumb to identify the disabled reader as one who is two or more grade levels *retarded* in reading relative to his schoolmates who have been exposed to the same educational system as he. In severe reading *disability*, a child has at no stage of his schooling been able to achieve at grade level. There is no single cause of *reading disablement*. The different causes lead to the same final result, namely *impairment* or *arrest* of *maturation*. (Editor's italics.)

In part, of course, the problem is stylistic—writers do not want to use the same words over and over again and they therefore resort to synonyms, but this is exactly what truly scientific discourse must not do. It is also true that shifts occur in criteria. In the passage just quoted, 'defective' implies making mistakes or having gaps in competence. 'Retarded' reading implies not achieving up to some predetermined standard.

The fact that 'severe reading disability' has been studied by medical men has had two outcomes as far as terminology is concerned. It led first to the use of the term 'word blindness', by analogy with colour blindness. Secondly it led to the coining of many terms taken from Greek and Latin, and hence to the implication that certain specifiable 'conditions' could be isolated. Most of these terms are now of historical interest only. For a more detailed discussion of the issues concerned with reading disability and of the implications of the various terms used the reader is referred to section 3 of this volume. The terms likely still to be met in current literature, however, are listed here with a brief indication of their meaning:

1 *Dyslexia*—severe difficulty in learning to read. *Dysgraphia*—severe difficulty in learning to write. These terms, when used at all, are increasingly coming to be used as descriptive of a child's state and not as diagnostic of the reasons for it. They may however be preceded by 'specific' (see above) or by 'specific developmental' (indicating that the condition is an anomaly of development—a departure from normality in maturation). The term dyslexia, used in isolation, is becoming less common, and the Tizard Report (see above and pages 127–129 of this volume) will probably hasten this process. The report suggests, instead, the use of 'specific reading difficulties'. Children are said to have these when their 'reading abilities are significantly below the standard which their abilities in other spheres would lead one to expect'.

2 *Word blindness* This term is often synonymous with specific dyslexia or specific developmental dyslexia or specific reading disability. It is *not*, however, synonymous with specific reading difficulties as used in the Tizard Report, because it has a connotation of causation which the writers of the Tizard Report do not want their term to carry. The use of word blindness has been recently revived (Franklin 1962) but it is disliked by many people because of the way in which it suggests an irremediable condition (see Reid 1968).

3 *Specific language disability* This is sometimes used to indicate a constitutional difficulty with all language skills, of which reading is one. It can therefore be regarded as the name of a predisposing factor to reading disability and the term is used particularly of children who have shown language difficulties of some kind or another before starting school.

4 *Syndrome* This is a medical term meaning a collection of symptoms which collectively define a medical condition. If it is the case that not all the symptoms are present in every case manifesting the condition, the syndrome may be described as 'variable'. The notion of a 'variable syndrome' is used frequently in some of the discussions of dyslexia, but many people do not agree that the concept of a syndrome is appropriate (Rutter, Tizard and Whitmore 1970).

This is by no means a complete glossary of terms. But many of the more esoteric ones have almost disappeared, and the aim here has been rather to clarify some important terminological distinctions than to provide a comprehensive review. Those interested in studying the terminology in more detail are referred, though with a cautionary note, to Gunderson (1969) *Reading Problems: Glossary of Terminology*. The cautionary note is necessary because Gunderson fails to be entirely consistent over the term retardation. But her list is in general a useful source of help, especially with terms that have a medical provenance.

So far problems of measurement have only been hinted at. This next section goes on to discuss these and their relationships to the problems of definition in greater detail.

The measurement of backwardness and retardation

From among the plethora of definitions of reading ability referred to in the previous section, two fundamental concepts stand out—those of backwardness and retardation. In slightly different ways both are fundamental in that they relate to a negative discrepancy between a child's expected and his observed ability in reading—a discrepancy which is an overt and general indication of the need to remedy some specific defect or defects. How is this discrepancy between expectation and observation to be measured?

Backwardness

1a *As difference between chronological and reading age*
The simplest way of assessing backwardness is to employ some test of reading ability (appropriate to the child's age) which has been standardized to record the various levels of reading ability in terms of reading age (RA). The first step in standardizing such a test is to administer it to all children in a carefully selected reference group spanning the appropriate age-range. The various 'raw' or original test scores for all children of a particular chronological age (CA) are then accumulated and averaged (usually the median is employed) over all these raw scores. This average raw score is next set as equivalent to the chronological age of the children concerned and this in turn is equated to, and so defines, the expected reading age. This operation is repeated at all chronological ages and the average raw scores (which will tend to increase with age) are tabulated alongside the corresponding reading ages. For example, the two upper lines in Table 1 show a portion of a typical table.

TABLE 1   *Reading ages and quotients*

Test score	25	30	34	37	39
RA ($y:m$)	9:0	9:3	9:6	9:9	10:0
RQs at CA:9:0	100	103	106	108	111
9:3	97	100	103	105	108
9:6	95	97	100	103	105
9:9	92	95	97	100	103
10:0	90	92	95	97	100

The test performance of an individual child can now be assessed by relating it to that of the children in the reference group. Backwardness is expressed by the simple difference between chronological age and reading age. For example Tom (chronological age 10:0) scored 25 on the test and hence has a reading age of 9:0. He is therefore backward by 12 months.

1b   *As ratio of reading to chronological age (reading quotient)*
Instead of reporting Tom's backwardness as the simple difference between his chronological and reading ages, we may choose to employ their ratio— the 'reading quotient' (RQ): RQ $= 100$ (RA/CA). The ratio is multiplied by 100 to remove decimals and the result is expressed to the nearest whole number. The child whose test performance is just at the average for his age-group clearly has a reading quotient of 100. Children with reading ages below their chronological ages, have reading quotients less than 100. For instance, Tom's reading quotient is 100 (108/120) $= 90$.

Frequently, the standardization table relating test raw score to reading age is extended so that the equivalent reading quotients can be read off directly, as shown in the lower part of Table 1.

To obtain Tom's reading quotient, enter the table with his test 'raw' score (25) and his chronological age (10:0) and so obtain his reading quotient, 90. Mary (test score 39, chronological age 9:3) has a reading quotient of 108.

The quotient method is perhaps slightly more informative than the simple difference method and is the one more frequently used.

Notice that although Tom's reading quotient of 90 suggests some degree of backwardness, it does not place him in the category of 'backwardness' as defined (page 24) by the Ministry of Education pamphlet (reading quotient below 80). Notice also that for children at the upper limit of backwardness (as defined in the pamphlet), the gap between chronological and reading ages is larger for older children than for those younger. A ten year old child with a reading age of eight years is backward by 24 months; a fourteen year old with a reading age of 11:2 is backward by nearly 34 months. Both have the same reading quotient of 80.

The reading quotient has the virtue of simplicity, but its use is attended by some problems, not the least of which is the variation from one chronological age to another in the proportion of children designated arbitrarily as backward (for example, those with reading quotients below 80).

2   *Standardized reading score*
The use of a different type of measure, designated a 'standardized reading score' (SRS), obviates some of these difficulties. As with the reading quotient, standardized score is a measure derived from the raw scores of a reference group of children on a reading test, but is based on more sophisticated statistical techniques.

For a full description of the method by which standardized scores are derived, a standard textbook should be consulted (for example Lewis

A. E. G. Pilliner and Jessie F. Reid

(1967), Vernon (1956)). Briefly, the raw scores on the reading test of all children of a fixed age in the reference group are in effect ranked, the ranks expressed as percentiles, and the percentiles in turn converted into standardized scores which are 'normally' distributed about some mean with some standard deviation, both arbitrarily assigned (usually 100 and 15 respectively). This procedure is repeated for all the ages concerned. As a result, a child with a test raw score which places him at the median (50th percentile) for his particular age-group is assigned a standardized score of 100; and since on average older children score higher than younger children, the older the child, the higher his raw score must be in order to 'earn' him a standardized score of 100. Similar arguments apply to other standardized scores corresponding to other positions on the percentile scale. In this way, age is 'built in' to the standardization. A diagram may help to make this clear:

FIGURE 1   *Standardized reading score*

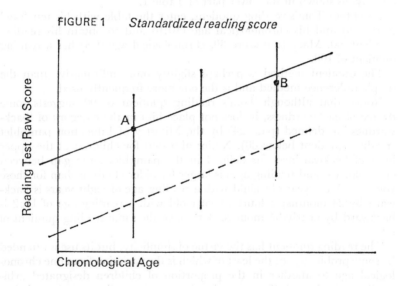

Chronological Age

All children on the full line (which slopes upwards with increasing age) are at the medians for their respective age-groups and hence by definition all have the same standardized reading score, 100. Therefore, any child with this standardized score is superior in test performance to 50 per cent of children in his age-group, and superior also, by virtue of the age allowance, to all the 50 per cent of children of other ages with standardized scores less than 100. Thus the younger child at A is superior in this score to the older child at B, although the latter has the higher raw score. Similarly, all children on the dotted line are at the 16th percentile and hence by definition have a standardized reading score one standard deviation lower, that is $(100 - 15) = 85$. Therefore any child with the latter standardized score is superior in performance to 16 per cent of all children in his own age-group and superior also (because of the age allowance) to all the 16 per cent of children of other ages with standardized scores of less than 85. Further lines are drawn in the same way to complete the standardization.

Suppose, then, we wish to select some predetermined proportion of children for special treatment and we believe that those scoring worst on the test are also those most in need of treatment. Standardization in the manner described enables us to specify a standardized reading score which will be the upper limit of performance of that predetermined proportion. Moreover, because of the built-in age allowance we shall know that the specified standardized score will cut off the same proportion at all age levels. Thus if we choose to label the poorest 16 per cent on the test 'backward readers', then we shall specify that standardized score which 16 per cent of the population sampled will not exceed—in this case 85. We shall further expect the proportion at each age level to be a constant 16 per cent.

Retardation

1a *As difference between mental age and reading age*
As already indicated, the concept of retardation is different from that of backwardness. The major advantage of chronological age as a base line is its ready availability. But children of the same chronological age differ markedly in their mental development. A dull child's reading, though below average for his age, may be commensurate with his mental capacity or potential—he is backward, but not retarded. Perhaps it is more logical to base expectation on mental rather than chronological level, as Kellmer Pringle has maintained (see page 24).

However, children's mental levels cannot be obtained from their birth certificates. They must be assessed by a test of mental ability. Estimating a child's reading retardation therefore involves testing him not once but twice. The test of 'intelligence' used must not be one based on material which has to be read, yet it must be of a type from which reasonable prediction about academic progress can be made. The tests used most by psychologists at the present time are the Wechsler Intelligence Scale for Children (wisc) and the Stanford–Binet.

Standardization of a test of mental ability or intelligence in order to derive 'mental ages' (mas) proceeds in exactly the same way as in the case of a reading test used to derive reading ages (see page 28).

With the child's mental age and reading age both in hand, the simplest way of expressing the extent of his reading retardation is as the straight difference between them. Thus if Tom who has a reading age of 9:0 is now found to have a mental age of 9:6, the extent of his *reading retardation* is 6 months.

A. E. G. Pilliner and Jessie F. Reid

1b *As ratio of reading to mental age (achievement quotient)*

Alternatively, retardation may be expressed as the ratio of reading age to mental age, which has been called the 'achievement quotient' (AQ): AQ = 100 (RA/MA). For Tom, this is 100 (108/114) = 95 which, being below 100, suggests some slight degree of retardation. Tom's achievement quotient is thus 5 points higher than his reading quotient of 90 (see page 29). The discrepancy arises because his mental age (9:6) is below his chronological age (10:0) so that his mental ability is below the average of his age level. The reader is invited to form his own judgment as to which of the two measures, one of backwardness (RQ), the other of retardation (AQ), furnishes the clearer or more useful picture of Tom's reading accomplishments.

2 *As difference between standardized scores in reading and intelligence*

More sophisticated procedures for assessing retardation make use of standardized scores in both reading and intelligence. The method previously described (page 29) of obtaining standardized scores on a reading test (SRS) can be employed to obtain corresponding standardized scores on an intelligence test (SIS). To simplify interpretation, it is desirable that both should be on the same scale. We shall suppose that for both tests the mean and standard deviation are 100 and 15 respectively.

Each child then has two standardized scores, one measuring his intelligence, the other his reading ability. The simple difference between them (SIS–SRS) is frequently used as a measure of retardation which seems on the face of it a reasonable indicator of the extent to which a child's reading ability is commensurate with his intellectual ability. It does not differ in *principle* from the use of the difference (IQ–RQ) already described.

In fact, all such procedures are open to serious objection. Their use implicitly assumes that reading and intellectual ability 'ought' to correspond completely—that ideally the correlation between the two measures should be perfect. However, there is no more reason to assert this than to postulate a perfect correspondence between the same children's physical heights and weights. Indeed, there is possibly less reason, for height and weight can be measured with a degree of precision the psychologist cannot emulate.

3 *As difference between actual and predicted standardized reading scores*

Moving from the ideal to the real world, we employ a procedure which establishes empirically the relationship which actually does exist between standardized scores in intelligence and reading in a reference group of children. Intelligence is used to *predict* reading. The reader is again referred to a textbook for a fuller exposition than is possible here of the statistical principles involved. Meanwhile, Figure 2 may help to illustrate the following facts.

FIGURE 2   *Prediction of SRS by SIS* *****

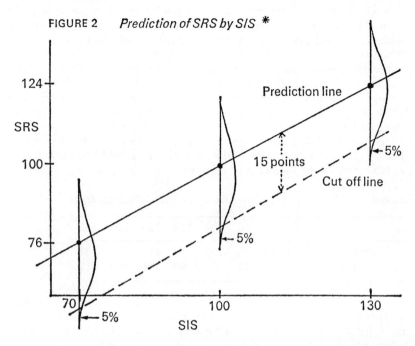

In predicting reading score from intelligence score, both on the same scale:

1   There is a *tendency* for more intelligent children to obtain higher scores on the reading test than children less intelligent.
2   An above-average intelligence score predicts a reading score *lower* than itself (in the diagram sis 130 predicts srs 124), and a below-average intelligence score predicts a reading score *higher* than itself (sis 70 predicts srs 76).
3   Children with the same intelligence score have differing reading scores distributed more or less symmetrically about the predicted score, the majority clustering around it and the rest tailing off in both directions.

---

* The specification for Figure 2 is: SIS $= x$, SRS $= y$, $\bar{x} = \bar{y} = 100$, $s_x = s_y = 15$, $r_{xy} = 0.8$ so that $b_{yx} = 0.8$ also.
Regression equation is: $\hat{y} = 100 + 0.8\,(x - 100) = 0.8x + 20$.
Standard error of prediction is: $s_{y.x} = 15\sqrt{(1 - 0.8^2)} = 9$.
Cut off for lower 5 per cent tail at: $1.65 \times 9 = 15$.
Equation for upper limit of selected 5 per cent group is:
$\hat{y} = (\hat{y} - 15) = 0.8x + 5$. For a child to qualify for selection, $(x - y)$ must exceed $(x - \hat{y})$, that is $(x - y)$ must exceed $0.2x - 5$ (see Table 2, page 34).

At each of the three intelligence levels shown (there will of course be more than this), the reading scores are distributed approximately normally with a standard deviation which can be calculated—in this case about 9 points.

For the present purpose we will not concentrate on children whose reading performances put them above the prediction line. Of the children below it, those towards the lower end of each tail are presumably most in need of special attention. Where we draw the dotted line separating these children from the rest is a matter of judgment. Let us suppose that the best available evidence suggests the lowest 5 per cent. Then the dotted line should be drawn parallel to the prediction line and 15 points below it. A table such as the following facilitates the selection process.

TABLE 2   *Selection of lowest 5 per cent at different intelligence levels*

sis:	70	80	90	100	110	120	130	140
Predicted srs:	76	84	92	100	108	116	124	132
Select below srs:	61	69	77	85	93	101	109	117

It will be seen that to qualify for selection the discrepancy (sis–srs) must be larger for brighter children than for those duller. For the very bright child (sis 140) the difference must exceed 23 before he qualifies. At the other extreme (sis 70), the difference need only exceed 9.

Some problems

The main problems which arise when attempting to identify children as either backward or retarded are as follows.

1   The procedures described above under 'Backwardness' 1a and 1b are essentially the same, but different from that under 2. Therefore the set of children identified as backward by 1a or 1b will not be the same as that identified by 2, though there will be considerable overlap.

2   Similar considerations apply to the several procedures for identifying retarded readers. Procedures 1a and 1b under 'Retardation' are essentially the same, but different from 2 and again from 3. Each will pick out different though overlapping sets of children. Procedure 2 under 'Backwardness' and procedure 3 under 'Retardation' are to be preferred as most statistically sound.

3   No test of mental ability or scholastic accomplishment is perfectly reliable. All measurements obtained with such tests are subject to error. It follows that not all decisions made as to backwardness or retardation are the best ones. Some children will be wrongly caught in the net, others will wrongly escape it. Borderline uncertainty is all the

more troublesome when retardation is assessed, for decision in this case depends on a difference between *two* fallible test scores. This difference is therefore liable to increased error.

4 It is important moreover not to assume uncritically that the tests used are valid measures of reading and mental ability. To the extent that they do not measure what they purport to measure, they invalidate the outcome of the selection procedures. Before being taken into general use, a procedure therefore needs *ad hoc* validation on a pilot scale with groups of children whose reading accomplishments have already been established by other means.

5 In the assessment of retardation, some children may be missed because their poor reading appears commensurate with their measured intelligence which, however, is itself depressed through some physical or psychological malfunction, remediable by appropriate treatment. The verdict of the intelligence test should therefore be treated with caution. This applies particularly when the intelligence test contains items liable to reflect weaknesses in, for instance, spacial perception or auditory memory.

6 Each of the procedures outlined in this chapter is normative: each has present average performance as its reference point. Gearing the measures to the average in this way might be taken to imply that present average performance is satisfactory. But such norms simply reflect what is and not what might be. We must keep in mind that not only the poorest children, but many of those who are progressing relatively quite well, could be helped, especially in the later stages, to develop their reading skills to greater effect.

In short, any procedure employed in assessing backwardness or retardation in reading should be seen as a guide to assist judgment and not as a substitute for it.

References

*BURT, C. L. (1937) *The Backward Child* London: University of London Press

DEPARTMENT OF EDUCATION AND SCIENCE (1972) *Children with Specific Reading Difficulties* (Tizard Report) London: HMSO

DONALDSON, M. (1956) The relevance to the theory of intelligence testing of the study of errors in thinking Unpublished PH.D dissertation, University of Edinburgh

DONALDSON, M. (1963) *A Study of Children's Thinking* London: Tavistock Publications

FRANKLIN, A. W. (1962) *Word Blindness or Specific Developmental Dyslexia* London: Pitman

*GRAY, W. S. (1956) *The Teaching of Reading and Writing: An International Survey* Chicago: Scott Foresman

A. E. G. Pilliner and Jessie F. Reid

GUNDERSON, D. V. (1969) Reading problems: glossary of terminology in *Reading Research Quarterly* IV, 4

KELLMER PRINGLE, M. L. (1956) The backward child—dull or retarded? in *Times Educational Supplement* 12th October

MINISTRY OF EDUCATION (1950) *Reading Ability* Pamphlet 18 London: HMSO

*MONEY, J. (1966) (ed) *The Disabled Reader* Baltimore: Johns Hopkins Press

REID, J. F. (1968) Dyslexia: a problem of communication *Educational Research* 10, 2 reading 3.2 in this volume, page 130

RUTTER, M., TIZARD, J. and WHITMORE, K. (1970) *Education, Health and Behaviour* London: Longman

SCHONELL, F. J. (1942) *Backwardness in the Basic Subjects* Edinburgh: Oliver and Boyd

VERNON, P. E. (1956) Dullness and its causes *Times Educational Supplement* 26th October

VERNON, P. E. (1960) *Intelligence and Attainment Tests* London: University of London Press

1.3 The scope of the reading problem

JESSIE F. REID

Centre for Research in Educational Sciences,
University of Edinburgh

First publication

Introduction

Firm quantitative evidence about the extent of backwardness and retardation in reading is valuable and even sometimes necessary. It is
needed by those who form educational policy, and by those who plan
provision. It is needed to inform the public, correct misconceptions and
counter complacency. The most important results from studies conducted
during the postwar years are reviewed in this paper.

Evidence up to 1966

Some of the earlier evidence is conveniently summarized in an appendix
by Cane (1966) to *Standards and Progress in Reading* (Morris 1966). Her
book is itself a detailed followup of a survey of reading in the county of
Kent, published a few years earlier (Morris 1959). Cane's summary is
here given in full. It will be evident how confusions in terminology and
definition have helped to invalidate much of the work on which Cane
reports.

Surveys—1946–64
During the period 1946–60, a number of local authorities conducted
surveys to ascertain reading standards and the incidence of backwardness. Their findings are difficult to compare or combine for the
following reasons:

1 Different criteria of reading ability were adopted: individual
   tests of word recognition in some areas, group tests of reading
   comprehension in others.
2 The borderlines chosen to ascertain backwardness were in-
   consistent: in some cases a reading quotient below 80 or 85 was

chosen; in others the criterion was based on the relation between attainment and mental age.

3 The terms 'retardation' and 'backwardness' were used ambiguously.

4 In some cases reading and intelligence tests not similarly standardized were used.

5 There was considerable variety in the sampling methods used, and in the age and sex of testees.

6 The tests used were differently normed and constructed and were not always consistently applied.

However these postwar surveys revealed that:

1 The war had had a deleterious effect on reading attainment.

2 Standards varied in different parts of England and Wales and were generally better in urban than rural districts.

3 There was a sizeable proportion of children with reading difficulties at different age and intelligence levels in all areas.

4 Reading ability, on average, had improved, particularly during the last nine years, but special provision for remedial treatment was still urgently needed.

5 Local authorities were becoming more ambitious in their surveys and were considering other factors besides the age, sex and intelligence of testees.

For the reasons already outlined, local estimates varied a good deal and naturally were not representative of conditions over the country as a whole. In 1948, therefore, the Ministry of Education decided to discover the national norms for two age-groups (10+ and 14+) and compare them with corresponding prewar norms, in so far as evidence about the latter was available.

Because of the considerable hazards involved in this inquiry conclusions were couched in cautious language. Apparently the proportion of backward readers in English and Welsh schools was larger than the estimated 10 per cent before the war, but total illiteracy among school leavers was less serious than had often been stated. The main value of the investigation, however, lay in the establishment of standards on a new and unpublished test against which subsequent progress could be measured.

The 1952 Ministry of Education survey of reading standards reported that 30 per cent of school-leavers could be classed as 'backward readers', 'semiliterate' or 'illiterate'. The 1956 survey showed some improvements for school leavers: the percentage of children in the three lowest reading categories was reduced to 25 per cent; the same survey placed 21 per cent of the eleven year olds in these categories. The 1961 survey of reading standards in the fourth year of secondary modern schools, conducted for the report *Half our Future*, confirmed the improvement shown by the juniors of 1956: only 20 per cent of the secondary modern school leavers studied in 1961 showed a reading standard as low as that shown by 30 per cent of the age-group sample studied in 1952. This progress was certainly impressive, but the percentage of 'backward readers' was still considerable.

Wiseman (1964) and his associates reported the abilities of children in the final year of secondary schools in the greater Manchester area for the academic year 1951: tests of reading comprehension, verbal intelligence and mechanical arithmetic, were selected for use. 'Backwardness' was defined as a standard score of 85 or below. Considerable variation of backwardness in reading from one school to another was found. The percentage of reading backwardness in secondary modern schools ranged from 10.1 to 37.7 per cent, and in all-age schools up to 75.0 per cent. Six years later, the mean percentage of reading backwardness in Manchester city schools was found to be 14.2 per cent in the case of secondary modern schools and 27.9 per cent in the case of all-age schools. During the period 1951-7, the percentage of superior 14 year old readers in the City of Manchester area increased from 3.1 to 7.7 per cent, whilst the percentage of backward, semiliterate and illiterate readers of the same age, decreased from 31.3 to 26.1 per cent (Wiseman, 1964; p. 131).

(Extracted from J. M. MORRIS (1966) *Standards and Progress in Reading* Slough: National Foundation for Educational Research Appendix 1 by B. S. Cane, pp. 465-6.)

The DES reports were brought up to date by a further study in 1964 of the reading ability of eleven year olds and fifteen year olds, using the same unpublished test as before. The results appeared as *Progress in Reading 1948-1964* (DES 1966), in which G. F. Peaker, the statistician responsible for the sampling techniques and the assessment of results, provided an integrated account of the way in which standards had moved over the sixteen years covered by the successive surveys. The results showed a steady upward trend at all parts of the range, equivalent to an overall advance (i.e. over the sixteen years) of 17 months of reading age for 11 year olds, and 20-23 months of reading age for 15 year olds, and was if anything greater towards the upper end of the ability scale. It was also evident that the lowest 10 per cent continued to constitute a core of almost illiterate children leaving the primary school.

Further evidence on a nation-wide basis about progress in reading, this time of 7 year old children, was provided by the first report of the National Child Development Study, 1958 Cohort (Kellmer Pringle *et al* 1966). Information was obtained for 11,000 of the 17,000 children born between 3rd and 9th March 1958. Reading progress was assessed by the Southgate

Group Reading Test (Word Recognition) and by teachers' ratings. Results showed that 40 per cent of the group could be classified as 'good' readers (scoring 28–30), while 18 per cent were 'poor' readers (scoring 15 or less). Teachers rated 50 per cent as 'above average' or 'superior readers', and 26 per cent 'below average', including some 3 per cent of nonreaders. The results indicated a proportion of around 20 per cent of children with poor attainments in reading on leaving the infant stage. A further report on this cohort (Davie 1972) provides more evidence of the correlation between social class and reading attainment. A study conducted by Morris for the NFER in the county of Kent (Morris 1959) gave similar results.

In 1968, the Inner London Education Authority conducted its own survey of reading attainment in 8 year olds (Little et al 1972). The test used was one version of a sentence completion test designed by the NFER for their streaming project (SRA). In the summer of 1971, the other version (SRB) was given to the same children who were then 11 +. The results for 1968 showed that mean reading quotients ranged from 93.4 in smaller classes of the lowest EPA rank, to 104.2 in larger classes of the highest EPA rank. Immigrant children did much less well than nonimmigrant, with means of 92.4 in smaller classes and 93.7 in larger classes, against 99.7 and 101.6 for the nonimmigrants. A group mean of 93 or thereabouts is consistent with a proportion of around 25 per cent scoring less than 85 so that the poorer ILEA schools repeat a pattern found elsewhere.

In April 1972 the NFER (Start and Wells 1972) produced further data for England and Wales, again on the attainment of 11 year olds and 15 year olds, and again using the unpublished Watts–Vernon test together with another similar test NS6. The results from this survey show that:

As measured by the WV Test there is a high probability that the reading comprehension standards of juniors had declined somewhat since 1964, and on the combined basis of both WV and NS6 the mean scores of juniors and seniors had undergone no significant rise or fall since 1960/61. The almost linear increase in reading comprehension that existed from 1948 to 1964 has not been maintained and there are significant differences between the reading scores attained in this survey and those that would have been predicted from the previous trends.

The writers point out that several factors combined to throw some doubt on the accuracy of these results. They included the possible 'ageing' of the test content, a large proportion of noncooperating schools, and uncertainty over the incidence of absence on the part of poor achievers. But the report ends with the observation that reading standards in 1972 were no better than they were a decade earlier.

Studies with special emphasis on problems

In the followup to the earlier Kent survey, in which Morris (1966) selected ten schools for intensive study, the author makes some comments on reading standards of second year juniors. She notes that in none of the schools selected for special study was there any child engaged on a reader suitable for children beyond the normal junior range and that all schools had pupils reading books designed for younger children:

> In the schools initially classified as 'bad' according to our set of predetermined criteria, only 9 per cent were reading books of a standard commensurate with or above their chronological ages. Twenty-five per cent of the children were retarded by one year and 16 per cent were having serious difficulties, being still at the infant primary stage of reading after two years in junior classes.

A study by Clark (1970) looked at reading problems in a complete year group of 1,544 children from a Scottish local authority. The survey had two aims: first, to look at reading levels in the year group as a whole and second, to look at characteristics of children with reading quotients of 85 or less, especially those whose measured intelligence suggested that they could perform at a higher level. Results for 7 year olds using the Schonell Graded Word Reading Test, yielded mean scores above average on the existing norms. When the criterion of a reading quotient of 85 or less was used by Clark to select those who were, after two years at school, not yet beyond the earliest stages of learning to read, 236 children, or 15.3 per cent of the total group (18 per cent of boys and 12.5 per cent of girls), were brought into this category. Of these, 8 boys and 7 girls were unable to read any word on the Schonell Graded Word Reading Test. One year later, 230 of these children were tested again, this time on the Southgate Word Recognition Test. Out of this group 120 were found to be still without 'adequate reading skill for the simplest classroom needs' (page 60).

One year later all children from this group with an IQ of over 90 on either the Verbal, Performance or Full Scales of the Wechsler Intelligence Scale for Children were examined extensively. Of this subgroup, 6.3 per cent were found to be backward in reading but only 1.2 per cent of them backward by more than two years. It should be noted however that only children regarded as 'at risk' at the age of 7 were followed up.

A somewhat similar study of an age-group, this time on the Isle of Wight, is reported by Rutter, Tizard and Whitmore (1970). Their study was concerned principally with retardation, that is with achievement relative to potential. The authors describe in detail the statistical means they used to arrive at an estimation of reading potential. This involves taking into account, by means of a formula, the child's score on a shortened form of the wisc and his chronological age. For a discussion of the rationale of this method, see Reid and Pilliner (1972) (page 32 in this volume). Rutter *et al* define severe reading retardation as 'an attainment either on reading accuracy or reading comprehension which was 28 months or more below the level predicted on the basis of each child's age and short wisc IQ.' Reading backwardness was defined in similar terms as an attainment in reading accuracy or comprehension on the Neale test, which was 28 months or more below the chronological age. They were therefore implying a fairly severe criterion of deficit and on the basis of this they found 86 children severely retarded in reading, i.e. 3.7 per cent of 9 and 10 year olds. 155 (6.6 per cent) were identified as backward in reading and there was considerable overlap between the two categories. The writers comment that direct comparison with other studies is difficult because of the way they selected their cases. It would seem, however, that both the areas which were the subject of these latest detailed surveys showed a lower incidence of reading problems than over the country as a whole and lower than the area studied by Morris.

Conclusions

If surveys of backwardness are based on nothing more than the numerical results of standardized tests, all they can do is to show how the proportion of children scoring below a specified point compares with the proportion in the standardization population. They are therefore useful in showing whether any particular area in a country has a greater or lesser proportion of backward readers than would be expected on the basis of national norms. Observations at intervals over a period of time can show whether there has been a movement in one direction or another and the extent of the change. To find out how bad, in functional terms, the backward children thus isolated really are, one has to look at a criterion not in terms of a standardized score but in terms of content—how much the children can actually do. Thus, Clark (1970) notes that the children in her survey who were backward by her criterion at the age of 7 were recognizing less than 10 words on Schonell's Graded Word List. That is in concrete terms, they were able to recognize less than 10 of the words: tree, little, milk, egg, book, school, sit, frog, playing, bun, flower, road, clock, train, light, picture, think, summer, people and something. In the latest DES survey and in the NFER followup the poorest children, aged 11, were taking 10 minutes to complete correctly around 7 very simple sentence completion tasks. The backward 9 year olds in the survey by Rutter et al were making around 14 errors on the first two passages of the Neale Analysis of Reading Ability, that is on sentences like 'A black cat came to my house' and 'The milkman's horse had wandered in the fog.' It is therefore clear that these are not just children towards the lower end of a distribution of attainment: they are children who, in the words of Clark, 'lack independent reading skill'. Clark (and Morris, who makes a similar point) are right to emphasize that this should be one of the measures by which the severity of the reading problem is judged.

Why does this failure happen? What can be done to amend it, and—more importantly—to prevent it? These are the questions around which studies of concomitant conditions, diagnosis, treatment and prevention must be gathered.

References

*CLARK, M. M. (1970) *Reading Difficulties in Schools* Harmondsworth: Penguin

*DAVIE, R., BUTLER, N. R. and GOLDSTEIN, H. (1972) *From Birth to Seven* London: Longman

DEPARTMENT OF EDUCATION AND SCIENCE (1966) *Progress in Reading 1948–1964* London: HMSO

*KELLMER PRINGLE, M. L., BUTLER, N. R. and DAVIE, R. (1966) *11,000 Seven year olds* London: Longman

LITTLE, A., MABEY, C. and RUSSELL, J. (1972) Class size, pupil characteristics and reading attainment in V. Southgate (ed) *Literacy at All Levels* London: Ward Lock Educational reading 2.4 in this volume page 86

MORRIS, J. M. (1959) *Reading in the Primary School* London: Newnes

*MORRIS, J. M. (1966) *Standards and Progress in Reading* Slough: National Foundation for Educational Research

RUTTER, M., TIZARD, J. and WHITMORE, K. (1970) *Education, Health and Behaviour* London: Longman

START, K. B. and WELLS, B. K. (1972) *The Trend of Reading Standards* Slough: National Foundation for Educational Research

2 The social, cultural and environmental correlates of reading failure

Introduction

The search for concomitants of severe backwardness in reading has been the concern of many investigators. Interest in social and cultural correlates dates from the early work of Burt, whose extensive surveys opened up this field of study. Interest in the notion of intrinsic or developmental reading disability arose at the turn of this century and was at first pursued mainly by medical specialists. (Section 3 relates to this aspect of reading failure.)

Over the last fifty years a few general concepts have guided the course of research into social and emotional aspects of reading failure, but the particular terms in which they have been embodied and investigated have changed with changing social conditions and with advances in—or at least extensions to—the areas of academic theorizing and research which bear on them.

One of these general concepts is that of *social underprivilege*. In Burt's work this was seen largely in material terms—poverty, malnutrition and its associated diseases, poor hygiene, bad housing, unemployment and so on. But over the intervening years, there have been improvements in living standards, in child care and in preventive medicine in general. At the same time, the disciplines of social and clinical psychology have contributed a great deal to our knowledge of nonmaterial determinants of learning and maturation, and the newer disciplines of sociology and psycholinguistics have given us many ideas with which to think about and try to make sense of the way a child grows up in a community. More recent studies of environmental correlations of reading failure concern themselves with features of family life and attitudes, with the interaction of home and school, with emotional satisfaction and deprivation, and with the role of language, in so far as these are connected on the one hand with socioeconomic level (nowadays defined in accepted ways in terms of father's occupation), and on the other hand with failure in the acquisition of literacy.

Another general concept which has received perhaps less attention in the literature, but which is always prominent in the minds of those working in a clinical setting with the backward and retarded reader, is that of interference with learning through environmentally caused emotional disturbance. The aggressive or antisocial child, the child whose relationships with his parents are troubled, the rejected child, the child confused and afraid because he has a broken home—these can appear at any level of the socioeconomic scale. Here, however, evidence is much more complicated, partly because of the difficulty of assessing the correct chronology of events, i.e. the time of onset of disturbance in relation to the associated educational failure. Emotional disturbance can often be understood as resulting from failure rather than causing it; but something which makes its first appearance as a result can later become a contributory factor, or at least an impediment to recovery. In either case, emotional aspects of reading failure can certainly not be ignored when remedial provision is being planned.

The third general concept is that of the unfavourable learning environment. This can be thought of in terms of 'methods'; it can be thought of in terms of school conditions in a much more comprehensive sense; it can be thought of in terms of attitudes and human relationships; and it can be thought of in terms of what one might label 'intelligibility to the learner'—of what Brandis and Henderson (1970) have called 'cultural discontinuity' (or its opposite) existing between the home and the school. In many ways, of course, the ideas in these groups overlap with or relate to one another.

The papers included in this section deal with some social and cultural correlates, with school conditions and relationships, and with emotional disturbance. Special emphasis has been given to recent speculation on, and study of, linguistic problems of social origin.

Reference

* BRANDIS, W. and HENDERSON, D. (1970) *Social Class, Language and Communication* London: Routledge and Kegan Paul

2.1 The effect of motivational and emotional factors on learning to read

M. D. VERNON
Emeritus Professor of Psychology, University of Reading

Reprinted from M. D. Vernon (1971) *Reading and its difficulties* Cambridge University Press, pp. 95–115

Conditions in the social environment

Difficulties in learning to read are often associated with children's social background. However, we are concerned here not so much with social factors as such, as with their relationship to cognitive and motivational differences in children which appear to affect reading achievement. Thus differences in socioeconomic status would seem to be related both to differences in intelligence, knowledge and linguistic competence; and also with variations in motivation. These variations stem at least in part from the different types of parent–child relationship occurring more frequently in certain social classes than in others.

One of the few facts connected with variation in reading achievement on which there is little disagreement is that it is highest in the upper *socioeconomic classes*, and decreases steadily as social class declines. This is well illustrated in Eisenberg's (1966) distribution of reading achievement (see Figure 1), in which socioeconomic status is lowest in the ordinary schools in the Metropolitan area and highest in the independent schools. In the three areas, the percentage of children retarded by two or more years in reading was 0, 3 and 28 respectively. Similar data have been obtained in British studies. Kellmer Pringle *et al* (1966) grouped the reading achievements of 11,000 seven year old children into three categories, good, medium and poor, on the basis of their scores on the Southgate test of word recognition. It then appeared that 7.1 per cent of those with parents in Occupational Classes I and II (Registrar General's classification), 18.9 per cent in Class III and 26.9 per cent in Classes IV and V were poor readers. Douglas (1964) found significant differences in word recognition and sentence completion among over 5000 eight year old children between those in upper-middle, lower-middle, upper-working and lower-working classes. These differences increased slightly in the same

47

M. D. Vernon

children by eleven years, the middle class children improving more than the working class.

Goodacre (1967) obtained a somewhat different result with 3000 children in infant schools, on the NFER test of sentence completion. The mean test score of children in lower working class areas was significantly lower than that of all other children. But there was no significant difference between children in middle class city schools and those in upper

FIGURE 1 *Reading achievement of children in different socioeconomic areas* *

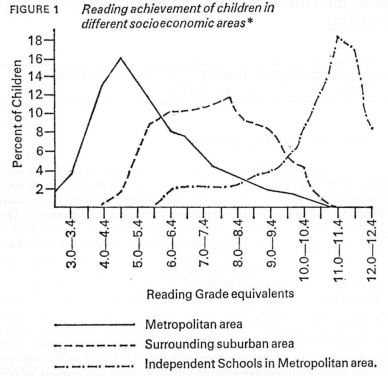

Reading Grade equivalents

———————— Metropolitan area

— — — — — — Surrounding suburban area

—.—.—.—.—. Independent Schools in Metropolitan area.

working class schools. However, for such young children a written sentence completion test might not give very reliable results.

It should be noted that the effects of differences in socioeconomic status are so generally accepted as sometimes to be exaggerated, even by teachers. Thus Goodacre (1968) found that teachers in infant schools expected that middle class children would reach a substantially higher level of reading achievement than would working class children, whereas as we noted the difference in tested achievement was sometimes small. The teachers overestimated the reading ability of middle class children and underestimated that of working class children.

There is a variety of factors associated with differences in socioeconomic

*(After Eisenberg (1966) p. 6)

status which may affect school achievement, including achievement in reading. Wiseman (1964), studying the variations in different areas of Manchester of various indices of social disorganization such as over-crowding, infant mortality, illegitimacy, etc, found significant correlations of 0.3–0.7 between these and reading achievement. However, these were lower than those obtained in London by Burt (1937), indicating a decrease of differences in the effects of poverty indices since that date. Though extreme poverty, malnutrition and disorganization in the home still exist, and may have a direct effect in depriving children of the physical energy essential for adequate school achievement, other factors in the home such as maternal care have begun to assume more importance (Wiseman 1964). It should be noted that Wiseman found 'lack of home care' to be associated with absence of superior attainment in reading rather than with backwardness. However, Ingram and Reid (1956) obtained a high incidence of broken homes and parental disharmony in seventy-eight cases of severe reading disability, although the proportion of cases in social Classes I and II was relatively higher than that in Classes IV and V.

There may be genetic factors which vary in different social classes and which affect reading achievement, of which the principal is *intelligence*. There is little doubt that the average intelligence of the lower social classes is less than that of the higher. There is of course extensive disagreement as to whether, and to what extent, these differences are the consequence of genetic endowment or of environmental pressures, or of both; and it is impossible here to discuss this controversy. We have noted that some association is commonly found between intelligence and reading ability. However, the evidence as to the association between class differences in intelligence and in reading achievement is somewhat more doubtful. Thus the investigation of Morris (1959) of over 7,000 Kent schoolchildren aged 7–11 years gave a correlation of 0.68 between socioeconomic class of schools and children's performance on the Watts–Vernon sentence completion test. But there was an even higher correlation of 0.71 between socioeconomic class and nonverbal intelligence test scores; and when reading test scores had been adjusted for differences in intelligence, the correlation of reading with socioeconomic class decreased to the non-significant figure of 0.20. Douglas (1964) showed that the variation with social class of scores on reading tests and on a nonverbal intelligence test were very similar. Morris, in a later study (1966), investigated three schools with high average reading scores in socioeconomic catchment areas classed I or II, and two schools with low scores in areas classed V. A group of 100 children from these schools who were 'poor' readers was compared with a group of 100 who were classed as 'good' readers. The majority of those in the first group (80 per cent) were children of manual workers; whereas 63 per cent of those in the second group were children of nonmanual workers. Again, the mean score of the latter on the non-verbal intelligence test was much higher than that of the former. But the overlap was considerable; many of the poor readers had high nonverbal intelligence. Lovell and Woolsey (1964) studied the performance on the Watt–Vernon reading test and the NFER nonverbal intelligence test of 1800 children aged 14–15 years. Among those with IQs of 90 or above who were backward readers with RQs below 80, 8.9 per cent were in Classes I and II, as compared with 11.1 per cent of children of these classes in the total group; whereas in Classes III, IV and V the proportion of backward readers exceeded the proportions belonging to these classes in the total sample. It appeared therefore that lower social class was associated with backwardness in reading independently of intelligence. But Lovell and Woolsey considered low social class to be a predisposing factor rather than a causal factor in reading backwardness.

Clearly homes in different socioeconomic classes show marked *cultural differences* which are likely to affect the children's linguistic ability, and this in turn is related to reading achievement. Even if the child's early speech develops spontaneously, his vocabulary and more complex language patterns are closely related to the language of the adults with whom he is in contact. The differences of language patterns between middle and working class parents were dramatically described and emphasized by Bernstein (1958). He hypothesized that working class parents employ a 'public language', consisting mainly of short grammatically simple sentences, often unfinished. Syntax is rigid, sentences are mainly in the active voice, there are few subordinate clauses, adjectives and adverbs are limited. Phrases are often repeated, and strung together in a disconnected manner by conjunctions. There are no overtones of finer meaning, though these may be indicated in part by gestures and intonational pattern. By contrast, the 'formal language' of the middle classes is not only more subtle and complex, but also more logical and individual. Thus middle class children become aware of a wide range of interpretations, meanings and precise discriminations in speech. This is the language mainly used by schoolteachers and in school books other than very early ones. The working class child is not only unfamiliar with this language, and finds it difficult to understand; but he may even feel that it threatens his basic ideas. Bernstein himself showed that boys of 15–18 years, with unskilled and semiskilled parents, scored within the normal range on a nonverbal intelligence test, Progressive Matrices, but were in most cases below normal on the Mill Hill Vocabulary test.

Again, Whipple (1961) found that American children of low socioeconomic status employed in their spontaneous utterances a smaller and less variable range of words than did children of higher status; and used words which differed from those considered normal for 6–7 year old children and from those appearing in these children's reading books. The children of low socioeconomic status used shorter sentences, often incomplete, fewer compound and complex sentences, and more ungrammatical constructions. Deutsch (1965) found that Negro and white children of low socioeconomic status were particularly deficient in the more advanced uses of language, in abstract categorizing. As the level of language complexity increased, the negative effects of social disadvantage were enhanced. Moreover, these effects appeared to be cumulative; they were more marked in children of 10–11 years than in those of 6–7 years. A similar accumulating deficit on the Illinois Test of Psycholinguistic Abilities was found by Schwartz, Deutsch and Weissman (1967) in young socially disadvantaged children who were not given 'enriched' schooling, by comparison with those who did receive such schooling. Jensen (1967) also noted the inability of the severely culturally deprived, such as many American Negro children, to use language in conceptual reasoning; they were inferior even in the verbal labelling of objects.

Newson and Newson (1968) showed that it was not only the linguistic structure of speech which varied in different social classes, but also the manner in which speech was employed. They observed that conversation between mothers and children aged four played a vital part in furthering the children's intellectual development. Such conversation did occur in all social classes. But middle class mothers employed speech to a greater extent than did working class mothers in controlling their children, explaining, persuading and reasoning with them, and formulating general principles of behaviour such as: 'If you tell lies, no one will ever believe you.' The working class mothers, especially those in Occupational Class V, more often gave brief specific commands and prohibitions and reinforced these with smacking when the children disobeyed. Therefore the middle class children were better able than the working class children to become aware of the use of language as an integral factor in understanding and directing their behaviour in accordance with general concepts of socially accepted behaviour. This in turn would tend to bring home to them the nature and value of verbal conceptualization.

There are other cultural characteristics and uses of language which may affect reading. Fraser (1959) obtained correlations for children aged twelve between school achievement and the education of parents and their reading of books and magazines, which were in general greater than were correlations with IQ. Malmquist (1958) found a significant relationship between backwardness in reading and the education of both father and mother. The fathers and mothers of poor readers had in most cases received only elementary education, whereas those of a high proportion of good readers had reached matriculation standard. Morris (1966) showed very marked differences between good and poor readers in the number of adult books and newspapers in the home, and in the frequency of parental membership of public libraries. The parents' education and reading are of course likely to affect the type of language they use.

Another influential factor is parents' reading aloud to their children. Thus Durkin (1966) found that mothers of children who could already read by the time they entered school at six years read aloud to their children and read much to themselves. Often the children had been given books. This tends to happen more frequently in middle class than in working class families. Again, Newson and Newson (1968) found that middle class parents, fathers as well as mothers, more often told their children stories at bedtime than did working class parents.

The deleterious effects of various environmental factors on intelligence and on school achievement were studied by P. E. Vernon (1965, 1969), in an investigation of the variations in performance of intelligence and of other tests.

Not only were differences in socioeconomic status of British boys investigated, but also the much greater degrees of *deprivation* experienced by boys living in other cultures—Jamaican, African, Canadian Indian and Eskimo. The information on deprivation was obtained through interviews with the boys. It was quite clear that both intelligence (*g*) and verbal ability (*v*) were lower among these children, all of them to a greater or less extent economically and culturally deprived, than among British children. However, some groups, for instance the Jamaicans and Uganda Africans, were relatively less retarded in spelling and on memory tests than on tests of reasoning and vocabulary, because they had been drilled in rote learning at school. Vernon analysed and assessed the following environmental factors as contributing to good intelligence and, in some cases, educational achievement.

1 Reasonable satisfaction of biological needs.
2 Stimulating environment and encouragement of exploration and experiment.
3 Linguistic stimulation, encouragement of linguistic and conceptual development.
4 Demanding but democratic family atmosphere, showing tolerance and lack of rigidity, and emphasizing self-control, responsibility and interest in school work.
5 Cultural stimulation in the home; parents' education; books, etc in the home; parents' cooperation with the school and aspirations for the child.
6 Regular and prolonged schooling, also emphasizing individual initiative and responsibility and discovery methods rather than rote learning.
7 Wide and adventurous leisure activities.

There was a general correspondence between the total number of adverse conditions and the inferiority of test performance, though particular factors affected some test performances more than others. The cultural stimulation supplied by the home was most closely related to allround ability. But in children like the Uganda Africans from homes where little English was spoken, or where it was largely a form of pidgin English, as with many of the Jamaican children, all tests involving the use and understanding of language were badly performed. However, performance on the Piaget type of test was affected also. And it was difficult to differentiate the effects of different adverse factors at all precisely, since in most cases so many were operating. In all these groups the majority of children were living in conditions of insecurity and want.

Werner, Simonian and Smith (1967) carried out an investigation of the reading achievement and performance on Thurstone's tests of Primary Mental Abilities of 10–11 year old children living in Hawaii. Many of these, and especially those of low socioeconomic status, were brought up in homes in which pidgin English was spoken. The children of low socio-economic status were inferior to those of higher status in reading achievement and in most of the Primary Mental Abilities. A correlation of 0.71 was obtained between reading grade and the total score on the Primary Mental Abilities tests; and of 0.69 between reading grade and V (verbal ability). Lower correlations were obtained with P (perceptual speed) and S (space); and with Bender test scores. Thus Werner *et al* concluded that when there were gross language deficiencies, these produced much more effect on reading than did perceptual deficiencies. However, it is possible that in this group also poor living conditions were partly responsible for reading backwardness.

Jensen (1967) considered that children's intelligence was not greatly affected by environmental factors within the normal range; though their effect on school achievement was greater. But severely adverse environmental circumstances, such as those suffered by many American Negro children, caused considerable impairment of intelligence, and even more of school achievement. Their cultural deprivation particularly affected their language abilities.

Effects on children's motivation of the home environment

Up to this point we have considered the relationships between environmental conditions and school achievement, particularly in reading, as if the effect of adverse conditions on school progress were a direct one. And so indeed it may be in the case of great poverty and malnutrition. The children are too weak, too lacking in energy and too prone to disease, to be able to work well. But except in circumstances of such physiological deprivation, the main effect of environmental factors may be upon the children's own cognitive abilities and on their *motivation to learn*. Of course poverty, hunger and insecurity impair motivation, as well as physical energy. No individual whose mind is dominated by craving for food or by fear of danger, illness or homelessness can take much interest in school activities, or make much effort to work hard. Though we are inclined to believe that the effects of poverty described by Burt are no longer operative in this country, they may in fact be more persistent than we suppose. Indeed, recent reports by Shelter confirm this.

But in default of these circumstances, or even in addition to them, as in some of the children studied in P. E. Vernon's investigations, there are many aspects of home life, and particularly of the relationship between parents and children, which may stimulate or inhibit school progress through their effects on the children's motivation to work and learn. One factor here would appear to be the closeness of the relationship between parents and children. The inferiority in reading achievement in the lower social classes may be due in part to the fact that the parents seem less close to their children, and do less to stimulate them to learn to read, than do parents in the higher social classes. Thus Milner (1951) found that among a group of six year old children, the majority of those who showed the best language ability came from middle class homes, and of those with the poorest language ability from lower class homes. The difference was due partly to the lack of books and of reading aloud in the latter, and of opportunity for frequent conversation with adults in adequate speech patterns. But also the middle class children had closer, warmer and more affectionate relations with their parents, who were permissive and encouraging to them.

The significance of *parental encouragement* was perhaps first noted by Fraser (1959) in relation to the general school achievement of twelve year old Scottish children. She obtained a correlation of 0.66 between parental encouragement and school achievement, a higher correlation than with any other aspect of home life. However, parental encouragement was estimated by the teachers; and it is possible therefore that these estimates were affected by the teachers' observations of the children's school behaviour. Thus Goodacre (1968) found that infant teachers tended to derive estimates of differences in home background from the children's desire to learn to read, and from whether or not the parents provided their children with books. Their actual contacts with the parents were rather slight. There was also the tendency to overestimate the attributes of middle class homes and underestimate those of working class homes.

Douglas (1964) also studied the effects of parental interest and encouragement, though the same doubts must be felt about his findings since these were based on teachers' assessment of parental interest. However, the assessments had some objective basis in, for instance, the frequency of visits paid to the school, by fathers as well as mothers; and general and medical care, and conscientiousness in taking children to clinics when recommended to do so. The degree of interest was highest in upper middle class parents, and decreased steadily down to the lower working class. But also, within each social class, the children with the most interested parents had the highest test scores; and this difference was greater for reading and arithmetic than for nonverbal intelligence. Indeed, there was an overlap in score between the children of the least interested parents in a particular class, and the children of the most interested parents in the class below it. Moreover, the children of the most interested parents improved their scores between the ages of eight and eleven years, whereas children of the least interested parents did not. When the relationships of test scores to standard of home and size of family were allowed for, the relationship to parental interest was still considerable.

Kellmer Pringle, Butler and Davie (1966) attempted to make estimates of parental interest as objective as possible by asking head teachers: 'Have the parents taken the initiative to discuss the child, even briefly, with you or any member of your teaching staff?' The children were then classified according to whether their parents had 'approached' or 'not approached' the teachers. The percentage of 'approached' among the 11,000 seven year olds decreased from 71 in Class I to 46 in Class V. Fourteen per cent of parents of poor readers fell into the 'approached' class; 41 per cent of medium readers; and 45 per cent of good readers. Moreover, in each social class there was a higher proportion of good readers in the 'approached' than in the 'not approached' class, although the differences were not significant in every social class. Incidentally, it should be realized that failure to make these approaches may be due in part to lack of interest and encouragement on the part of the teachers, probably more towards working class than middle class parents. But as we have seen parental interest and approaches are not governed solely by social class membership.

Douglas (1964) also investigated directly the relationship between parental interest and encouragement, and children's motivation and application to their school work. The teachers were asked to estimate whether the children were hard workers, average workers or poor workers. The frequency of hard workers varied with social class, from 26 per cent of upper middle class children to 7 per cent of lower working class children. Among children of interested parents, 70 per cent were hard workers, as against 33 per cent of those with uninterested parents. However, clearly a fair proportion of the latter did work hard in the absence of parental encouragement. Hard workers scored higher on the tests, and especially on those of school achievement, than did less hard workers. Moreover, the former improved their test performance between eight and eleven years; whereas the poor workers decreased in score, whether they received parental encouragement or not. However, a later study (Douglas, Ross and Simpson 1968) of some of the same children at fifteen years showed that hard workers with interested parents had improved their scores since eleven years, whereas those with uninterested parents had deteriorated.

It is generally considered that reading achievement is increased by strong *achievement motivation*. (It has been argued by critics of the author's book, *Human Motivation* (Vernon 1969), that there is considerable doubt as to the existence of achievement motivation as an independent entity. This objection may be valid. Nevertheless, the term may be employed to refer to a class of behaviour which is frequent in and characteristic of Western civilization.) Thus Zimmerman and Allebrand (1965) compared the Thematic Apperception test stories of 9–10 year old backward readers, retarded by at least two years, with those of good readers. The stories of the latter stressed achievement and effort in work; but these themes were absent from the stories of the backward readers. Undoubtedly the motive to achieve is related to parental stress on achievement; and such encouragement is more frequent in the higher than in the lower social classes.

But parents of children with high achievement motivation, while advocating achievement and independence and rewarding children when they show these, are also permissive rather than authoritarian in their discipline. In other words, the child is attracted rather than forced by pressure to achieve; and this is reinforced by his identification with his parents and his desire to be like them. Thus if the parents are themselves well-educated and successful in life, the children are further stimulated to achieve by this identification. Moreover, educated parents tend to show greater encouragement to their children to work well in school than do less educated parents (Douglas, Ross and Simpson 1968). Himmelweit (1963) compared the attitudes to school work of middle class and working class boys of 13–14 years, and found that the former were more concerned than were the latter with their school achievement and with higher educational and vocational prospects. They were more responsible, and possessed a higher and firmer system of values. Although the middle class parents were more concerned than were the working class with their sons' progress, and exerted more supervision over their work and leisure activities, they were also closer to their children in personal relationships. Any tendency to increase of anxiety in the children through parental pressure was relieved by this contact, and the feeling that they could talk to their parents about their aspirations and difficulties. The working class children, less often urged by their parents to achieve in school, were left largely to fend for themselves without parental guidance. However, in this respect 'upwardly mobile' working class parents were more like middle class than other working class parents. Now it is true that the interactions between parents and children are likely to be somewhat different at 13–14 years than at the age at which children begin to learn to read. But the findings of Milner emphasized the importance of these interactions.

Further evidence was supplied in a study by Kent and Davis (1957). On the basis of interviews with the parents of eight year old children, they divided the parents into four classes: demanding, overanxious, unconcerned and normal. These differences were unrelated to social class. The children of demanding parents, who put much pressure on the child to succeed, possessed higher Stanford–Binet IQs than did those of normal parents, and tended to be higher on the WISC Verbal than Performance scale; but they were not significantly higher on the WISC mean IQ nor on reading test scores. It would appear that parental demandingness, which often caused the children to be emotionally disturbed and overanxious to succeed, did lead to a greater development in verbal reasoning; but this did not affect reading. The children of overanxious parents, though not significantly inferior generally to the normals, were somewhat deficient on the practical side; WISC Performance IQs were lower than Verbal. Finally, the children of unconcerned parents, though too few in number to give entirely valid results, were inferior to the normals on the Stanford–Binet IQ and in reading age, which averaged only 6.4 years. The majority showed signs of emotional disturbance, which appeared in apathy, lack of effort and of spontaneity. Highfield and Pinsent (1952), in a study of difficult school children of 6–9 years, found that children of rigid punitive parents tended to be restless and distractible, and to need control in school. The children of lax indifferent parents were apathetic and listless, and required stimulation rather than control.

Other studies have indicated that children with relatively good verbal ability may have parents who afford them much verbal stimulation, but at the same time may be demanding and overprotective. On the other hand, children with parents who stimulate independence tend to have higher nonverbal than verbal ability. Bing (1963) carried out a study of the upbringing of and maternal behaviour towards ten year old children in two groups. In the first, verbal ability as measured by Thurstone's Primary Mental Abilities Tests, was significantly higher than nonverbal; in the second group, the reverse. Relatively higher verbal ability was associated with verbal encouragement in early childhood, a plentiful supply of books, punishment for poor school achievement, restriction on freedom and some degree of overprotectiveness. The mothers, when present while their children were being tested, tried to help the children, encouraged and put pressure on them to succeed, but discouraged them when they failed. Higher nonverbal ability was associated with opportunity for exploration and experiment. However, we cannot infer that the demandingness of the former parents and their emphasis on dependence necessarily promote good verbal achievement, including reading; or whether it is merely that the child is more proficient in verbal than in practical activities, practical ability being promoted by inculcation of independence. P. E. Vernon (1969) obtained some evidence that poor performance on tests of practical ability, such as Kohs Blocks, was associated with lack of encouragement of initiative in the home, which seemed to affect the capacity to act purposefully in performing such tests. But performance on purely perceptual tests such as Gottschaldt's embedded figures was unrelated to home circumstances, though deficient in some cultures. The causes of this deficiency were not clear.

However, it would seem that there is good evidence for the effect on reading achievement of lack of stimulation in the home. Again, Collins (1961) studied a group of primary school backward readers in whose homes maternal and cultural conditions were generally poor. The children lacked curiosity and vivacity, and interest in their work; and there was a general low level of value on culture and aspiration for success.

Motivation and the school environment

It would thus appear that interest and desire to achieve play an important part in stimulating children to learn to read. Those who inevitably find it difficult, through lack of intelligence, linguistic ability or favourable cultural influences in the home, may require *special stimulation in the school*. It is currently maintained that *free activities* in the school appealing to the child's natural interest, and methods of *discovery* and experiment, are more stimulating than are more formal methods emphasizing rote learning, in that the former improve the children's initiative, interest in school work and effort to learn. Indeed, we noted that P. E. Vernon considered the former methods to constitute one of the factors favourable to intellectual development and educational achievement. Such methods appear to be employed successfully in the new discovery techniques of learning mathematics and science. On the other hand, their use in teaching reading would seem to be more difficult. Once the child has mastered basic reading skill, clearly he can discover much through reading. But in the early stages, there would appear to be little room for experiment or original thought, since the scope of these is limited by the necessity for learning printed letter shapes and their phonic associations. Thus Southgate (1970) considered that discovery methods were inappropriate to the teaching of reading because the irregularity of English spelling prevented children from generalizing phoneme pronunciation (as for instance from 'mat' to 'mate'). However, more regular schemes of grapheme–phoneme correspondence, such as those of ita and Gattegno's *Words in Colour* (Gattegno 1962) gave better opportunity for discovery. Indeed, it has been noted that one advantage of ita is that children can learn from it themselves, with less instruction from the teacher than is necessary with the ordinary alphabet.

Though Southgate (1970) advocated the use of a carefully structured method of teaching reading such as she described, the results of experimental inquiries into the relative efficacy of *formal* and *informal methods* have been somewhat variable. Morris (1959) obtained a correlation of 0.4 between reading achievement in children of 7–11 years, and the employment of a formal approach and systematic instruction in reading in the infant school. But later (1966) she stated that this association was affected by other factors and was not significant. Anderson, Byron and Dixon (1956) showed that the average age of learning to read was lower in a school which employed early teaching of reading by formal methods than in a school which laid more emphasis on informal methods and encouraged individual activities. However, once the children in the latter school had learnt to read, they soon overcame their initial delay, and caught up those in the former. Gardner (1942, 1950) also found that children taught by progressive methods were able to read as well as those taught by formal methods at 9–10 years. Kellmer Pringle and Reeves (1968) compared the reading achievement of children in the second, third and fourth years at two junior schools, one in which they received a traditional formal education and the other in which a progressive approach was employed. Allowing for differences in intelligence between the two groups, there were no significant differences on the Neale Reading test. Curiously enough, the most able children profited more by the formal approach than by the informal.

Lovell (1963) gave the Vernon Graded Word Reading test and the

NFER nonverbal intelligence test to over 1300 children of 10–11 years in eleven matched pairs of schools. Each pair contained one school employing formal teaching methods with the traditional curriculum, and one school using informal teaching encouraging the children's interests and creative activities. There was no significant difference in average reading achievement between the children in the two types of school. But the spread of achievement was greater in the schools with formal teaching; 14 per cent of the children had RQs below 80, as against 9.5 per cent in the informal schools. Thus it would seem that the amount of backwardness was greater in the schools using formal methods. Even if early reading teaching does not readily lend itself to informal teaching, this teaching may stimulate interest which may produce at least an adequate level of reading achievement. Morrison and McIntyre (1969) stated that studies had shown that children preferred the use of discovery methods, and were therefore presumably better motivated. These methods were less effective in the acquisition of routine skills than in more complex tasks where the employment of ideas is important. Nevertheless, the development of spoken language can well involve experiment and discovery, and in turn benefit reading.

The children's motivation may be particularly important in connection with what has been called *reading readiness*. It would appear that readiness to begin formal reading instruction depends in the first place on the child's level of development in conceptual reasoning, linguistic ability and visuo-spatial perception. A certain competence in performing these cognitive processes is essential, and without it children may experience great difficulty in learning to read. Indeed, it seems likely that many children do not attain this competence during their first year at school, and would profit from the postponement of formal reading teaching till the second year. Moreover, they would benefit from increased opportunity for free activity. However, children of superior intelligence and linguistic ability may well be able to understand and learn from formal reading teaching as soon as they enter school. This depends also on previous experience, especially in linguistic activities and in the use of books. We noted that Durkin (1966) found that children who could already read when they first went to school were accustomed to the use of books; and that their parents had read aloud to them and sometimes actually taught them.

Thus undoubtedly children vary considerably in the age at which they are ready to learn to read, and it may be difficult to estimate their readiness. In some schools in the USA children are given tests of 'reading readiness', adequate performance on which is claimed to demonstrate that the children possess the cognitive capacities necessary to enable them to learn to read. But these tests have not been standardized for British children. Goodacre (1970) pointed out that their correlations with subsequent reading achievement were only of the order of 0.4–0.6. Indeed, tests other than those of actual letter discrimination and recognition appear to have little predictive value.

Moreover, it would seem that readiness depends also on the children's motivation, their interest in reading and their desire to learn, as is generally recognized by English infant teachers (Goodacre 1970). Interest may develop only slowly in those from uncultured homes with uninterested parents. Desire to learn may be created by the example of other children; and in this connection Stauffer (1968) has suggested that group teaching may be superior to individual teaching in that children in a group stimulate one another. But in infant classes in poor neighbourhoods, particularly in the slums of large towns, the majority of children may have comparatively little desire to learn, and thus the effects of social conformity and imitation may be negative rather than positive.

Another factor of considerable importance is the child's capacity to attend to what the teacher says and does. Jensen (1967) noted that socially disadvantaged children were often unable to focus and sustain their attention on the teacher, and quickly became distracted and restless. He considered that middle class children developed the capacity for sustained attention through their interaction with the mother, through observing and responding to what she did and said. This had not occurred in children who had not experienced a close individual relationship with the mother, as was frequent with socially disadvantaged children. Moreover, their capacity for attending might even deteriorate during their first year at school. They did not really understand what the teacher was saying and doing. The tasks she set were too difficult for them and they were unable to perform them successfully. Failure was negatively reinforcing, and the children became more and more confused, inattentive and discouraged, and might develop an aversion for school activities.

Clearly therefore readiness to learn to read may depend as much on the teacher's capacity to stimulate interest as on the children's cognitive abilities, and her task of arousing and maintaining interest as well as giving instruction may be exceptionally severe. She may find it best to postpone the difficult processes of phonic analysis, which require more concentration and energy than does simple look-and-say. The slow start in the early stages of reading which is almost inevitable in these circumstances may produce an apparent initial backwardness. But this is greatly preferable to a widespread failure among children who are not motivated to respond to this instruction, and therefore simply do not grasp what they are required to do. As we have noted, such failure has a negative reinforcing effect, decreasing positive motivation still further and even producing resistance.

It has been established by Morris (1966) that reading achievement is related to the *skill of the teacher*; and that children taught by untrained, inexperienced and unskilful teachers tend to be especially backward in reading. Now teaching skill obviously involves the knowledge of correct methods in all their details and variations and the ability to communicate these. But is some additional capacity necessary to stimulate and motivate? Perhaps this is relatively unimportant for normal, lively, curious and reasonably intelligent children. But for the apathetic and uninterested, the anxious and overprotected, constant encouragement and stimulation may be necessary, and above all the capacity to make reading materials and activities interesting. Teachers may regard these as truisms, but if as we noted reading is difficult to make the subject of discovery and experiment, it may not be easy to create interest.

A study by Sampson (1969) showed that teachers were well aware of the importance of incentives in learning to read. One teacher, fortunately exceptional, wrote: 'My children are not really interested in anything.' The majority thought that most children were eager to learn, but that success was the most important factor in encouraging effort, and that children were greatly disheartened when they failed. Thus encouragement and praise, even of small efforts, were important. But also frequent attempts were made to appeal to children's individual interests. Additional ways of stimulating interest were through provision of attractive books and of subsidiary games, for instance of word matching. The value of these for severely backward readers was strongly emphasized by Stott (1964). Morris (1966) found that the selection and supply of books and other reading materials was most inadequate in junior school classes in which there were many backward readers.

Several teachers in Sampson's inquiry noted the importance of good social relations between teacher and children. The ability to establish sympathetic, friendly and understanding relationships may be one of the most significant factors in teaching skill. Obviously this is more difficult in large classes of children, especially if many are apathetic and unforthcoming. Thus Morris (1966) showed that the junior school teachers of backward readers were less skilled in breaking up classes into small suitably occupied groups and in giving individual attention where needed.

Yet clearly the teacher must herself possess the ability to encourage and stimulate. Harvey *et al* (1966) found that with teachers who were flexible in their ideas, perceptive of the children's needs and warm in their relations with them, the children were significantly more interested, active and higher in achievement than with teachers who were relatively rigid, authoritarian and intolerant. Washburne and Heil (cited by Morrison and McIntyre 1969) showed that the interaction between teachers and children varied with the characteristics of the children as well as those of the teachers. In general teachers who were warm but also businesslike and orderly in their treatment of the children were more effective than those who were conscientious but anxious. Children who in themselves were hard workers did comparatively well with all types of teacher; those who were docile conformers worked best with warm, exuberant and independent teachers. Children who tended to oppose authority, though on the whole they performed badly whatever the type of teaching, were more responsive to the businesslike and orderly than to the others. However, as Morrison and McIntyre pointed out, we need to know far more about the effects of social interaction between teachers and children, and how

M. D. Vernon

different types of children are best motivated. And if more information were available, then it might be possible to train teachers more effectively to exercise the most suitable treatment.

References

ANDERSON, I. H., BYRON, O. and DIXON, W. R. (1956) The relationship between reading achievement and the method of teaching reading *University of Michigan School of Education Bulletin* 7, 104

BERNSTEIN, B. (1958) Some sociological determinants of perception *British Journal of Sociology* 9, 159

BING, E. (1963) Effect of childrearing practices on development of differential cognitive abilities *Child Development* 34, 631

*BURT, C. (1937) *The Backward Child* London: University of London Press

*COLLINS, J. E. (1961) The effects of remedial education *Education Monograph* University of Birmingham Institute of Education

*DEUTSCH, M. (1965) The role of social class in language development and cognition *American Journal of Orthopsychiatry* 35, 78

*DOUGLAS, J. W. B. (1964) *The Home and the School* London: MacGibbon and Kee; Panther (1971)

DOUGLAS, J. W. B., ROSS, J. M. and SIMPSON, H. R. (1968) *All Our Future* London: Davies; Panther (1971)

DURKIN, D. (1966) *Children Who Read Early* New York: Teachers' College, Columbia University

EISENBERG, L. (1966) The epidemiology of reading retardation and a program for preventive intervention in J. Money and G. Shiffman (eds) *The Disabled Reader* Baltimore: Johns Hopkins Press

FRASER, E. (1959) *Home Environment and the School* London: University of London Press

GARDNER, D. E. M. (1942) *Testing Results in the Infant School* London: Methuen

GARDNER, D. E. M. (1950) *Long Term Results of Infant School Methods* London: Methuen

GATTENGO, C. (1962) *Words in Colour* Reading: Educational Explorers

*GOODACRE, E. J. (1967) *Reading in Infant Classes* Slough: National Foundation for Educational Research

*GOODACRE, E. J. (1968) *Teachers and their Pupils' Home Background* Slough: National Foundation for Educational Research

GOODACRE, E. J. (1970) The concept of reading readiness in M. Chazan (ed) *Reading Readiness* University College Swansea Faculty of Education

HARVEY, O. J., PRATHER, M. S., WHITE, B. J., ALTER, R. D. and HOFFMEISTER, J. K. (1966) Teachers' belief systems and preschool atmospheres *Journal of Educational Psychology* 57, 373

HIGHFIELD, M. E. and PINSENT, A. (1952) *A Survey of Rewards and Punishments in Schools* Slough: National Foundation for Educational Research

HIMMELWEIT, H. (1963) Socioeconomic background and personality in E. P. Hollander and R. G. Hunt (eds) *Current Perspectives in Social Psychology* Oxford: Oxford University Press

INGRAM, T. T. S. and REID, J. F. (1956) Developmental aphasia observed in a department of child psychiatry *Archives of Diseases in Childhood* 31, 161

JENSEN, A. R. (1967) The culturally disadvantaged: psychological and educational aspects *Educational Research* 10, 4

*KELLMER PRINGLE, M. L., BUTLER, N. R. and DAVIE, R. (1966) *11,000 Seven Year Olds* London: Longman

KELLMER PRINGLE, M. L. and REEVES, J. K. (1968) The influence of two junior school regimes upon attainment in reading *Human Development* 11, 25

KENT, N. and DAVIES, D. R. (1957) Discipline in the home and intellectual development *British Journal of Medical Psychology* 30, 27

LOVELL, K. (1963) Informal vs. formal education and reading attainments in the junior school *Educational Research* 6, 70

LOVELL, K. and WOOLSEY, M. E. (1964) Reading disability, nonverbal reasoning and social class *Educational Research* 6, 226

MALMQUIST, E. (1958) *Factors related to reading disabilities in the first grade of the elementary school* Stockholm: Almqvist and Wiksell

MILNER, E. (1951) A study of the relationship between reading readiness in grade one school children and patterns of parent–child interaction *Child Development* 22, 95

MORRIS, J. M. (1959) *Reading in the Primary School* London: Newnes

*MORRIS, J. M. (1966) *Standards and Progress in Reading* Slough: National Foundation for Educational Research

*MORRISON, A. and McINTYRE, D. (1969) *Teachers and Teaching* Harmondsworth: Penguin

NEWSON, J. and NEWSON, E. (1968) *Four Years Old in an Urban Community* London: Allen and Unwin

*SAMPSON, O. C. (1969) A study of incentives in remedial teaching *Reading* 3, i, 6

SCHWARTZ, S., DEUTSCH, G. P. and WEISSMAN, A. (1967) Language development in two groups of socially disadvantaged young children *Psychological Reports* 21, 169

SOUTHGATE, V. (1970) The importance of structure in beginning reading in W. K. Gardner (ed) *Reading Skills: Theory and Practice* London: Ward Lock Educational

STAUFFER, R. G. (1968) Individualized and group type directed reading instruction in G. Natchez (ed) *Children with Reading Problems* New York: Basic Books

STOTT, D. H. (1964) *Roads to Literacy* Glasgow: Holmes

VERNON, P. E. (1965) Environmental handicaps and intellectual development *British Journal of Educational Psychology* 35, 9

VERNON, P. E. (1969) *Intelligence and the Cultural Environment* London: Methuen

M. D. Vernon

WERNER, E. E., SIMONIAN, K. and SMITH, R. S. (1967) Reading achievement, language functioning and perceptual-motor development of 10 and 11 year olds *Perceptual Motor Skills* 25, 409

WHIPPLE, G. (1961) The culturally and socially deprived reader in H. M. Robinson (ed) *Controversial Issues in Reading and Promising Solutions Supplementary Education Mongraph* no. 91

WISEMAN, S. (1964) *Education and Environment* Manchester: Manchester University Press

ZIMMERMAN, I. L. and ALLEBRAND, G. N. (1965) Personality characteristics and attitudes towards achievement of good and poor readers *Journal of Educational Research* 59, 28

2.2 A summary of environmentalist views on language deprivation and reading failure

DAVENPORT PLUMER
Graduate School of Education, Harvard

Reprinted from F. Williams (1970) (ed) *Language and Poverty*
Markham, pp. 292–301

Language 'codes' and 'styles'

More sociolinguistic than psycholinguistic in approach is a body of research literature which refers not only to social-class distinctions in language but in its uses and manner of uses. This literature expands the view of language to its functioning in social systems, and such systems may range all the way from parent–child communication to the uses of language within a given subculture.

Bernstein's restricted and elaborated codes
Bernstein is most frequently linked with his contributions to the idea that different classes have their own language codes—i.e. the particular ranges of linguistic selection characteristic of communication within given social structures. Bernstein theorizes that members of the lower classes (or in Great Britain, the working classes) have access only to a style of language (restricted code) characteristic of their social structures but different from that of the middle class and the language used by the schools (elaborated code). Obviously this distinction carries substantial implications concerning social mobility, educational intervention programmes and the like.

Much of the empirical research into this theory has been focused upon isolation and definition of the two codes. This work dates back to studies conducted on the language and IQ of teenage boys from different social classes (see Bernstein 1961, 1962). Although this research has been carried further by Bernstein and his associates (see esp. Lawton 1968), three fundamental problems are yet to be resolved. The first refers to a suitably objective definition of the linguistic distinctions between restricted and elaborated codes (see Bernstein 1961, pp. 297–9; 1964; 1965; 1966; and 1967, pp. 94–5 for his attempts at this). The definitions of these distinctions have varied substantially according to researcher and project. The items listed by Lawton (1963, 1968) differ from Bernstein's lists, and all of these differ somewhat from distinctions described by Loban (1966b) and Robinson (1965). Thus when we speak of restricted and elaborated codes we are, in fact, referring to a varying configuration of characteristics rather than a consistent set. Part of this problem is that Bernstein's statement of the characteristics that constitute both codes is imprecise—for example one characteristic is 'a discriminitive selection from a range of adjectives and adverbs' (Bernstein 1967, p. 95).

A second major problem—more important than inconsistency or imprecision but probably underlying both—is the lack of consistent theoretical grounding for the individual items or the full code. This problem is illustrated in Lawton's (1968) treatment of passive verbs. Bernstein found (1962) that his middle class subjects used a higher proportion of passive verbs than did his working class subjects. This finding was later supported for both writing and speech by Lawton (1963). This is an interesting finding only if it can be related to something else—a theoretical notion of some set of empirical data like reading performance, family size, disciplinary pattern, or a developmental scheme showing the use of passive verbs at certain ages. When Lawton (1968) attempts to give some theoretical account for this finding he refers to three grammarians with divergent points of view and concludes (p. 119): '. . . although it might be argued that in theory anything could be expressed in English without ever using the passive voice, in practice its absence or low frequency is probably symptomatic of a limited control over language use.' This kind of support (and this is not atypical) is insufficient to establish the significance of the individual feature or its relation to the rest of the features of the code.

That there are class-related differences in speech and writing has been clear for some time. What is needed now is greater attention to what these differences mean. Does the difference in the proportion of passive verbs signify, for example, a developmental lag? Is it related to verbal or non-verbal IQ? How does it relate to the other revealed differences in language or language usage? In short, what do we know when we have found such a difference in the proportion of passive verbs used?

A third problem is the representative–optimum argument. Although Lawton (1963, 1964) reported class differences roughly similar to those earlier found by Bernstein—i.e. restricted code used by lower-class subjects, elaborated by higher—attempts to get at the heart of the social implications of this thesis have been inadequate. That is, the main problem is whether a lower-status person can use an elaborated code, or even whether he has one. As Robinson (1965) has argued, the earlier findings may show only a choice (representative) in codes typical of the lower-status speaker, rather than what he actually can do (optimum). Lawton (1968) has more recently concluded that when pushed, working class boys will attempt a linguistic adjustment toward an elaborated code, but that (p. 140) 'they lack practice and therefore facility'. Data and interpretations reported by Williams and Naremore (1969) tend to support this position, although these researchers have yet another definition of the code differences.

Despite these problems, Bernstein's theories are richly suggestive, particularly in the way he explains the social and family-group patterns of organization and communication that give rise to the two codes.

A recent study by Bernstein and Henderson (1969) deals with the orientation towards use of language for various kinds of socialization. The subjects were working class and middle class mothers who were asked questions about the relative difficulty that a mother who could not talk would encounter in socializing her children in interpersonal relations and in certain rudimentary skills. The results showed both groups wanting to use language more for interpersonal socialization than for teaching children skills. However, the differences between the groups are marked. Bernstein and Henderson (1969, p. 21) conclude:

> The results show that the middle class, relative to the working class, place a greater emphasis upon the use of language in dealing with situations within the person area. The working class, relative to the middle class, place a greater emphasis on the use of language in the transmission of various skills.

These preferences are not due to a difference in the relevance of the skill area as opposed to the person area for the two groups, but rather to different implicit learning theories which in turn shape the language codes of the children of the two groups (Bernstein and Henderson 1969, p. 13):

> It would appear then that the difference in the response of middle class and working class mothers to the relevance of language in the acquisition of various skills is more likely to arise out of differences in the concept of learning than out of differences between social classes in terms of the value placed upon the learning of such skills. The socialization of the middle class child into the acquisition of skills is into both operations and principles which are learned in a social context which emphasizes *autonomy*. In the case of the working class child his socialization into skills emphasizes operations rather than principles learned in a social context where the child is accorded *reduced autonomy*.

Although it is clearly impossible to do more than suggest the richness of Bernstein's views on language and education, we can at least note the kinds of research needs that his work has generated. First, we need to consider the feasibility of teaching elaborated code. What is the optimum age for this teaching to begin; what aspects of the code should come first? Second, we need to study the families that may characteristically use the two codes. That is, we need to look naturalistically at families of different

Davenport Plumer

social classes and describe the social relations within them. Such a study would emphasize those topics that have appeared in Bernstein's and his colleague's theoretical work and interview research—mother's control behaviour, socialization in the areas of skill training, and learning about interpersonal relations. This research would produce a much needed picture of the specific conditions in the two types of homes which give rise to different codes and the educational assets and liabilities associated with them.

Family language styles
Bernstein has not been alone in studying language and communication within family structures. Some pertinent ideas have been reported in papers by Dave (1963), Strodtbeck (1965) and Gordon and Wilkerson (1966). However, the best known recent study which deals with social-class differences in family language styles was conducted by Hess and his colleagues in Chicago.

As reported in various places (Hess and Shipman 1965, Hess, Shipman, Bear and Brophy 1968, Olim, Hess and Shipman 1967), the project involved administering a variety of tests to Negro mothers selected from a range of social strata; among the data were interview and selected verbal-task materials. The researchers cite four major correlations that support Bernstein's notion of language as the mediating variable between a mother's social-class orientation and her child's perceptions and abilities. First is a significant relationship between a mother's control behaviour and her language. If she uses status-normative controls—if she presents rules in an assigned manner where compliance is the only rule-following possibility—then she will also use imperatives frequently and she will use a restricted code in telling her child a story in an experimental situation. Second is the correlation between a mother's status-normative, imperative controls and her child's performance on the Binet, the Sigel Sorting Task and a block-sorting task. The performance of the children with status-normative mothers was significantly lower on seven out of eight tasks than that of children whose mothers used so-called cognitive-rational controls. The third major correlation related mother's language styles to children's performance on the cognitive tasks above. Again the relationship is in the expected direction, the children of elaborated code mothers doing significantly better than children whose mothers used the restricted code. Finally, the researchers report that the mothers who use elaborated code, cognitive-rational controls, and who use instructions rather than imperatives are most likely to be members of the middle class, while the mothers who use less option-opening language and controls are to be found in the lower two classes in this sample.

Although the language measures used in this study are not always clear and uncontroversial, the research as a whole suggests that Bernstein's point about the importance of a mother's control behaviour and speech patterns certainly merits more intensive investigation. However, the emphasis on the options which the mother's control behaviour opens for the child raises the additional question that will be harder to investigate but which is vital to any plans for systematic remediation. The question centres on the relation between the kinds of real options that exist in the life of the child, the way these options are reflected in the behaviour of the family, the extent to which the child can select among options for his own behaviour, and the language of the mother which sets up these options. Stated another way, this question concerns the relation between so-called fate control, which seems to be positively correlated with academic success (Coleman *et al* 1966), and the speech codes characteristic of those families in which there exists this sense of fate control.

The rough scheme in Figure 1 suggests one way of visualizing this

FIGURE 1

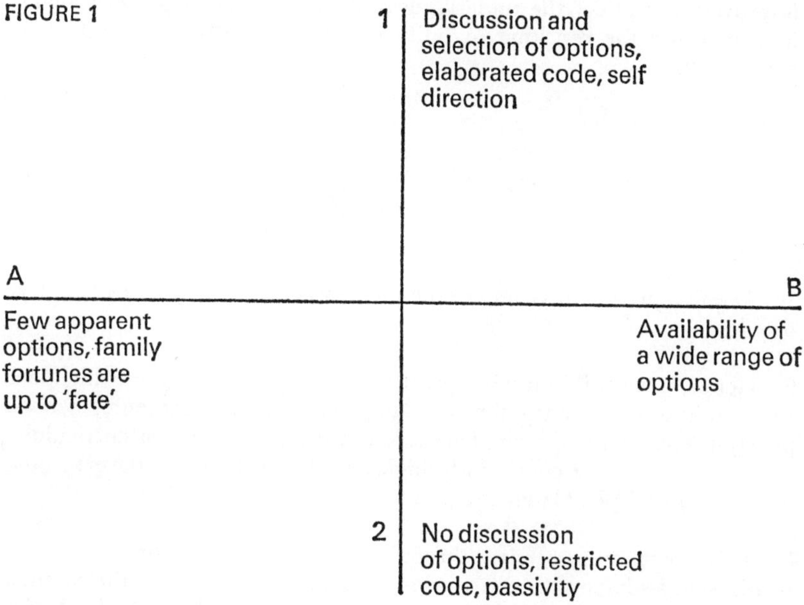

	1	Discussion and selection of options, elaborated code, self direction

A		B
Few apparent options, family fortunes are up to 'fate'		Availability of a wide range of options

	2	No discussion of options, restricted code, passivity

relationship, based on the way a family would perceive its ability to shape its own destiny and the way that perception might be related to its customary patterns of speech performance.

From the research discussed above, the apparent conclusion seems to be that quadrants A2 and B1 would represent social-status extremes and also either end of the restricted–elaborated code spectrum. This is a conclusion we can infer from the work of Bernstein and Hess (see also Strodtbeck 1965). It is, of course, important to investigate in detail the possible exceptions represented by quadrants A1 and B2—the elaborated code speakers with few viable options and the restricted code speakers with many options. On a much broader scale, Stodolsky and

Lesser (1967) have proposed that some of the alleged relationships between language, school success, and life style should be studied by means of a very direct, large-scale experiment.

Would poor people, given jobs and money (and the counselling necessary to see and act upon options) change in their behaviours relevant to the child's educability? Would parental behaviours such as cognitive level, teaching style, values and attitudes change with a change in economic conditions?

Without these two kinds of studies a great deal of time and money may be spent ministering to a symptom—the child's inability to use the elaborated code—that may itself resist treatment and may, even if improved, not affect the underlying problem, that is, poor performance in school and the resulting inability to make a satisfying, dignified life for himself.

Implications

A book with the title *Language and Poverty* must consider the implications of research in quite broad terms. Let us begin with four conclusions that emerge with considerable force from this research.

1 The five preschool years are the most important in a child's language development.

2 Hence, poor children who spend these five years in homes which lack the conditions necessary for full language development enter schools poorly prepared for the challenges of the traditional school curriculum. There is, in short, a consistently high correlation between poverty (and often race) and poor language performance.

3 This correlation persists throughout a child's schooling. In other words, schools have at best a very modest impact in terms of their ability to educate poor children. That is, a poor child who begins school with submedian tests scores will, in all likelihood, end his school career even further below the median score for his age and grade. The Coleman report (1966) indicates that this is true for middle class as well as lower class children. Irrespective of the child's social status, schools do not account for much of the variance in achievement scores.

4 Finally, there are exceptions to the poverty cycle (and to the prosperity cycle). The poor children who 'make it' may be genetically superior, or they may have had an unusually supportive environment. Thus far, however, research has not been able to distinguish between these causes or to specify in detail the characteristics of a supportive environment.

These four points can be incorporated into a circular relation as shown in Figure 2—a version of the poverty cycle. This circular representation of the problem recommends itself because it invites multiple solutions, and because it represents the magnitude of the problem. Cohen (1968, p. 339), reviewing the Plowden Report on primary education in Great Britain, comments forcefully on both of these points:

Thus, if the Council (which sponsored the research) is to be faulted, perhaps it should not be for making such policy suggestions as it did,

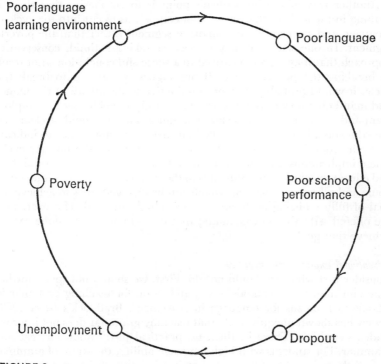

FIGURE 2

but rather for not more fully exploring the other lines of inquiry and policies which seem to be suggested in its data. Chief among these were the findings on school social class, and quasi-experimental research to more directly and competitively test various policy alternatives.

The Council's report invites one other reflection on the relation between research and policy in this area. It is that efforts to provide equality of educational opportunity will be enormously costly, in whatever terms we choose to compute cost. In the last analysis it is the low social and political priority assigned to equality of opportunity in both England and America—not the absence of adequate research—which is the chief obstacle to effective policy. The pity is not that the Plowden research was less than perfect, or less than conclusive, for given the constraints of time it is remarkably good and useful. The pity is that were the research much more perfect and conclusive we would be little closer to schools that would remove, rather than reflect, the educational consequences of social and economic inequality.

Another way of putting Cohen's point is to emphasize that there is nothing in the logic of this review that compels us to cut into the cycle of language and poverty at the language segment rather than the poverty segment. In one sense we may be seen as taking a timid, conservative approach that may—even if carried to a successful conclusion—not result in breaking the poverty cycle. If our highest priority is to break this cycle, it would probably be more productive to devote all of the money and man-hours now devoted to language study to achieving full employment and an adequate income for all families. Thus it should be clear that the educational implications spelled out below are not meant to indicate that education is the way, or the only way, to break the poverty cycle. These implications are offered to an audience of professional researchers and educators whose commitment is to those aspects of a child's immediate home and school environment which can be changed so as to achieve the goal of fully realizing each child's intellectual potential. However, they are offered with the understanding that educational effort alone cannot achieve that goal.

Educational implications: negative
Consider first what we should not do. First, we should not spend further time and money on methods, texts, and so on for teaching grammar in schools as a means for language improvement. Braddock's (*et al* 1963) review has shown unequivocally that teaching grammar does not improve students' writing. There is, then, no practical justification for teaching grammar. For students with high language ability, the study of grammar does little serious harm, except that it takes time from more valuable activities. My own observations suggest that children in inner-city schools suffer most from studying grammar simply because they study it more. In many such schools, sophomores, juniors, and seniors spend half to three-quarters of their language–arts time studying grammar—that is, between sixty and ninety hours a year that they could be using more profitably. Assuming these sixty and ninety hours were to be suddenly made available for some other purpose, how should they be used? What would an English teacher teach during that time?

One negative answer is clear; this time should not be spent on attempts to change disadvantaged students' dialect. Students do not drop out of school because of dialect problems unless, of course, they leave out of frustration with the school's efforts to change their dialect. However, they do leave because they can't read. Hence, one simple recommendation: drop grammar study and let students read, or teach them to read better, for sixty to ninety hours per year. This may be a difficult change to bring about, given the expectations of parents, students and teachers with respect to grammar study. Until such a change has been accomplished, however, no school should, in good conscience, apply for Federal or other money for a compensatory language programme.

A third, and perhaps obvious, change that should not be made is that suggested by Davis (1965) to make school less verbal, less language-oriented for the children who come to school with underdeveloped language skills. The implication of lowered teacher expectations makes this suggestion difficult to accept in light of recent research on expectations (Rosenthal and Jacobson 1968). It is difficult to imagine how the sixty to ninety hours we might allocate to a nonverbal programme might be spent, but any alternatives that come to mind would do little to help the language-poor student.

Educational implications: positive
We have emphasized the need to focus on reading. The emphasis must be on basic reading skills, not a peripheral issue like developing taste. A student will not come to share a teacher's taste by being required to read a nineteenth century novel. He may simply not read. Whether or not the student reads should be the final judgment. To this end, he might be encouraged to read Brown's *Manchild in the Promised Land* (1965), Miller's *The Cool World* (1964), or magazines on karate or automechanics. Children learn to read by reading; thus, the school must somehow provide them with books they can and will read. *Hooked on Books* (Fader 1969) presents one way of getting around a small (under $10 per pupil in many school systems) book budget. A school should exhaust these approaches before looking into a compensatory or remedial reading programme.

What else does this review suggest about school practice? The most prominent theme running through all of the literature on language development is that children learn language through verbal interaction with more mature speakers. They learn language by using it. This does not mean simply listening to more mature speakers—otherwise poor children who have attended school regularly and listened to television more than middle class children would be on a par with their middle class counterparts.

To improve language performance by using language, a student has to talk, write and read in school. The younger the child, the more he should be allowed and encouraged to talk to mature speakers. The interaction must be frequent, structured and systematic, though not necessarily without humour or 'soul', as the Bereiter (1965) dialogues often appear to be. This kind of interaction is hard to achieve. However, older students

73

and nonprofessional adults can be trained to work with young students as tutor-conversationalists. Several programmes based on Vygotsky's (trans. 1962) theories about dialogue being the germ of inner thought have been tried and these should provide a basis for programmes adapted to the particular needs of a given school (see, for example, Blank and Solomon 1968, Bereiter 1965, Karnes 1966, 1969).

Schools, no matter who their clientele, are at a disadvantage when attempting to supplement or enrich a child's home experience. The child enters school as the period of fastest language development is ending. If a school is to offset any disadvantage in the child's home language environment, it must concentrate on providing for his language development not just in a single class but throughout the day. An excellent language–arts class can be wiped out by two periods of sitting and listening, even to a well-intentioned, competent teacher. Every class or activity must develop the child's language ability in some way. If it does not, the school cannot hope to overcome the effects of a language-poor environment.

The kinds of changes proposed may help to overcome some of the language disabilities stemming from a language-poor home environment. They will, however, be seen by the child and his parents as irrelevant if the child's schooling appears to lead nowhere except onto the front doorstep and into the street. If the disadvantaged child and his parents do not see schooling as a means of achieving equal opportunity, if the society is not able to demonstrate the relevance of education, its relation to a man's life chances, then no educational changes are sufficient to alter the charge that education is irrelevant to the lives of disadvantaged children.

References

BEREITER, C. and ENGELMANN, S. (1966) *Teaching Disadvantaged Children in the Preschool* Englewood Cliffs, New Jersey: Prentice-Hall

BERNSTEIN, B. (1961) Social class and linguistic development: a theory of social learning in A. H. Halsey, J. Floud and A. Anderson (eds) *Education, Economy and Society* New York: Free Press

BERNSTEIN, B. (1962) Social class, linguistic codes, and grammatical elements *Language and Speech* 5, 221–40

BERNSTEIN, B. (1964) Aspects of language and learning in the genesis of the social process in D. Hymes (ed) *Language in Culture and Society* New York: Harper and Row

BERNSTEIN, B. (1965) A sociolinguistic approach to social learning in J. Gould (ed) *Penguin Survey of the Social Sciences* Harmondsworth: Penguin

BERNSTEIN, B. (1966) Elaborated and restricted codes: their social origins and some consequences in A. Smith (ed) *Communication and Culture* New York: Holt, Rinehart and Winston

BERNSTEIN, B. (1967) Social structure, language and learning in J. P. DeCecco (ed) *The Psychology of Language, Thought and Instruction* New York: Holt, Rinehart and Winston

BERNSTEIN, B. and HENDERSON, DOROTHY (1969) Social class differences in the relevance of language to socialization *Sociology* 3, 1–20

BLANK, MARION and SOLOMON, FRANCES (1968) A tutorial language program to develop abstract thinking in socially disadvantaged pre-school children *Child Development* 39, 379–89

BRADDOCK, R., LLOYD-JONES, R. and SCHOER, L. (1963) *Research in Written Composition* Champaign, Illinois: National Council of Teachers of English

BROWN, C. (1965) *Manchild in the Promised Land* New York: Macmillan

COHEN, D. (1968) Children and their primary schools *Harvard Educational Review* 38, 329–40

COLEMAN, J. S. *et al* (1966) *Equality of Educational Opportunity* Washington DC: US Government Printing Office

DAVE, R. H. (1963) The identification and measurement of environmental process variables that are related to educational achievement Doctoral dissertation, University of Chicago

DAVIS, A. (1965) *Social Class Influence upon Learning* Cambridge, Massachusetts: Harvard University Press

FADER, D. N. and SHAEVITZ, M. H. (1969) *Hooked on Books* Oxford: Pergamon

GORDON, E. W. and WILKERSON, D. A. (1966) *Compensatory Education for the Disadvantaged* New York: College Entrance Examination Board

*HESS, R. D. and SHIPMAN, VIRGINIA (1965) Early experience and the socialization of cognitive modes in children *Child Development* 36, 869–86

HESS, R. D., SHIPMAN, VIRGINIA, BEAR, ROBERTA M. and BROPHY, J. (1968) *The Cognitive Environments of Urban Preschool Children* Chicago: University of Chicago Press

KARNES, M. B. *et al* (1966) Activities for developing psycholinguistic skill with preschool culturally deprived children Mimeographed Urbana, Illinois: Institute for Research on Exceptional Children

KARNES, M. B. (1969) A new role for teachers: involving the entire family in the education of preschool disadvantaged children Mimeographed Urbana, Illinois: University of Illinois College of Education.

LAWTON, D. (1963) Social class differences in language development: a study of some samples of written work *Language and Speech* 6, 120–43

LAWTON, D. (1964) Some class language differences in group discussions *Language and Speech* 7, 182–204

LAWTON, D. (1968) *Social Class, Language and Education* London: Routledge

LOBAN, W. (1966b) *Language Ability, Grades Seven, Eight and Nine* Washington DC: US Government Printing Office

MILLER, W. (1964) *The Cool World* New York: Fawcett

OLIM, E. G., HESS, R. D. and SHIPMAN, VIRGINIA (1967) Role of mother's language styles in mediating their preschool children's cognitive development *The School Review* 75, 414–24

ROBINSON, W. P. (1965) The elaborated code in working class language *Language and Speech* 8, 243–52

Davenport Plumer

ROSENTHAL, R. and JACOBSON, LENORE (1968) *Pygmalion in the Classroom* New York: Holt, Rinehart and Winston

STRODTBECK, F. L. (1965) The hidden curriculum in the middle class home in J. D. Krumboltz (ed) *Learning and the Educational Process* Chicago: Rand McNally

*VYGOTSKY, L. S. (1962) *Thought and Language* Eugenia Hanfmann and Gertrude Vakar (ed) and trans. Chichester: Wiley

WILLIAMS, F. and NAREMORE, RITA C. (1969) On the functional analysis of social class differences in modes of speech *Speech Monographs* 36, 77–102

2.3 Language development and reading attainment of deprived children

M. L. KELLMER PRINGLE
Director, National Children's Bureau

Reprinted from M. M. Clark and S. M. Maxwell (1969) (eds) *Reading: Influences on Progress* United Kingdom Reading Association, p. 25, and from 'A study of deprived children, part 2: Language development and reading attainment' written with Victoria Bossio *Vita Humana* (1958), 1, pp. 142–70

Introduction

The term 'deprivation' is commonly used to denote three different conditions: first, the child who is living in residential care, either for long periods or permanently, is deprived of normal family life; second, if a child is unloved and rejected by his parents, especially his mother, he is likely to suffer emotional deprivation; and third, the child who is growing up in a home which is culturally and educationally extremely unstimulating will be handicapped by environmental deprivation. Of course these three conditions are not mutually exclusive, but at the present there are no estimates available to indicate the likely number of children within each of these categories or how many may be affected by two or all three types of deprivation. The overall number of children in care (using the term in the technical sense of the word) is by no means negligible—over 70,000 or as high as the total number of children suffering from physical handicap. If we add to this the other two groups of deprived children this figure may well have to be trebled.

It is generally accepted now that each of these three conditions may be detrimental to emotional and social development. Far less is known about the likely effects of deprivation in all its forms on language development, intellectual growth and educational progress. Yet these are just as important for a child's all-round development and adjustment.

The reasons which led me to undertake a series of investigations were threefold: first, there had been comparatively little systematic study of the language development and scholastic attainment of children living in residential care; secondly, teachers of such children were of the opinion that many of them showed serious learning problems in school; and thirdly, in recent years there has been growing awareness that in this scientific and technological age a nation's reservoir of intelligence is among its most important raw materials. It has become essential to search for 'pools of unrealized ability'.

If we need to find and train more teachers, more social workers, more technicians and so on, then potential ability can neither be wasted nor ignored. And language development is basic for general intellectual development. Similarly, it is now recognized that children whose language development remains stunted will later on also become seriously backward educationally. Of course the most critical period for the fostering of language and speech is during the preschool years. Since all children whose language development remains needlessly limited will inevitably be under-functioning both intellectually and educationally, they represent a waste of potential ability.

Subjects and procedure

In the study to be described here, a comprehensive inquiry was made into the development and achievements of some unselected samples of children aged eight, eleven and fourteen years, who were living in residential care. Wherever possible, comparisons were made with the abilities and attainments of children who lived with their own families. In addition, three hypotheses were tested regarding the results of deprivation: namely, that its effects would be more marked if

1 the first separation from the mother occurred at an early age
2 deprivation had been severe (i.e. no contact whatever with the family)
3 the period of residential care had been prolonged.

All the children were given both the Verbal and Performance Scales of the Wechsler Intelligence Scale for Children. Language development was assessed further by means of the Mill Hill Scale Oral Definitions Form and (in the case of the eight year olds) the Watts English Language and Vocabulary Test for Young Children. Reading was assessed by the Schonell Graded Reading Vocabulary Test (eight and eleven year olds) and the Schonell Silent Reading Test B.

Results

The main findings were marked backwardness in language development in general and reading in particular found not only among both boys and girls but also at each of the three age levels studied.

1 More than two-thirds of the total sample had language quotients below 85 (the expected proportion in a normal population being roughly 16 per cent).
2 Severity of retardation was positively related to the age at which separation took place.

3 Retardation was positively related to the severity of the deprivation.
4 Mean verbal quotients on wisc were significantly lower than mean performance quotients, and verbal scale quotients were positively related to age of first separation and severity of deprivation. The performance scale showed no such correlation.
5 Sixty-two per cent of the total sample were backward in reading (reading quotient less than 85) and 40 per cent were retarded (reading quotient less than intelligence quotients).

Discussion of the findings

Language development
The findings support the hypothesis that deprived children are backward in language development. It seems very likely that this is, at least to some extent, functional and due to adverse environmental factors. Prior to separation the majority of children live in homes where verbal stimulation is minimal: overworked and underprivileged mothers, often burdened with too many pregnancies or forced by economic necessity to go out to work, have little time and energy available to encourage the baby in his early experiments with sound and to elicit continued trial and effort by taking delight in his prespeech vocalizations. Similarly, once the child is beginning to speak, there is likely to be less verbal stimulation in the form of nursery rhymes, stories, songs and general conversation. When the child enters an institution, the staff–child ratio as well as the training of the staff are of paramount importance. Too low a staffing ratio, frequent staff changes and overemphasis on child training as against child development, are all likely to have a retarding effect on the growth of language. Our results suggest that young children deprived of normal family life tend to have very limited knowledge of everyday activities which take place in the home and that they are not even sure of the name for the various parts of their own bodies. The all too common absence of father figures, especially in homes for preschool children, is also reflected in their ignorance of male personal effects and apparels. Probably the older children can more readily widen their experience as their growing independence increases the opportunity for outside contacts.

The extent of backwardness in language development was considerably larger than that in intelligence or reading attainment; similarly, it was greater than the incidence of unsettledness and maladjustment, shown both at the day school and at the residential home. These results support Gesell's (Gesell and Amatruda 1947) and Goldfarb's (1945) assertion that the effects of deprivation tend to be more detrimental to a child's language development than to any other aspect of his developing personality. If that is so, it is likely that assessing the intelligence of deprived children by predominantly verbal tests inevitably results in an underestimate. This view is supported by our findings on the wisc where all three age-groups obtained significantly higher scores on the Performance Scale. There are

M. L. Kellmer Pringle

a number of possible hypotheses, which are not mutually exclusive, to account for the differential results on the Verbal and Performance Scale of the WISC. First, as a group our sample of deprived children was of low average intelligence and Wechsler states 'that subjects of superior intelligence generally do better on the verbal, and subjects of inferior intelligence do better on the performance part'.

Secondly, the abilities measured by the verbal subtests (especially information, arithmetic and vocabulary) depend to some extent on opportunities and stimulation given at home and at school. The majority of children in care come from homes with a culturally and educationally low level; their schooling is often irregular, including frequent changes. Thirdly, when in care and living in a residential home, opportunities for outside contact tend to be rather limited and the staff ratio of one adult to ten or more children further reduces opportunities for discussion and verbal stimulation. Fourthly, once a child is able to read he can increase his vocabulary and enlarge his knowledge by the use of books. Since the incidence of backwardness and retardation in this subject was quite considerable in our sample, this avenue too is closed to many. Lastly, the severe degree of backwardness in language development found in our sample may well be the most important single factor.

1 *Age and sex differences* Though the eleven year olds achieved the highest mean language quotient, it was only slightly above the mean of the fourteen year olds, whereas the youngest group received a significantly low score. To some extent this may be a reflection of differences in intelligence. Ability to read may also play a part, since eight year olds, even if progressing satisfactorily in this subject, are unlikely to have reached a level where through their reading they are able to enlarge their vocabulary.

2 *Differences according to the three criteria of deprivation* Our results support the hypothesis that backwardness in language development is more marked in children who have been separated from their mothers for the first time at an early age. To some extent, however, this may also be linked with the fact that the 'early entrants' were found to be intellectually more backward than children whose separation took place at a later age.

It is difficult to account for the fact that length of institutional residence has not resulted in differences of language development. It may be that for language development it is the preschool period (i.e. before the age of five years) which is of greatest importance; moreover, if children enter an institution after that age and without seriously impaired language development, it is likely that they will be able to acquire reading skills more readily and thus enlarge their vocabulary through reading even though they may remain in a home. The results obtained from the reading test would seem to lend some support to this hypothesis.

80

Continued contact with the family seemed to be related to the children's language development since backwardness in this aspect of growth was most marked where no contact had been maintained. Thus, considering the evidence from the three criteria of deprivation together, it would seem that the important factors are the time when the mother–child relationship is first severed and the nature of the contact maintained subsequently. Maybe what matters most is the opportunity to develop early a close personal relationship with the mother or mother-substitute and for this relationship to continue even though the child cannot live in his own home. For example, McCarthy (1952) strongly supports the view that language development depends to a considerable extent upon the child's identification with his mother. If contact with her or a mother-substitute is maintained, then the child continues to strive to communicate his thought and experiences; thus continued personal interest and contact seem to provide the requisite motivational forces which stimulate this learning process.

Reading attainment
Educational attainments show the responses a child is making in a more formal and structural learning situation. To obtain a comprehensive picture of a child's scholastic level it might seem desirable to give a full range of attainment tests covering the basic subjects. Practical considerations of time, however, precluded the use of more than one or two attainment tests. Reading was chosen since it is the most fundamental skill and the basis of all academic learning. Backwardness in this subject almost inevitably leads to difficulties with most other aspects of school work.

A very serious degree of backwardness in comprehension reading was found in our sample of deprived children. Though completely comparable statistics are not available, it seems that the incidence of backwardness and retardation in this subject is at least twice as high among our sample as in the ordinary school population. Results from a national survey of normal children carried out in 1948 (Ministry of Education 1950), showed that reading backwardness among eleven year olds amounted to 23 per cent and among fifteen year olds to 30 per cent. A retest in 1956 (Ministry of Education 1957) indicated that the incidence had decreased to 21 per cent and 25 per cent respectively. Thus our two comparable age groups of deprived children contain at least twice the proportion of backward readers. No national surveys have been carried out to ascertain the incidence of retardation in reading. However, regional investigations (Kellmer Pringle 1965) indicate that among seven to nine year old children it ranges from 11 per cent to 23 per cent; while among children aged 9–12 years the incidence of reading retardation ranges from zero to 12 per cent (City of Leeds Education Committee 1953). Again the incidence is twice as high in our samples.

There are a number of possible hypotheses, which are not mutually

M. L. Kellmer Pringle

exclusive, to explain the deprived child's inferior attainment. Retarded speech development and a limited vocabulary inevitably handicap him in learning to read. Moreover, in the deprived child's home little interest is usually taken in books and in education generally. Because of these circumstances, he is less ready for school when he starts at the age of five years, than are his more fortunate contemporaries. Thus right from the beginning, the methods and materials used for the majority are unsuited to his needs. (Just as success begets further success, so failure begets further failure.) Soon he will be labelled backward. (In any case, he is aware of the fact that others are doing much better than he, which results in a loss of confidence and diminished effort, which in turn lead to further educational difficulties.) Frequent absences and changes of school are also likely to hinder progress in reading. The deprived child tends to come from families where there are frequent minor ailments, where he is kept at home to look after younger siblings or to run errands, or where he himself may play truant. Removal from home usually means a change of school and all that this involves, such as developing new loyalties, adjusting to a different school atmosphere and possibly also to different teaching methods. Lastly, there is research evidence to show that children who have emotional difficulties tend to do badly at school, partly because of preoccupation with their problems (Monroe 1932, Gates 1941, Schonell 1942, Burt 1946, Vernon 1957).

1 *Age and sex differences* Once again, the eleven year olds achieved significantly higher mean scores than the other two age groups. Their superior achievement in reading may in part, if not wholly, be due to their superiority in most other aspects which were measured. It will be remembered that this group was relatively superior in intelligence, language development and emotional adjustment.

Since the boys achieved higher mean intelligence and higher mean language quotients than the girls, one would have expected the latter to have also lower attainments in reading. However, this was not the case. Girls consistently scored higher than boys though this difference did not reach a statistically significant level. Deprived boys, despite their relative superiority, tended to be more backward in reading than girls. Thus the same sex difference, though to a less severe degree, seems to exist among ordinary pupils.

2 *Differences according to the three criteria of deprivation* Our findings lend some support to the hypothesis that early first separation has an adverse influence on later reading achievement. However, the link here is likely to be indirect: early first separation appears to have an adverse effect on intellectual and language development and this in turn exercises a detrimental influence on reading ability. A similar indirect influence is likely to be responsible for the fact that severity of deprivation was also associated with poorer attainments in reading. On the other hand, length of insti-

tutional residence did not seem to affect the level of attainment in this subject.

3 *Reading backwardness and emotional adjustment* Since learning to read depends to a considerable extent upon intellectual and language development, one would expect deprived children to be more backward in reading attainment. Once allowance has been made for these limitations or disabilities, one would not necessarily expect to find a more serious degree of retardation than among the ordinary school population. However, this was the case. Thus it seems that additional adverse factors were influencing the learning process, such as a lack of motivation, a poor relationship with the teacher and emotional maladjustment. We were only able to assess the extent of the last mentioned factor. Nor can we judge from our findings whether the high incidence of unsettledness and maladjustment among the poor readers was due to their learning difficulty or whether the learning difficulty was causing the maladjustment. There is a great deal of evidence (Monroe 1932, Gates 1941, Schonell 1942, Fernald 1943, Burt 1946, Vernon 1957, Seglow *et al* 1972) to support both these explanatory hypotheses. If one accepts the close interrelationship between educational and emotional difficulties, it becomes apparent that deprived children are caught in a vicious circle. The very circumstances preceding and eventually leading to separation are likely also to lead to a high incidence of maladjustment; maladjustment militates against successful learning; unsuccessful learning results in a sense of failure and frustration, thus further increasing the likelihood, and possibly also the degree, of maladjustment.

Summary and conclusions

The results of the individual intelligence testing showed that the majority of our sample of deprived children fell within the average range of ability, although the mean IQ was considerably below 100. Moreover, the proportion of educationally subnormal and dull children was considerably higher, and that of bright and very able children considerably lower than among the ordinary school population. In language development and reading attainment the deprived children were also markedly backward. In addition, they tended to differ from ordinary children in many of their personal attitudes and reactions and a considerable proportion showed symptoms of maladjustment, both in the residential home and at school. Social competence was the only developmental aspect in which the deprived equalled ordinary children.

Regarding the three criteria of deprivation, it was found that early first separation from the mother resulted in significantly greater ill-effects on the various developmental aspects which were measured; similarly, complete deprivation, i.e. no contact whatever with the family or relatives, had a significantly deleterious effect. Sheer length of institutional residence, on the other hand, did not result in any significant differences.

The eleven year olds were superior to the two other age groups in all respects except social competence. It may be that at this age children are better able to accept separation from their parents and to adjust to institutional life than when they are younger or during adolescence. This hypothesis receives some support from developmental psychology since for normal children the latency period is considered to be a time of relative calm and settledness. However, our sample is too small to draw this inference with any certainty.

Lastly, boys tended to be superior in general ability and language development, while girls were relatively better readers and socially more competent. These trends were not statistically significant.

Hitherto the various aspects studied have largely and necessarily been analysed and discussed separately. Yet it is likely that our findings are the end product of a chain of adverse conditions which interact and reinforce one another and which affect the lives of deprived children long before they come into care. Among these conditions the following are probably of considerable importance: poor intellectual and possibly poor emotional endowment; unstimulating and impoverished cultural conditions; a lack of educational standards and ambitions; a family which may be broken in spirit if not in reality; poverty, ill health and unemployment. Thus a vicious circle is produced: impoverished and often unhappy home conditions leading to backwardness in intellectual and language development as well as to emotional maladjustment, which in turn result in unsatisfactory school adjustment.

Since at home the child's early learning efforts are often met with little interest and encouragement, he is likely to be discouraged and to accept low standards of achievement. When he starts school, these attitudes are transferred to classroom learning; moreover, possessing only a limited speaking vocabulary, educational difficulties are likely to follow. The teacher, very understandably, is disappointed at the child's lack of responsiveness and progress and yet this disappointment is likely to make the child feel even more hopeless and insecure; hence further lack of progress and apathy follow. Removal to a children's home means usually also a change of school, so that the child has to make new adjustments all round. Institutional life can hardly be expected to have beneficial effects on a backward, discouraged and insecure child; on the contrary, existing difficulties may be still further aggravated.

Incidentally, our findings shed some light on the reasons why teachers and houseparents commonly believe that most deprived children are very dull: children's ability is judged by what they say and by what they are able to do. Since deprived children tend to suffer from a severe degree of language and educational retardation, they give the impression of lacking ability, when in many cases they have lacked mainly appropriate stimulation and opportunity.

References

*BURT, C. (1946) *The Backward Child* London: University of London Press

CRELLIN, E., KELLMER PRINGLE, M. L. and WEST, P. (1971) *Born Illegitimate* Slough: National Foundation for Educational Research

EDUCATION, MINISTRY OF (1950) *Reading ability: some suggestions for helping the backward* (Pamphlet no. 18) London: HMSO

EDUCATION, MINISTRY OF (1957) *Standards of reading, 1948–1956* (Pamphlet no. 32) London: HMSO

*FERNALD, G. M. (1943) *Remedial Techniques in Basic School Subjects* New York: McGraw-Hill

GATES, A. I. (1941) The role of personality maladjustment in reading disability *Journal of Genetic Psychology* 59, 77–83.

GESELL, A. and AMATRUDA, C. S. (1947) *Developmental diagnosis; normal and abnormal child development; clinical methods and pediatric applications* New York: Hoeber

GOLDFARB, W. (1945) The effect of psychological deprivation in infancy and subsequent stimulation *American Journal of Psychiatry* 102, 18–33

KELLMER PRINGLE, M. L. (1965) *Deprivation and Education* London: Longman

SEGLOW, J., KELLMER PRINGLE, M. L. and WEDGE, P. (1972) *Growing Up Adopted* Slough: National Foundation for Educational Research

LEEDS EDUCATION COMMITTEE (1953) *Report on a survey of reading ability* Leeds: Education Department

MCCARTHY, D. A. (1952) Language and personality development *The Reading Teacher* 6, 28–36

MONROE, M. (1932) *Children who cannot read: the analysis of reading disabilities and the use of diagnostic tests in the instruction of retarded readers* Chicago: University of Chicago Press

SCHONELL, F. J. (1942) *Backwardness in the Basic Subjects* Edinburgh: Oliver and Boyd

VERNON, M. D. (1957) *Backwardness in reading: a study of its nature and origin* Cambridge: Cambridge University Press

2.4 Class size, pupil characteristics and reading attainment

ALAN LITTLE, CHRISTINE MABEY and
JENNIFER RUSSELL
Research and Statistics Group, Inner London
Education Authority

Reprinted from Vera Southgate (1972) (ed) *Literacy at all levels*
Ward Lock Educational, pp. 205–11

The desirability of reducing class sizes in our primary schools is one of the few educational topics on which there is widespread agreement amongst professionals, administrators, politicians and parents. One reason for this consensus is, perhaps, that this is one fact which it is relatively simple to change (given adequate numbers of teachers, money to pay them, the classrooms or sufficient space to accommodate them) and the change is directly observable. Yet there has been comparatively little recent research on the link between class size and the attainment of young children. Furthermore the majority of investigations have indicated that class size does not in itself appear to be an important factor in influencing the speed of learning (Thouless 1969).

There are three fairly recent English studies to which reference should first be made. In chronological order they are: first, the investigations of Joyce Morris in Kent during 1954–7, reported in *Reading in the Primary School* and *Standards and Progress in Reading* (Morris 1959, 1966); second, the investigation by Stephen Wiseman in Manchester in 1964, reported in volume II of the Plowden Report (HMSO 1967); third, the National Child Development Survey which covered the whole of Britain—the part with which we are concerned is the survey of the children in 1965 when they were seven years old (Davie 1970).

Morris found that there was a tendency for children in large classes in top infants and juniors to have better reading attainments. She suggested that the reasons for this were partly the urban/rural difference (larger schools are in the towns, large classes are found in large schools) and also the policy of putting the less able children in smaller classes. As part of the evidence presented to the Plowden Committee, Wiseman considered children in a 25 per cent sample of Manchester primary schools (controlling for school size, type and socioeconomic level). Although these children were 10+ at the time of his investigation, he had available test results throughout the junior school. He found a small but positive association between size of class and educational attainment (holding parental occupation constant); in other words the larger the class, the better the reading.

The National Child Development Survey is a study of a complete cohort of children born in one week in 1958. The children were traced again in 1965 when they were seven years of age and amongst other measures the relationship of class size to reading attainment at the end of infant school was considered. Even taking account of school size, length of schooling, parental interest and occupation, it was still the case that the children in larger classes had higher attainments. Davie suggested that this was partly due to the difference between urban and rural schools and also that 'small' was not small enough—that is, classes might have to be as small as 20–25 before attainment was improved. The research of Marklund in Sweden has particular relevance in this context (Yates 1966). He considered attainment of thirteen year olds, both in a national sample and from south Stockholm, examining class sizes of 16–20, 21–25, 26–30, 31–35. Attainment was highest in the classes of 26–30 and lowest in the classes of 21–25 and when classes were combined, the attainment in classes of 26–35 was significantly higher than that in classes of 16–25. He concluded that a reduction in class size would not *in itself* lead to improved attainments especially as having made 281 different comparisons between the class sizes, all but 59 were not significant (and of these 37 favoured the larger classes and 22 the smaller).

A certain amount of fresh evidence is available from a literacy survey covering all the ILEA junior and junior-infant schools. The testing took place in October 1968 when all children in the authority's schools born between 2nd September 1959 and 1st September 1960 were given a sentence completion reading test. The test was designed by the National Foundation for Educational Research for their streaming project: it has two parallel versions, SRA and SRB. SRA was used in this study. In the followup study of the same cohort immediately prior to transfer to secondary schooling (i.e. summer 1971) SRB was used. Further information relating to the children's backgrounds and educational experience was also collected. The aspects that concern us here are the size of the classes that the children were in at the time of the survey (normally pupils at the beginning of the second year juniors), the children's countries of origin, the occupational status of the fathers or guardians, as well as the teachers' knowledge and judgment of the homes and the children. Furthermore, we had access to an index of the educational priority ranking of the school which provides some idea of the social and physical problems affecting the schools in comparison with the rest of the authority.

Our first finding was striking: there was an increase of reading attainment with increase in class size—from a mean reading quotient of 90.7 in classes of 30 or under to 100.5 in classes of over 40. However, many of the children in smaller classes were those whom headteachers thought

A. Little, C. Mabey and J. Russell

required special help (though not necessarily a remedial class). Also in London more of the denominational schools have large classes, and these schools have higher mean reading scores (99.2 in Roman Catholic schools and 96.9 in Church of England schools compared with 94.3 in county schools). In addition children who were reported as having had some remedial help in the school they were attending at the time of survey tended to be in smaller classes. Further, the LEA has a policy of allocating more resources (including teachers) to schools in most need. We therefore propose to look more closely at certain of the characteristics of pupils in classes of 31–34 and of 35–40 pupils and to exclude from the analysis children who had any specific remedial help with reading during the previous 14 months, whether in remedial classes, withdrawn groups or individual remedial help. However, it must be pointed out that although class sizes of 31–34 are probably realistic current improvements on existing sizes, they may not be sufficiently small to have significant impact on pupil performance. What these results may indicate is the likely results of current policy in primary school staffing. In our sample the mean size of the 31–34 groups was 32.4 pupils, and of the 35–40 group, 37.5 pupils; a difference of 5 pupils or a 14 per cent reduction.

As it is ILEA policy to allocate more resources to the schools considered to be most in need, that is schools with a high EPA ranking, we compared schools of similar ranking on an EPA index. We found small but consistent differences favouring classes of 35–40. For example, in the most disadvantaged areas the mean reading quotient of pupils in classes of 31–34 was 93.4, compared with 94.1 in classes of 35–40. Figures for schools in the most privileged areas were 102.4 and 104.2. It can be seen from Table 1 that the smaller classes tend to be in schools of higher rank but

TABLE 1   *Reading scores and percentage of children in classes of different sizes and in schools of different EPA ranks*

EPA rank	Class size			
	31–34		35–40	
	RQ	%	RQ	%
1–99	93.4	11.6	94.1	6.3
100–299	94.8	18.9	96.5	19.3
300–599	99.1	36.5	99.5	30.6
600–875	102.4	32.9	104.2	43.8
N	(98.7)	3,783	(100.6)	11,826

the marginal difference in attainment in favour of the larger classes still occurs. We next considered the kinds of pupils in the schools—the proportion of immigrants and the proportion of children from lower socioeconomic backgrounds. The same tendency for the children in the larger classes to have a higher mean reading score irrespective of nationality or social class emerges. From Table 2 it can be seen that the differences

TABLE 2 *Reading scores and percentages of children in classes of different sizes*

Nationality	Class size			
	31–34		35–40	
	RQ	%	RQ	%
Nonimmigrant	99.7	86.1	101.6	87.1
Immigrant	92.4	13.9	94.7	12.9
N	(98.7)	3,764	(100.7)	11,814
Social class	*Class size*			
	31–34		35–40	
	RQ	%	RQ	%
Nonmanual	104.6	24.8	105.9	29.9
Manual	96.8	75.2	98.5	70.1
N	(98.7)	3,764	(100.7)	11,814

are small but consistent and favour the larger classes. Probably the safest conclusion is that reduction of class size on the scale currently envisaged may have little impact on reading.

In themselves nationality and social class are rather unsatisfactory ways of categorizing children and their families. In our survey (in an attempt to assess the support the children had from their families) the teachers were asked if they considered the homes to be culturally stimulating, if they felt the parents were interested in the children's education, and whether or not parents had discussed their child's education with the teacher. When class background was controlled, sixteen comparisons were made between small (31–34) and large (35–40) classes; all the differences were small and all favoured the larger classes. As a detailed example, Table 3 gives the results for cultural stimulus of the home.

But the main reason for reproducing this table is to contrast the impact of cultural stimulus with reduction of class size. The difference in the mean reading score of children from stimulating and unstimulating home backgrounds is a year and a half or more (15–17 points). Contrast that with the differences between 'small' and 'large' classes which although real are very small; in most cases there is less than two points between the mean reading scores of the two class sizes under consideration. In other words, although we have found an almost consistent difference in favour of the larger class size, this difference is perhaps educationally insignificant. The indications from our evidence are that for these class sizes, one of which is over the target number of 35 and the other (31–34) within the

TABLE 3 *Reading scores and percentages of children of different social class in classes of different size according to cultural stimulus of the home as this was rated by the teacher*

Nonmanual	Class size			
	31–34		35–40	
	RQ	%	RQ	%
Stimulating	111.3	41.2	111.5	42.5
Average	101.0	50.2	103.5	49.7
Unstimulating	94.9	8.6	95.9	7.8
N		859		3,254
Manual	Class size			
	31–34		35–40	
	RQ	%	RQ	%
Stimulating	106.6	11.0	108.1	10.8
Average	98.9	55.3	100.2	62.9
Unstimulating	90.3	33.7	91.9	26.3
N		2,545		7,301

range of realistic short-run improvements in class sizes, the actual class size in itself is not the most important factor in reading performance. More important influences would seem to be pupil characteristics, the homes they come from and the support they receive.

Conclusions

Our main findings have been that little or no differences exist between the reading standards of children in relatively small classes compared with those in larger ones and even when social class, length of education, immigrant status and the educational priority status of the schools are controlled, little difference can be found. If anything, children in large classes do marginally better than their counterparts in smaller ones. Given the extent to which this conflicts not only with professional opinion but also with lay views on the desirability of smaller classes, some mention of the limitations of the analysis is necessary. Only one measure of educational performance has been used (a group test of reading). Had other tests of reading been used, or other tests of basic skills (numeracy) or tests of personality skills and development, different results might have been obtained. Furthermore, the measure was used at a single age—an age after the basic skill of reading has normally been acquired. Perhaps had the tests (or similar ones) been used during the period of learning to read (infants and first year juniors) different results might have been forthcoming. Obviously the full force of these points is made when taken together: testing various skills covering the full range of the curriculum at successive ages. However, Wiseman had available information on different attainments at successive ages and still found the attainment to be slightly superior in the larger classes. These results suggest that we ought to begin collecting more information on basic skill performance, resource inputs, and teaching strategy before placing the priority upon reduction of class size as current educational policy implies.

A further note of caution must be sounded. In this paper we have assumed that all teachers are equally effective, the only variable being the numbers of pupils in their classes. This is obviously naïve, and might well be a factor in producing the results we have found. For example, internal school policies might result in the deployment of the weaker and younger teachers with smaller groups and the more experienced and skilled teachers being given the larger teaching groups. A parallel policy could be the allocation of more advanced readers to the relatively larger classes and less advanced to the smaller ones. Both of these points assume that there are considerable variations of class sizes within schools (i.e. some below and some above 35 in terms of our present analysis).

But in 45 per cent of ILEA junior schools such differentiality was impossible because the school had only one class in the relevant age range. In another 35 per cent of schools there was no difference in the sizes of parallel classes or a difference of one or two pupils. Eight out of ten schools did not make use of improved staffing ratios to create relatively large and small teaching groups. In fact, in schools that had the opportunity to have parallel classes in the same age band only one in eight had a difference of six or more pupils and at least a third of these would have been eliminated from our analysis. But there are possible arguments consistent both with our findings and the desire to reduce class size in the hope that it will affect pupil performance. However, they open an area of discussion that is seldom mentioned in the debate about class sizes and the need for more teachers, which is deployment of these teachers within the school and the deployment of teacher time and teaching strategy within the classroom. American research on the 'more effective school' suggested that for the first couple of years, a drastic reduction in class size in the early years of elementary school produced no improvement in pupil performance, largely because teachers taught smaller groups in exactly the same way as they had been teaching the larger groups, and with the same effect (or lack of it). This observation suggests that thought should be given to ways of using improved pupil–teacher ratios and not restricted to pressuring for their reduction and, allied to this, ways of teaching pupils from different home backgrounds, different motivations etc.

This brings up a further point, the extent to which schools with relatively large classes were already deploying teacher resources outside the traditional classroom, whereas schools with relatively small classes made use of extra teaching resources to reduce class size. In the relevant academic year (1967–68) schools with the larger classes had a pupil-teacher ratio of 1 teacher to 26·6 pupils whereas the schools with smaller classes had the teacher ratio of 1 to 24·6. Therefore the difference between the two groups of schools was not in how staff was deployed but in the amount of staff available. There is another indication of the same point: pupils who had received special help for reading were eliminated from each analysis. Just over 30 per cent of pupils in the smaller classes and just under 30 per cent in the larger classes received such help. In other words the incidence of providing additional teacher support for reading was virtually identical in the two groups of schools. Therefore, differential deployment of the existing staff does not seem to be a distinguishing characteristic between the two groups of schools.

But how far need classes be reduced to improve performance? This paper has examined the types of reductions that are likely in primary schools in the near future. Perhaps significant improvements in performance will only be achieved with even more drastic reductions (classes of 15, 20 or 25). Our lack of relationship might be because the reductions we have examined, although currently politically relevant, are not educationally significant. In principle this is a strong argument and obviously should be seen in relation to the deployment of teachers and the changed teaching strategy mentioned above. It also raises an even more profound organizational question: given the current impracticality of teaching groups of 15 or 20 in primary schools throughout the day, how far can team teaching, family grouping, integrated day, create such teaching situations for part of the teaching day by staff deployment? There is the obvious danger of small group situations within large classes being used as an alternative to improvements in pupil–teacher ratio; this is not what is wanted. The strain of teaching large groups of children is probably considerable (and perhaps the best argument for smaller classes is reduction of that strain) but what we are suggesting is that smaller teaching groups can be achieved by organizational changes within the classroom; also one of the reasons why the existing reduction in class sizes has not produced improved pupil performance, has been the failure to modify teaching practice in such a way as to utilize the possibilities of existing class sizes.

What then is our main argument? Reduction of class sizes on the scale currently envisaged, i.e. primary classes of 30–35, may not directly improve pupil performance, in so far as this has been measured by reading skills. Paradoxically our evidence shows that it might be linked with lower performance—a finding which is consistent not only with previous English educational research but also Scandinavian research. The solution is not simply more teachers. Some thought and consideration must be given to how the educational opportunities offered (at considerable human expense) in smaller teaching groups can be utilized, and how such smaller groups can be contrived within existing staffing ratios. Briefly, staff utilization and deployment should be given as much professional attention as staff numbers.

Finally, the magnitude of the differences found in the scores of children coming from interested and stimulating homes and the scores of children from unstimulating and uninterested homes, surely suggest that the social and psychological factors are of greater immediate significance than the types of reductions in class size we are currently envisaging. Perhaps the best way to utilize and deploy improved staffing ratios would be to attempt to influence parental interest and involvement, and pupils' attitude towards work and school rather than reduce class sizes. However, as Bernstein and Davies have pointed out, this may be a sociologically naïve recommendation because such attitudes and relationships are the consequences of other aspects of the structure of a complex industrial society unamenable to change through education.

References

*BERNSTEIN, B. and DAVIES, B. (1969) Some sociological comments on Plowden in R. S. Peters (ed) *Perspectives on Plowden* London: Routledge and Kegan Paul

DAVIE, R. (1970) *The Child, the School and the Home* Unpublished paper presented to the British Association

MARKLUND, S. (1962) Scholastic attainment as related to size and homogeneity of classes Abstracted by the author in A. Yates (1966) (ed) *Grouping in Education* Hamburg: UNESCO Institute for Education, pp. 248–50

MORRIS, J. M. (1959) *Reading in the Primary School* London: Newnes

*MORRIS, J. M. (1966) *Standards and Progress in Reading* Slough: National Foundation for Educational Research

THOULESS, R. H. (1969) *Map of Educational Research* Slough: National Foundation for Educational Research

WISEMAN, S. (1967) The Manchester Survey in *Children and their Primary Schools, Volume II*, Appendix 9 London: HMSO

2.5 Reading retardation and antisocial behaviour—the nature of the association

M. RUTTER and W. YULE

Reader in Child Psychiatry; Lecturer in Psychology,
Institute of Psychiatry, University of London

Reprinted from M. Rutter, J. Tizard and K. Whitmore (1970)
Education, Health and Behaviour Longman, pp. 240–49, 254–55

Severe reading retardation is frequently associated with antisocial behaviour. In this paper some possible explanations of the association will be explored. That delinquency and antisocial behaviour tend to be accompanied by educational failure is no new observation; it has been noted in many investigations over the last half century (for example, Burt 1925; Fendrick and Bond 1936; Glueck and Glueck 1950; Gibbens 1963), and some workers have actually included scholastic failure among the indices of maladjustment or emotional handicap (Rogers 1942a, Bower 1960). In the present study reading retardation was found to be as common among antisocial and aggressive children who were not overtly delinquent as among those who had transgressed the law, but from other work it appears not to be a feature (at least not to the same extent) of delinquency which starts for the first time during adult life (Robins and Hill 1966).

It is curious, therefore, how little interest this association has aroused in those concerned with the study of delinquency. Several of the most comprehensive reviews of delinquency do not even mention it (Bovet 1951, Gibbens 1961, P. D. Scott 1965) and the matter has also received very little recent attention from writers on reading disability.

Yet the issue is of very considerable theoretical importance. Determination of the *nature* of the association between antisocial behaviour and reading backwardness might shed important light on the etiology and mode of development of the two conditions. Also, as Blau (1946) pointed out, the elucidation of which disorder is primary and which secondary is crucial from a practical viewpoint. If the reading retardation is the basic defect and the behaviour disorder a secondary consequence of educational failure, an educational approach to treatment may be indicated. On the other hand, if the emotional disturbance is primary and the reading difficulties a secondary feature, a psychiatric approach to therapy may be preferable.

In fact, it is exceedingly difficult to decide what leads to what, which is the cart and which the horse (Gibbens 1962, Money 1962, Critchley 1968), and a study of the literature is not much help. Some writers hold that the emotional disorder is primary (e.g. Blau 1946, Pond 1967), others maintain that the basic problem is a constitutional defect in reading ability (e.g. McCready 1926, Orton 1937, Critchley 1962) while still others have put forward an intermediate position (e.g. Monroe 1932). Unfortunately, in most cases these views amount to little more than a statement of faith, without any systematic attempt to evaluate the evidence.

It is of course most unlikely that the same mechanism will explain *all* cases and, furthermore, it is probable that in many cases there will be multifactorial determination. However this is no reason to dodge the issue and either avoid any interpretation of the findings or assume all causes are *equally* important. If progress is to be made, it is essential to examine the evidence in an attempt to elucidate the direction and nature of the association and so to find which factors are the *most* important in most cases. This is the purpose of this chapter. In nonexperimental studies only possible and plausible causes can be determined, but some causes may be ruled out and by narrowing down the choice to a limited number of hypotheses, only a few variables may be left for which experimental tests can be devised (Robins, in press).

Much of the conflict over the nature of the association between reading retardation and antisocial behaviour stems directly from the fact that most investigations have been concerned with highly selected groups of children (Rutter *et al* 1967). The types of problem seen at any one clinic naturally reflect the services provided by the clinic and the factors influencing referral to it, and these will tend to bias any attempt to examine associations between different variables. This kind of bias can best be avoided by epidemiological investigations of total child populations, and so far as the present problem is concerned, by using methods of selecting children with reading backwardness and with antisocial behaviour which are independent of possible associations between the two. As the Isle of Wight survey fulfils these criteria it is appropriate to see what conclusions may be drawn from the study findings.

Summary of situation

The findings of the present study concerning the association between reading retardation and antisocial behaviour may be summarized as follows.

There were 4 per cent of children aged nine to ten years who were reading at a level *at least* twenty-eight months below that predicted on the basis of their WISC IQ and chronological age (Yule 1967a). The reading disability was specific in that it was not associated with a general retardation in intellectual functioning. However, while the reading backwardness was specific in relation to IQ, it was not educationally specific in that the backward readers were also severely retarded in arithmetic and spelling. Reading backwardness was three times more common in boys than in girls.

About 2 per cent of the children showed a clinically significant antisocial disorder and a little over 1 per cent had an antisocial disorder with prominent neurotic features. Of these two groups combined, half had committed frankly delinquent acts but only a small minority had appeared before the Courts. There was very marked excess of boys among these antisocial children. In contrast, there was a slight excess of girls among the 2 per cent with clinically significant neurotic conditions.

A very considerable degree of overlap was found between reading retardation and antisocial behaviour. Of the children who were severely retarded in reading a third exhibited antisocial behaviour. This rate is several times that in the general population even when sex differences are taken into account. The backward readers also showed a lesser increase in neurotic problems—this reflected a general tendency at this age (nine to ten years) for antisocial children also to exhibit neurotic symptomatology.

Similarly, of the group of antisocial children, over a third were at least twenty-eight months retarded in their reading (after IQ was partialled out). Again, this rate is many times that in the general population, after controlling for sex differences. Backwardness in reading was as common in the antisocial children who also showed neurotic problems as in those with 'pure' antisocial disorders but, in sharp contrast, the rate of reading retardation among neurotic children (who were not antisocial) was little above that in the general population.

Hypotheses

In general, hypotheses concerning the nature of the association between reading retardation and antisocial behaviour may be divided into those which suggest

1 that antisocial behaviour develops as a reaction to the educational failure implicit in reading difficulties
2 that retardation in reading is a consequence of the emotional or motivational difficulties which lead to antisocial behaviour
3 that both disorders are due to the same predisposing factors in the child or in his environment
4 various combinations of the above three types of hypotheses.

There are various ways of testing these hypotheses.

Possible approaches to the problem

Which comes first?
One approach to the question of the *nature* of the association between reading difficulties and behavioural disturbance is to consider which

developed first, on the rather questionable assumption that the condition that was present earliest in the child's life is likely to be the primary condition in an etiological sense. This could only be established with precision by means of longitudinal studies. It is very difficult to obtain accurate dates of onset in retrospect. However, if the time relationship was sufficiently clearcut it might be apparent even from a retrospective account (as in this study).

Psychogenic hypotheses concerning reading difficulties have been developed chiefly in relation to children who make satisfactory school progress at first and only later develop a failure to learn, of which the reading problem is but one part (Pearson 1952). The children in the Isle of Wight study did not fall into this group—it is evident that they had had difficulties in learning to read from an early stage. Some were still non-readers and, on average, they were reading only at the seven year level although aged nine or ten years. In contrast, the children's delinquent activities were of much more recent onset. But it is necessary to note that most of the antisocial children had shown some kind of emotional or behavioural abnormality well before they committed any delinquent act. Altogether, two-thirds of the antisocial children had disorders of at least three years' duration, which would put the onset in these cases at before the age of seven or eight years.

However, there was a slight (but not quite significant) tendency for the antisocial boys who were over two years retarded in their reading to have a shorter duration of disorder than those whose reading achievement was normal (40 per cent of the poor readers had disorders which had lasted less than three years compared with 21.7 per cent of the normal readers). Thus there is some suggestion that antisocial disorders may begin somewhat later when the disorder develops in association with a failure to learn to read.

Nevertheless, this still leaves a majority of the children in whom it was not possible to tell which came first. The matter is further complicated by the fact that reading develops on the basis of preexisting linguistic and perceptual skills so that when there is a failure to learn to read, the basic defects may often have been present well before the child attempted to read. Similarly, antisocial disorders often stem from earlier abnormalities in personality development so that the timing of the onset of the overt disorder will often not date the beginnings of emotional disturbance.

Malmquist (1958) found that of backward readers with nervous symptoms half were reported to have had no symptoms until after their first year at school. In these cases it was thought that the nervous symptoms represented the effects of reading disabilities. However, in that study also the timing of symptoms was based entirely on retrospective information.

What are needed are longitudinal studies of preschool children or children just starting school, in which the progress of those with defects of language or perceptual development (but *no* emotional difficulties) can be compared with those with emotional or behavioural problems (but *no* defects of language or perceptual development). Such a study has not yet been undertaken. There is some evidence to suggest that behaviour problems in nursery school often persist into later childhood (Westman *et al* 1967) and also some evidence that emotionally handicapped children tend to fall progressively further behind in academic achievement (Stennett 1966). But no one has yet made the crucial comparison of the behavioural and educational progress of children with these two types of deviance which would enable a determination of which condition is primary and which secondary in relation to etiology.

Effects of treatment
In 1936 Fendrick and Bond wrote:

> The crucial test for this association (between reading backwardness and delinquency) lies in the elimination of these school failures and then studying the effects in terms of delinquency. This attack is obviously a long-term project, but should merit attention.

A considerable variety of methods have been tried in the treatment of children with reading difficulties and behaviour problems. Drugs (Conners *et al* 1967) and operant conditioning methods (Becker *et al* 1967) have been shown, in controlled trials, to be effective in improving children's behaviour and attention to work in the classroom. However, in neither case were the effects on reading attainment or on antisocial activities directly examined. It has been said that remedial teaching is the answer (Roswell and Natchez 1964) but it has also been stated that psychotherapy must precede remedial teaching (Bills 1950, Lipton and Feiner 1956). Unfortunately, there have been very few attempts to compare the efficacy of different approaches to treatment.

Gates and Bond (1936) reported a study in which it was said that children who learned to read following special instruction 'were given a new lease on school life . . . better emotional and social adjustment and conduct usually accompanied, or followed, the improvement in scholastic ability'. Ratings of classroom adjustment and conduct showed twice as many gaining in the coached as in the uncoached group. This finding is consistent with the view that in some cases the reading problem was primary and the behavioural difficulties a maladaptive response to educational failure. However, insufficient details of the study are given in the paper to enable an adequate evaluation of their results, it is not clear how severe were the behaviour disorders in the children studied, and validation of the findings by other studies is required before very much can be concluded.

Margolin *et al* (1955) found that delinquents with reading retardation made somewhat better progress with remedial reading than with psychotherapy, but the best results were obtained in children who received both methods of treatment. However, the groups were very small and the differences were not statistically significant. Studies of the progress of maladjusted children in special schools have not examined the relationship between progress in reading and progress in behavioural adjustment (Roe 1965) or have been concerned with children who showed little retardation in reading (Petrie 1962).

The only systematic and controlled comparison was undertaken by Schiffman (1962). A sample of forty students was selected and divided into four equal groups. One group received remedial reading and psychotherapy, one group received remedial reading only, one group received psychotherapy only; the fourth group received no treatment. A gain in reading grade level was used as a criterion. Analysis of covariance showed that remedial reading was effective whereas psychotherapy was not. Unfortunately there were no measures of behaviour, so that although the study showed that remedial reading had more effect on reading than did psychotherapy, the effects on behaviour of this educational advance remain unknown.

Thus the studies offer slight support for the view that behavioural difficulties *may* sometimes develop as a secondary reaction following educational retardation, but it is uncertain how often this is the case in the more severe behavioural problems. Further studies comparing the effects of different methods of treatment in children with both an antisocial disorder and severe reading difficulties would be very rewarding.

Neurotic determination of reading difficulties
It might be thought that a detailed study of the psychopathology of children with both reading difficulties and antisocial behaviour would help elucidate the nature of the association between the two conditions. However, while it has often been suggested that retardation in reading is due to neurotic conflict or to an 'emotional block' (Blau 1946, Pond 1967) there is a quite remarkable variety of conflicting views on the nature of the supposed psychopathology (Anthony 1961). These views have not so far been systematically tested. Indeed, because of the highly speculative nature of some of the hypotheses and the absence of clear predictions arising from them, some clarification of the hypotheses would be needed before adequate evaluation could usefully be attempted. This is illustrated by the tendency to use opposite findings to support the same view. Thus, the fact that many backward readers show emotional disorder has often been used to support the view that reading backwardness is neurotically determined. On the other hand, it has also been said that 'the fact that some children with these specific defects seem to be relatively psychologically normal, is, I think, due to the apparent normality being equivalent to the *belle indifference* of the adult hysteric' (Pond 1967).

So far there is only very limited evidence which bears on the problem. Comparisons between reading retardation and neurosis show marked differences so that if reading difficulties are neurotically determined the process is likely to be rather different from that in most other neurotic conditions. Firstly, reading disability is very much commoner in boys, while neurotic disorders are about equally common in the two sexes, or slightly commoner in girls (Rutter 1965, Rutter and Graham 1966). Secondly, while neurotic disorders show a generally good prognosis (Rutter 1965, Robins 1966), reading backwardness has a very poor prognosis. Thirdly, reading difficulties are associated with antisocial behaviour rather than neurotic symptomatology. This is not a 'displacement' of neurosis, as it is the presence of antisocial symptoms and not the absence of neurotic symptoms which is associated with retardation in reading.

Reading backwardness was as frequent in children with a mixed neurotic and antisocial disorder as in those with a more 'pure' antisocial disorder. These findings pose difficulties for any view that backwardness in reading is due to a neurosis (Blau 1946) but, of course, they by no means rule out such a hypothesis. More specific testing is needed, and so far there have been very few attempts in this direction.

However, the nature of the association between reading retardation and antisocial behaviour may be further examined by determining whether the children with *both* conditions have more in common with children who show reading retardation alone or with children who show an antisocial disorder alone.

Backward readers with and without antisocial behaviour
Severe reading retardation has been shown in this and in other studies to be associated with a family history of reading backwardness, a delay in the development of speech, current articulation difficulties, or retardation in language, clumsiness, constructional difficulties, motor impersistence and imperfect right–left differentiation. These factors have often been listed as features of 'specific dyslexia' which has been regarded as a developmental disorder, constitutional or genetic in origin (Money 1962, Critchley 1964). While there is some doubt as to the validity of this concept, there are good grounds for considering that these abnormalities of functioning may often be of prime importance in the etiology of reading retardation. If this assumption is made, the relationship between antisocial behaviour and reading backwardness may be assessed by comparing the frequency of these developmental abnormalities in antisocial and in behaviourally normal backward readers (Table 14.1).

Table 14.1 shows the frequency of occurrence of these developmental characteristics in children whose scores on the parental and the teachers' questionnaire were below 13 and 9 respectively (the behaviourally 'normal' children), and in 'antisocial' children with scores above these points on either scale and with pattern of scores which was antisocial in type. On no characteristic was there a significant, or even a sizeable, difference between the antisocial and the behaviourally normal readers; the antisocial children shared the same developmental characteristics as the other backward readers. In view of this similarity in background, it seems un-

TABLE 14.1 *Comparison of antisocial and behaviourally normal children among backward readers*

| | Designation on basis of questionnaire scores* | | |
| | Normal | Antisocial | Statistical |
Characteristic	%	%	significance
History in parent or sib. of delay in learning to read	36.8	34.5	N.S.
Delay in development of speech	10.5	19.4	N.S.
Current articulation defect or retardation of language	24.4	22.6	N.S.
Clumsiness or constructional difficulty	12.2	22.6	N.S.
Motor impersistence	12.2	9.7	N.S.
Imperfect right–left differentiation	78.5	67.7	N.S.
TOTAL NUMBER IN GROUP	41	31	

* Children with a 'neurotic' designation on the questionnaire scores have been excluded from this comparison.

likely that the reading problem in the antisocial children was different in nature to that in the other backward readers. This suggests that either the antisocial difficulties developed as a response to reading backwardness or that both the reading problem and the antisocial behaviour arose on the basis of the same factors in the child.

It could be argued, however, that the concept of specific dyslexia requires the combination of several of these developmental abnormalities and that it is inappropriate to consider each feature in isolation.

The question may be reexamined by considering each child's developmental deviation score. This score is derived by giving one point each for an abnormality in language or speech, in motor coordination, in constructional tasks, in motor persistence, and in right–left differentiation, so that there is a minimum of 0 and a maximum of 5. Table 14.2 shows the lack of significant relationship between the developmental deviation score and antisocial behaviour.

Thus far there is no evidence to support the view that the reading backwardness is due to emotional factors. However, although developmental abnormalities of language, motor function and perception were frequently associated with reading retardation, there were several children who had no developmental abnormalities, no family history of backwardness in reading and did not come from a family of four or more children (a factor also found to be associated with reading difficulties). It might be thought that this would be the group which would show

M. Rutter and W. Yule

psychiatric problems (either neurotic or antisocial) to the greatest extent. However, this was not the case. Of the thirteen children who had none of these features, six had abnormal scores on the parental or teachers' questionnaire compared with thirty-nine of the seventy-three children with these features. It was not possible to isolate a group of children in whom the reading retardation seemed to be due to an emotional or behavioural disorder.

TABLE 14.2   *Developmental deviation score and antisocial behaviour*

| | Designation on basis of behavioural questionnaire scores* | | |
Developmental deviation score	Normal	Antisocial	Total
0	12	6	18
1	16	11	27
2	9	9	18
3	3	2	5
4	1	3	4
TOTAL NUMBER IN GROUP	41	31	72

* Children with a 'neurotic' designation on the questionnaire scores have been excluded from this comparison.

Up to now, it has been assumed that the language, motor and perceptual defects are physiologically rather than psychologically determined. However, it has sometimes been suggested that the delays in the development of speech and language, the clumsiness and the perceptual abnormalities, are due not to a neurological lesion or to a developmental immaturity of brain functioning but rather to an 'emotional block' (Pond 1967), that the motor awkwardness and even reversed cerebral dominance are due to 'inner emotional inhibitions arising from an infantile psychoneurotic condition' (Blau 1946).

While there is a paucity of evidence in support of these views, it must be said that the origin of the developmental delays is largely unknown. Developmental motor awkwardness may be associated with epilepsy or other evidence of an organic brain condition (Gubbay et al 1965), as may any of the other developmental abnormalities, but there is no satisfactory evidence to suggest that this is usually the case. On the other hand, the defects in language and motor development are evident in infancy (in this group of backward readers as well as in general) so that it would have to be very early emotional disorder in order to cause, for example, a delay in the age at which the infant can sit without support. There is no evidence to suggest that such an early emotional disorder exists, although it should be said that the matter has not been systematically investigated. Also, although adequate studies have not been carried out, clinical experience suggests that biological factors are more important than psychological factors in the prognosis of these developmental disorders.

Good readers and poor readers among antisocial boys

Girls were excluded from this part of the study as there were so few anti-social girls. A high proportion of the antisocial boys were severely back-ward in reading. But also about half the antisocial boys were reading quite normally. If it is argued that the reading backwardness is primary and that the antisocial disorder arises secondarily as a reaction to the educa-tional difficulties, there should be important differences between the anti-social children who were good readers and those who were bad readers. It would be expected that the bad readers should possess characteristics related to reading backwardness that the good readers with antisocial disorder did not possess. Furthermore, if some delinquents become antisocial as a response to educational failure, the antisocial children who are good readers will need to have *other* adverse background factors to explain their behavioural disorders—other adverse factors *not* shared by the backward readers.

Table 14.3 shows this comparison between the good readers and bad readers within a group of children, all of whom exhibit antisocial disorders. For this purpose, bad readers are those children whose reading is at least two years below that predicted on the basis of their age and intelligence. Good readers are those whose reading skills were better than predicted or less than twelve months below the predicted level. The mildly retarded readers were excluded from both groups.

The data in the table refer to psychiatric assessments based on informa-tion from parents. The teachers' questionnaire and the psychiatric inter-view with the child produced closely similar findings.

On the whole, the symptomatology of the good readers and the poor readers was remarkably similar (the table gives only the items which show the largest differences between the groups out of a total of thirty-two comparisons). About half the boys in each group had stolen in the last year and both groups showed fairly similar proportions of other types of antisocial and neurotic problems. There was slight tendency for the good readers to have more symptoms in relation to the home, but only for 'sleeping difficulties' was the difference statistically significant.

It has often been thought that reading failure leads to delinquency via truancy but this did not seem to be the case in the present sample. Few children had truanted or refused to go to school, and the good readers and poor readers did not differ in this respect. Furthermore, the average number of half days absent from school was the same for the good readers as for the poor readers. In the present study, absence from school was un-related to either reading backwardness or antisocial behaviour and Mitchell and Shepherd (1967) have shown that, in this age group, dislike of school is unrelated to the absence rate from school. The process of

TABLE 14.3 *Comparison of poor readers and good readers among antisocial boys*

Item	Good readers %	Poor readers %	Statistical significance
ANTISOCIAL SYMPTOMS			
Stealing	43.3	54.5	N.S.
Fighting	33.3	22.7	N.S.
Bullying	41.7	27.3	N.S.
NEUROTIC SYMPTOMS			
Worrying	33.3	13.6	N.S.
Misery	29.1	18.2	N.S.
SYMPTOMS IN RELATION TO HOME			
Disturbed relationship with parent(s)	29.2	18.2	N.S.
Eating difficulty	12.5	0.0	N.S.
Sleeping difficulty	45.8	9.1	<0.01
SYMPTOMS IN RELATION TO SCHOOL			
Very poor concentration	13.6	52.9	<0.01
Truanting	16.7	9.1	N.S.
School refusal or tears on arrival at school	12.5	22.7	N.S.
Mean no. half days absent from school in previous year	28.2	24.0	N.S.
FAMILY BACKGROUND			
Four or more children in family	33.3	65.0	<0.05
Broken homes	34.8	4.5	<0.01
TOTAL NUMBER	24	22	

educational failure leading to dislike of school, leading to truancy, leading to delinquency may be important among older children but it seems not to be so among nine to eleven year old children—at least not on the Isle of Wight.

There was, however, one very striking and significant difference in the symptomatology of the good readers and poor readers—over half the poor readers showed very poor concentration compared with only 13.6 per cent of the good readers. This item refers to *parental* reports of the child's behaviour at home, so that it is not merely an aspect of the child's performance at school in relation to his failure to read. It was also frequently reported for the backward readers who were not antisocial, and it may reasonably be supposed that poor concentration was important in relation to the reading retardation—although whether it was a cause or an effect remains a matter for conjecture at this stage.

To test the nature of the association between reading retardation and antisocial behaviour it is necessary to examine background factors which are associated with *either* of the two conditions but not both. Only limited background information was obtained in the present study and just two items met this requirement. Large family size was shown to be associated with reading retardation but not with antisocial behaviour, while a broken home was shown to be associated with antisocial behaviour but not with reading retardation.

Both these items differentiated the poor readers and good readers. Twice as many poor readers as good readers came from families with four or more children. This may be regarded as a social rather than a biological factor, and it is one not particularly associated with dyslexia as described by Critchley (1964) and others. It suggests that antisocial behaviour is associated with severe reading backwardness of all sorts, not just the variety termed dyslexia which is often thought to be due to constitutional causes. The finding also shows that with regard to family size, the antisocial children who were poor readers are similar to the poor readers who were not antisocial rather than to the antisocial children who were not poor readers.

Furthermore, a broken home was associated with antisocial behaviour in the good readers, but not in the poor readers. Again, in this respect the antisocial poor readers were similar to the poor readers who were not antisocial rather than to the antisocial children who were not poor readers.

Unfortunately in the present study there were very few items which differentiated children with antisocial disorders from those with reading retardation. However, with respect to the few items which did (very poor concentration, family size, and broken home) the children with *both* reading retardation and antisocial behaviour had more in common with children with 'pure' reading retardation than with a 'pure' antisocial disorder.

Summary

Severe reading retardation is very frequently associated with antisocial behaviour. A third of the children more than twenty-eight months retarded in their reading exhibited clinically significant antisocial behaviour and a third of the antisocial children were at least twenty-eight months retarded in reading. In their developmental features and their family characteristics the children who were both antisocial *and* backward in reading showed a closer resemblance to the children with 'pure' reading disability than to those with a 'pure' antisocial disorder. It is suggested that both reading difficulties and antisocial behaviour may develop on the basis of similar types of temperamental deviance but also that delinquency may sometimes arise as a maladaptive response to educational failure. Thus, the child who fails to read and who thereby falls behind in his school work may rebel against all the values associated with school when he finds that he cannot succeed there. These school values include obedience to authority and respect for property. Accordingly, in searching for alternative sources of satisfaction which run counter to what the school stands for, he may get involved in antisocial activities and so become delinquent. Some ways in which these hypotheses might be tested are outlined. The association between reading retardation and antisocial behaviour is an important one; further investigation is likely to be rewarding and the results might well throw light on the processes involved in the development of both conditions.

References

ANTHONY, E. J. (1961) Learning difficulties in childhood *Journal of the American Psychoanalytic Association* 9, 124–34

BECKER, W. C., MADSEN, C. H., ARNOLD, C. R. and THOMAS, D. R. (1967) The contingent use of teacher attention and praise in reducing classroom behaviour problems *Journal of Special Education* 1, 287–307

BILLS, R. E. (1950) Nondirective play therapy with retarded readers *Journal of Consulting and Clinical Psychology* 14, 140–9

BLAU, A. (1946) The master hand *American Orthopsychiatry Association Research Monograph* no. 5

BOVET, L. (1951) *Psychiatric Aspects of Juvenile Delinquency* WHO Monograph, no. 1

BOWER, E. M. (1960) *Early Identification of Emotionally Handicapped Children in School* Springfield, Illinois: Thomas

BURT, C. (1925) *The Young Delinquent* London: University of London Press

CONNERS, C. K., EISENBERG, L. and BARCAI, A. (1967) Effect of dextroamphetamine on children *Archives of General Psychiatry* 17, 478–85

CRITCHLEY, E. M. R. (1968) Reading retardation, dyslexia and delinquency *British Journal of Psychiatry* 115, 1537–47

CRITCHLEY, M. (1962) Developmental dyslexia: a constitutional dyssymbolia in A. W. Franklin (ed) *Word Blindness or Specific Developmental Dyslexia* London: Pitman

CRITCHLEY, M. (1964) *Developmental Dyslexia* London: Heinemann

FENDRICK, P. and BOND, G. (1936) Delinquency and reading *Pedagogical Seminary and Journal of Genetic Psychology* 48, 236–43

GATES, A. I. and BOND, G. L. (1936) Failure in reading and social maladjustment *National Education Association Journal* 25, 205–6

GIBBENS, T. C. N. (1961) Trends in Juvenile Delinquency WHO *Public Health Paper* no. 5

GIBBENS, T. C. N. (1962) Psychiatric aspects of crime in D. Richter, J. M. Tanner, Taylor Lord and O. L. Zangwill (eds) *Aspects of Psychiatric Research* London: Oxford University Press

GIBBENS, T. C. N. (1963) *Psychiatric Studies of Borstal Lads* Maudsley Monograph no. 11, London: Oxford University Press

GLUECK, S. and GLUECK, E. (1950) *Unravelling Juvenile Delinquency* New York: Commonwealth Fund

GUBBAY, S. S., ELLIS, E., WALTON, J. N. and COURT, S. D. M. (1965) Clumsy children: a study of apraxic and agnosic defects in 21 children *Brain* 88, 295–312

LIPTON, A. and FEINER, A. H. (1956) Group therapy and remedial reading *Journal of Educational Psychology* 47, 330–4

McCREADY, E. B. (1926) Defects in the zone of language (word deafness and word blindness) and their influence in education and behaviour *American Journal of Psychiatry* 6, 267–78

MALMQUIST, E. (1958) *Factors Related to Reading Disabilities in the First Grade of the Elementary School* Stockholm: Almqvist and Wiksell

MARGOLIN, J. B., ROMAN, M. and HARARI, C. (1955) Reading disability in the delinquent child: a microcosm of psychosocial pathology *American Journal of Orthopsychiatry* 25, 25–35

MITCHELL, S. and SHEPHERD, M. (1967) The child who dislikes going to school *British Journal of Educational Psychology* 37, 32–40

*MONEY, J. (ed) (1962) *Reading Disability; Progress and Research Needs in Dyslexia* Baltimore: Johns Hopkins Press

MONROE, M. (1932) *Children Who Cannot Read* Chicago: University of Chicago Press

OSWIN, E. M. (1967) *Behaviour Problems Among Children with Cerebral Palsy* Bristol: Wright

PEARSON, G. H. J. (1952) A survey of learning difficulties in children *Psychoanalytic Study of the Child* 7, 322–86

PETRIE, I. R. J. (1962) Residential treatment of maladjusted children: a study of some factors related to progress in adjustment *British Journal of Educational Psychology* 32, 29–37

POND, D. (1967) Communication disorders in brain-damaged children *Proceedings of the Royal Society of Medicine* 60, 343–8

ROBINS, L. N. (1966) *Deviant Children Grown Up* Baltimore: Williams and Wilkins

ROBINS, L. N. and HILL, S. Y. (1966) Assessing the contributions of family structure, class and poor groups to juvenile delinquency *Journal of Criminal Law, Criminology and Police Science* 57, 325–34

ROE, M. (1965) *Survey into Progress of Maladjusted Pupils* London: Inner London Education Authority

ROGERS, C. R. (1942a) The criteria used in a study of mental health problems *Educational Research Bulletin* 21, 29–40

*ROSWELL, F. and NATCHEZ, G. (1964) *Reading disability: Diagnosis and Treatment* New York and London: Basic Books

RUTTER, M. (1965) Classification and categorization in child psychiatry *Journal of Child Psychology and Psychiatry* 6, 71–83

RUTTER, M. and GRAHAM, P. (1966) Psychiatric disorder in 10 and 11 year old children *Proceedings of Royal Society of Medicine* 59, 382–7

RUTTER, M., YULE, W., TIZARD, J. and GRAHAM, P. (1967) Severe reading retardation: its relationship to maladjustment, epilepsy and neurological disorders in *What is Special Education?* Proceedings of the First International Conference of the Association for Special Education July 1966 London: Association for Special Education

SCHIFFMAN, G. (1962) Dyslexia as an educational phenomenon: its recognition and treatment in J. Money (ed) *Reading Disability: Progress and Research Needs in Dyslexia* Baltimore: Johns Hopkins Press

SCOTT, P. D. (1965) Delinquency in J. G. Howells (ed) *Modern Perspectives in Child Psychiatry* Edinburgh: Oliver and Boyd

STENNETT, R. G. (1966) Emotional handicap in the elementary years: phase or disease *American Journal of Orthopsychiatry* 36, 444–9

WESTMAN, J. C., RICE, D. L. and BERMANN, E. (1967) Nursery school behaviour and later school adjustment *American Journal of Orthopsychiatry* 37, 725–31

YULE, W. (1967) Predicting reading ages on Neale's analysis of reading ability *British Journal of Educational Psychology* 37, 252–5

2.6 Emotional and personality problems of severely retarded readers

HELEN ROBINSON
Emeritus Professor of Education, University of Chicago

Reprinted from Helen Robinson (1946) *Why Pupils Fail in Reading*
University of Chicago Press, pp. 76–90

The relationship between a child's emotional pattern and his reactions in the learning situation is being studied with increasing frequency by psychologists. These studies have led investigators such as Sherman (1939) to say:

> In many instances a given emotional pattern may be a distinct hindrance to learning a specific task or skill, whereas in others the emotionality of an individual may be a motivating force to greater effort. Thus the emotions must be taken into account in evaluating success and failure.

The effects of the emotions on learning and retention have not been studied extensively, nor have the effects on the emotions of failure to learn been adequately considered. Educators, psychologists and teachers are showing an increased awareness of this problem and the need for more information concerning it.

Sherman continued:

> The emotionality of an individual at the time he is learning a task has a definite influence upon his efficiency in the learning situation. His emotional balance or imbalance also has a definite effect upon his retention of the material that he has learned and upon his ability to recall and put into use that which he may have learned well previously.

Since it is so difficult to measure ease of learning in varying emotional states, the studies in this direction have been few. Carter (1936) selected words classified as 'pleasant', 'indifferent' and 'unpleasant' and showed them, with corresponding pictures, to children. He studied the recall of words when pictures were shown later and found that pleasant words were better learned than unpleasant or indifferent words and that unpleasant words tended to be better learned than indifferent ones. He noted a tendency to replace unpleasant and indifferent words with incorrect pleasant ones, indicating that pleasantness of association of words may be directly associated with the rate of learning the words.

Failure to learn what is expected may lead to frustration or fear-conditioning to such an extent that the sight of the material may cause a disorganized emotional response, which further inhibits concentration, perseverance and motivation.

Shame may result from failure in which there is a feeling of anxiety. Sanohara (1934) noted this in his study, and Sherman (1939) pointed out that pupils who are ashamed of their failures may develop defensive reactions.

Frustrations and their effect on learning were considered significant by investigators. Irritation and loss of interest were reported by Thorndike and Woodyard (1934) when frequent frustrations were introduced. Kendrew (1935) concluded that frustration disturbed the rate of work and of learning.

The knowledge of success and failure was found by Sullivan (1927) to affect the length of time required to learn nonsense syllables. Gilchrist's (1916) experiment induced him to conclude that praise led to improvement, while reproval led to poorer performance on tests.

While the studies were relatively few, they agreed that learning was more rapid when the stimulus was pleasant, when the subject had been successful and had been praised. However, learning was inhibited by indifferent or unpleasant associations and by failure and frequent frustration, with shame and reproval.

Emotional reactions and reading failure

During the last twenty years, failure in reading has frequently been attributed to emotional problems, and emotional problems have likewise been said to be created by reading failure. The experimental studies just mentioned would provide a basis for both opinions.

Children come to school with a variety of experiences and therefore different associations with different words. Whereas the child who has had unpleasant or indifferent associations with words may find learning to read a difficult task, the child who has had many pleasant associations may learn more quickly.

Since reading is required of the child who remains in school, the teacher is expected to present it to him over and over, with the result that he may have very frequent frustrations, resulting in loss of interest, lack of application, and lowered motivation. The teacher who discovers that a pupil is failing to progress in reading may reprimand him, thus adding to the difficulties he is already experiencing in learning to read.

It seems evident that emotional difficulties may cause reading disability in the beginning and that this disability may in turn result in frustration, which further blocks learning and again intensifies the frustration. The interaction and intensification become a vicious circle, leading to intense emotional maladjustments and complete failure to progress in reading.

The emotional maladjustment seen in a severely retarded reader, then, may be either the cause, the effect, or the result of the interaction of reading failure and emotional maladjustments.

Emotional and personality maladjustments as a cause

As early as 1917, some writers expressed the belief that emotionally unstable children were backward at school, their reading being fluent and expressive but full of guesswork and inaccuracy.

Woolley and Ferris (1923) listed among their school failures 'the psychopathic' children who frequently revealed 'flashes of genius' but were unable to learn as others did.

Hollingworth (1923) explained how this might operate to cause reading failure. She said that neurotic children, even though intelligent, were often deficient in reading because the mechanics of reading requires cooperation, following directions, and sustained effort. Neurotic children are characterized by inferiority in these areas, as well as in others. Where negativism, instability and illusion interfere with learning, these children fail to make progress, except when taught individually.

Fernald's view is:

> The blocking of voluntary action has long been recognized as one of the conditions that result in emotion. . . . The individual who fails constantly in those undertakings which seem to him of great importance and who is conscious of failure is in a chronic state of emotional upset.

She thinks that every child entering school is eager to learn to read and write and that as he sees other children learning while he is not, he always becomes an emotional problem because of this blocking of voluntary action. Of 78 cases of extreme reading disability treated in her clinic, all but four entered school with no history of emotional instability, and the upset occurred as the child showed repeated failure. The child learns to hate or fear the reading situation and everything connected with it such as books, papers, pencils etc. If this is his first group experience, he may react the same way to the social group. Such conditions promote the development of the 'solitary' child and the 'bombastic' child.

In a more recent report, Sherman (1939) stated that:

> Many neurotic conditions are found in children with reading disabilities. These children clearly fall in the therapeutic realm of the psychiatrist, and no reading therapy can be attempted until treat-

Helen Robinson

ment by a psychiatrist is completed. Neurotic children are especially sensitive to failure, and a reading disability may be a focal point of an individual's final reorientation from a neurosis to a normal condition.

These more severe personality difficulties, such as neurotic and psychotic conditions, and their relationship to reading failure might be more evident than the subtle ones, such as specific emotional blocks and unfavourable attitudes. However, a number of authorities have concurred in the belief that even minor emotional and personality difficulties may cause failure in reading.

A child who comes to school is faced with new problems of adjustment. Prescott (1938) enumerated some of these as follows:

. . . learning to get along with other children of many types; learning to get along with a group of parent surrogates in a variety of situations; establishing membership in a new social group; experiencing many situations where affection does not temper requirements; learning to accept and live with one's own peculiarities of appearance, physical handicaps, racial and religious differences in a group which recognizes and calls attention to them as undesirable differences from the group; learning and accepting new group standards of behaviour; learning new games and physical skills necessary to maintain status.

It is little wonder that with these problems at hand the child sometimes occupies himself in learning patterns of behaviour and developing security with the teacher and social group rather than attending to reading.

Concerning the relation of these problems to reading, Jameson (1939) stated:

This period is a difficult one for many children. When children's anxieties about themselves, about their positions in this new competitive group, are sufficient to cause some preoccupation, they often do not have the energy, the confidence, and the motivation to fortify themselves, to equip themselves to learn the complicated task of reading. When added to that situation are . . . significant organic and functional handicaps . . . the child fails in learning to read. Generally his failures have been accepted by him long before they are recognized by his parents and teachers, and his observation of the concern of these adults has intensified his awareness of his inadequacy.

Writers on causes of reading disability have recently recognized the effects of frustrating experiences in learning. Thus a child who has been frustrated in learning other tasks might be conditioned against reading. Dolch (1931) expressed such an opinion when he stated:

Probably more deficiency in reading can be traced to discouragement through failure, and the consequent attitude of antagonism toward reading, than to any other cause. Many children hate the reading lesson simply because it compels them to exhibit before their companions their ignorance or lack of skill. A child caught in this situation is very frequently scolded or held up to ridicule. If this condition is allowed to arise, a child may go on from year to year with scarcely any improvement because he never looks at a book unless he has to and then with a distinct aversion. When he is supposed to be reading, his attention wanders, so that very little reading is really done, and consequently no improvement of skill results.

Such frustration very often results in what the teacher frequently describes as the 'lazy' child. Usually this child is unmotivated and, as Ridenour (1935) pointed out, one of the first steps to undertake is to recognize his resistance to reading and to prepare him so that he wants to read.

Beyond this, Durrell (1932) found that when there were confusions created by exposing an immature child to reading too early,

> ... mental blocking, additional confusion, discouragement, withdrawal of attention, or meaningless activity induced by fear of failure or ridicule, the child often stays on the learning plateau a long time.

Studies

In addition to the opinions expressed by the writers referred to above, there have been a few experimental studies of emotional and behaviour reactions. Bird (1927) studied 100 children between the ages of four and six years and found that 30 had habitual personality handicaps that interfered with their learning. They were classified as follows: two showed introversion; eight were retarded by shyness, lack of self-confidence, dislike of scrutiny, or fear of the task; eight showed excessive dependence on commendation; two worked only for the instructor; four wished to win distinction by unusual behaviour; two were antisocial, as they teased, bullied, and disobeyed; and four had vagrant tendencies, such as flitting from one task to another and leaving unfinished work.

In studying the effect of short auditory span, Saunders (1931) discovered that those children who did not learn to read were not aggressive; they played alone and avoided social contacts until they were considered antisocial; and they developed behaviour problems. She also observed that these children were emotionally dependent on their parents.

A study of 13 children before and after entrance to Grade I led Castner (1935) to list eight traits as significant for reading failure. Two of the traits were instability and excitable personality, and he explained the effects by reporting that

> Many of these children are of the active, talkative, energetic, excitable type, not necessarily uncooperative in the interviews and examina-

tions, but showing fluctuations of attention and oftener a greater or less degree of instability.

Unfortunately, his number of cases was so small that conclusions could be only tentative.

Monroe and Backus (1937) have studied a great many retarded readers and have reported the following primary emotional factors as causes:

1 General emotional immaturity—the child is dependent on the mother and unaccustomed to responsibility; infantile in manner and interests. He may resist reading as a step to growing up.
2 Excessive timidity—has failed in social adjustment and is too shy to speak or attempt group activities.
3 Predilection against reading, since he has heard someone say it is 'hard' or he identifies himself with some person who does not read.
4 Predilection against all school activities.

In a recent summary of his studies of emotional and personality problems in relation to reading disability, Gates (1941) expresses the opinion that emotional problems are present in about 75 per cent of retarded readers but that in only one-fourth of these is it a cause of the disability.

Summary
The opinions of authorities in the field and the findings of a few experimental studies are agreed that emotional and personality problems might be a cause of reading failure. The severe maladjustments of the neurotic child are most evident; nevertheless, the minor adjustments which the child must make when he enters school are so many that he may not be prepared to devote himself to reading. Even though he is willing to learn, he may be hampered by emotional immaturity, lack of confidence and security, unpleasant or indifferent associations with words, or excessive timidity. Prescott (1938) believes that personality needs are so complicated that it is surprising that their frustration does not more seriously interfere with the work of the school.

Failure to make the first steps in adaptation to reading may lead to frustration and all its accompanying reactions, such as inattention, lack of motivation, confusion and lack of application to the task of learning to read.

Emotional and personality difficulties as an effect of reading failure

Authorities have agreed that continued failure in reading might create emotional tension due to frustration. Dislike for the subject, as well as everything surrounding it, might follow, and all manner of compensations have been noted. Social maladjustment and even delinquency and crime have been listed as results of the failure to learn to read.

Symptoms
Sherman (1939) made psychiatric studies of a number of severely retarded readers and listed their most common symptoms:

Indifference to the problem of failure and emphasis upon some skill or interest as compensation for school inadequacy.

Instances in which even a slight reading defect causes withdrawal from effort and, in some cases, results in emotional disturbances. Some of these children become behaviour and disciplinary problems as a result of these emotional upheavals.

Antagonism to academic problems and a defensive reaction to any activity relating to school.

Refusal to improve reading ability, as a bid for attention and as a mark of differentiation. In some instances children who have had reading difficulties have received a great deal of attention, not only from teachers, but also from their parents. In consequence, failure has become synonymous with personal attention, and as the result these children may at times unconsciously refuse to improve their reading level.

Daydreaming, incorrigibility, inattentiveness, shyness and negativism were listed by Kirk (1934) as personality traits which improved with remedial treatment in his high-grade mentally defective cases.

Gates (1936) has listed the symptoms of personality maladjustment of 100 random cases of reading disability as follows:

1 Nervous tensions and habits such as stuttering, nail-biting, restlessness, insomnia, and pathological illness—ten cases.
2 Putting on a bold front as a defence reaction, loud talk, defiant conduct, sullenness—sixteen cases.
3 Retreat reactions such as withdrawal from ordinary associations, joining outside gangs, and truancy—fourteen cases.
4 Counterattack, such as making mischief in school, playing practical jokes, thefts, destructiveness, cruelty, bullying—eighteen cases.
5 Withdrawing reactions, including mind-wandering and daydreaming —twenty-six cases.
6 Extreme self-consciousness; becoming easily injured, blushing, developing peculiar fads and frills and eccentricities, inferiority feelings— thirty-five cases.
7 Give up or submissive adjustments, as shown by inattentiveness, indifference, apparent laziness—thirty-three cases.

In only eight cases did the child develop a constructive compensation, such as drawing etc.

Daydreaming, seclusiveness, lack of interest, 'laziness', inattention, absent-mindedness, sensitiveness etc, were listed as causes for referring children with reading disabilities to Blanchard (1928).

Orton (1937) reported that his so-called 'strephosymbolics' showed a definite frustration reaction, although they might attempt to cover up their deficiency and evade demands for reading. However, some assumed a swaggering, boisterous attitude and insisted that they read well and liked it very much.

Preston (1940) made a careful and detailed evaluation of personality characteristics of 100 reading failures. She found that children who were '. . . bewildered, fearful, full of inhibitions, or "shut-in" on the one hand and antagonistic, rebellious or antisocial on the other', came from homes where they were overprotected and treated as infants until failure in reading caused a sudden change. She found that after reading failure a child might react in these ways: following initial bewilderment he would try to gain the limelight at any cost to offset his position in reading; adopt attitudes of suspicion and antagonism towards rivals and teacher, sometimes becoming almost hostile in character; after fourth to ninth year of failure, those of submissive make-up became 'shut-in' and moody with feelings of inferiority; the aggressive ones became increasingly antisocial.

Why reading failure appears to cause personality problems
Sherman (1939) concisely summarized this effect when he wrote:

A child may react with a deep sense of failure, not only because he realizes his inability to develop adequate reading efficiency, but also because he constantly has to face various social pressures. He must deal with the attitudes of his parents, who are greatly disappointed in his inability to learn, as well as those of his fellow pupils. He must deal also with the attitudes of the teachers, many of whom do not understand the difference between an inherent reading disability and an unwillingness to learn. The child with a reading disability must also deal with the reactions of his playmates, who certainly do not understand the complexity of a reading problem and who frequently tend to categorize the pupil with a reading disability as 'dumb' or backward or peculiar. Thus it is not unnatural that frustration and its consequences play an important role in the case of children who have reading difficulties.

He also pointed out that a feeling of anxiety might result from failure, and as a consequence, defensive reactions might develop.

Blanchard (1928) found that when reading failure continued, it resulted in a feeling of failure and that unless socially acceptable compensations were developed, personality and behaviour deviations were liable to arise. However, with substitution of success for failure, these compensations were no longer needed. Newell (1931) believed that the presence of emotional tension with anxiety and misunderstanding led to resentment and antagonism towards help.

The unfortunate attitude of parents was, in a measure, responsible for Preston's (1939) conclusion:

> Placing the blame on the child is rank injustice and is either felt as such by the victims, with the usual reaction of mankind against injustice, or if the burden of guilt is accepted by the child, his personality tends to be overwhelmed by guilt feelings with disintegrating effect, as time goes on.

Concerning the effect of threatened home security on the personality adjustment of the child she stated (Preston 1939):

> Reading failure causes not only a blighting insecurity in the school world which gives rise to serious maladjustments in the personalities of these normal children, but also an embarrassing, belittling insecurity in the social life of these children at school and sometimes in the home; adding to maladjustments which interfere with proper development and constituting a menace to future social adjustment. More serious still, home security . . . is undermined to an unhealthful, sometimes pernicious degree, and brings forth even greater maladjustments in the personalities. . . .

If reading disability were a cause of emotional and personality maladjustment in certain cases, then it would follow that treatment resulting in improvement of the former might result in improvement of personal relations. Damereau (1934) studied 22 cases of reading disability, all of whom were behaviour problems. All the cases received reading treatment, but in addition four received psychiatric treatment, seven received treatment from a social worker and six received both psychiatric and social treatment. After following these cases, she concluded that improvement in one area bore little relation to improvement in the other. Changes in behaviour occurred when tutoring was supplemented by social or social psychiatric assistance or when the child–parent relations were satisfactory. Thus if reading disability caused behaviour maladjustment, the removal of this disability did not seem to improve behaviour. From the evidence presented in her study, it is questionable whether one might say that the reading disability was removed.

Summary
There is no doubt that reading failure has led to frustration, discouragement, disinterest, inattention, and maladjustment, except in cases in which a satisfactory compensation of a socially approved nature has been established. Children's reactions seemed to be of three general types: first, aggressive reactions in which the child attacked the whole environment associated with reading; second, withdrawal when the child sought for satisfaction outside the reading environment, which included playmates;

third, lack of emotional affectivity where the child appeared responsive but evidenced no feeling tone to his responses. In some instances, at least, the treatment of the reading disability was not sufficient, and it was necessary to give added psychiatric treatment to obtain satisfactory readjustment.

Emotional and personality maladjustment as both cause and effect

If failure can cause emotional maladjustments, then those maladjustments inhibit further learning, which creates more emotional difficulty. The two interact, each making the other more intense. The reciprocal relationship was emphasized in the following statement by Tinker (1934):

> Nonreaders usually show an emotional reaction to the reading situation. In one type of case a neurotic constitution is the direct cause of the reading disability. It seems that many neurotics exhibiting impulsive responses, negativistic attitudes and illusions are unable to give the cooperation and sustained effort required in learning to read. For such cases prognosis is poor. Until their emotional adjustments are improved little progress in reading may be expected, even with individual teaching. It has been shown, however, that emotional maladjustments, especially emotional reaction to the reading situation, may be caused by reading disability. Lack of success during early attempts to read produces unfortunate emotional conditioning. Feelings of inferiority arise, and personality and behaviour deviations may occur.

Bennett (1938) summarized some of the more pertinent findings in this field and pointed out the implications referred to in this summary. After weighing the evidence, he concluded:

> There seems general agreement, however, that children with certain types of undesirable behaviour habits or personal characteristics, and children struggling with deep emotional conflicts face more than average likelihood that they will find the art of reading difficult to master. There seems equal agreement that a serious retardation in reading is quite apt to have detrimental effects upon the general development of the child's personality. Probably the relationship is often reciprocal, and in older and more seriously handicapped children each problem may require specific and intensive treatment. The nature of the difficulty seems similar if it is cause or effect.

Monroe (1932) found evidence of an interaction and intensification in her study, in which she compared the personality problems of reading-disability cases and other unselected cases. She concluded:

Whether the reading defect is caused by unfavourable behaviour or personality, or vice versa, is sometimes difficult to determine. A child may be resistant to learning through negativism and unfavourable emotional attitudes. In such a case reading would undoubtedly suffer along with other scholastic achievements. On the other hand, and probably more frequently, a child may develop the emotional and personality problems as a result of failure in learning to read. The emotional attitude may develop through the child's failure and then in turn may aggravate still further the retardation in reading.

Her implication, that a child whose learning difficulty was not confined to reading might have an emotional basis for the difficulty, was particularly significant. Tulchin (1935) concurred in this belief when he suggested that '. . . the more primary the emotional factors, the greater the stumbling block in treatment. . . . Also, when the emotional factors seem primary, disability and general lack of progress in other subjects as well as in reading are more likely to occur.'

Monroe and Backus (1937) listed as secondary emotional factors those which resulted from reading disability and which in turn further retarded the child's progress in reading. These were: aggressive opposition; withdrawal, either direct or truancy or daydreams; compensating mechanisms, such as getting satisfaction from achievement in other school subjects; defeatism, in which the child gave up and suffered from feelings of inadequacy; and hypertension, or development of anxieties, nervous mannerisms etc.

Studies of the interaction of emotional maladjustment and reading disability seemed quite limited, since most research workers did not consider it desirable to permit a child with severe reading disability to continue untreated while such observations were being made. Hence this section contains only opinions of authorities, without further evidence of the facts on which they based their opinions.

Summary
Expert opinion concurred in the belief that emotional and personality maladjustment might be both a cause and an effect of a severe reading disability. Studies were not available to substantiate these opinions.

A common cause for both reading disability and emotional maladjustment

A number of factors have been suspected as being basic to reading disability and emotional maladjustment. Wells (1935) pointed out that sometimes reading difficulties are a means used by children reacting to difficulties of home adjustment, just as stealing and tantrums may be another.

A common cause for both is suggested by Blanchard (1936) who said:

... the reading disability often arises from the same source of difficulty in emotional development, and in the same manner as the accompanying personality or behaviour problems or neurotic symptoms, such as fears, illness without physical basis, infantile regressions, and the like. ...

While sex conflicts are evident in many reading disability cases, even more pronounced in the material produced in treatment interviews are difficulties in establishing masculine identifications and in handling aggressive impulses, together with excessive anxiety and guilt over destructive, hostile and sadistic feelings.

Witty and Skinner reported that at least 50 per cent of their cases of subject matter disabilities at the Northwestern Psychoeducational Clinic had 'fears and anxieties' sufficiently serious to require therapeutic measures, and they stressed

success rather than failure, regular habits, home cooperation in the development of such character traits as initiative and self-direction, more effective social relationships, and a sense of security. Bad behaviour, we find, is generally a reflection of school and home situations which are limited in opportunity for varied experience and which are saturated with tensions resulting from efforts to make all children equally amenable. ...

Either a reading disability or a personality problem might be responsible for the other according to Hardwick (1932), who concluded that if the personality problem is basic to a reading failure, it must be treated before we can expect much gain in reading. However, if reading failure brings about emotional disturbances, the reading pressure must be alleviated before the emotional difficulty can be entirely cleared up.

Summary
A third factor or group of factors might be responsible for both reading failure and personality problems, according to opinions expressed by several writers. The home and family seem to have received major attention as such a cause.

Conclusions

Authoritative opinions and results of many studies agree, without exception, that a large number of severely retarded readers also evidenced emotional and personality maladjustments. There was likewise a strong implication that more severely retarded readers were subject to more severe personality problems.

Studies also indicated that words with pleasant associations were more easily learned. Thus the emotions might be definitely responsible for reading failure, especially if the child were not emotionally ready to begin the task of reading. Neurotic children should always be considered by the psychiatrist before reading is attempted, or failure might result. If a child had failed repeatedly in his attempts to learn to read, he might accept failure and lose all confidence in himself or he might rationalize the failure or he might refuse to accept it. In general, such children seemed to become aggressive, withdrawn, or to lose emotional affectivity.

In many cases, emotional maladjustments and reading failure seemed to interact, each adding to the seriousness of the other. This might become a vicious circle so that ordinary attempts at reading training would be unsuccessful. According to Sherman (1939):

> Whatever therapeutic programme is instituted, the initial step must be an evaluation of the emotional pattern of the child, first, because no therapeutic plan can be formulated without first recognizing a child emotionally, and second, because consistent motivation for improvement cannot be introduced if the child is distracted by personal problems.

This evaluation would have been equally useful if reading failure had been a symptom of some other basic factor, just as emotional maladjustments might be. Such factors have proved most difficult to locate and evaluate, although home conditions have received major attention.

The complexity of evaluation of human emotions might well be the reason for so many opinions expressed in the literature, with only a few studies to substantiate such views. Hence the psychiatric study of severely retarded readers should aid materially in evaluating these findings.

Behaviour disorders associated with serious reading retardation

Even beyond the milder personality and behaviour difficulties, there are indications that reading failure may cause delinquency. Gates (1941) pointed out that Chatfield, Director of Attendance and Child Welfare of New York City, was convinced that '. . . the continual frustration in school, produced by inability to read efficiently, frequently led to truancy and delinquency'.

A study by Fendrick and Bond (1936) summarized various opinions, one of which was that of Peyser, who believed school failures are more highly correlated with delinquency than are poverty, broken homes, physical and mental defects, or psychopathic conditions. In the case of 187 delinquents between the ages of sixteen and nineteen years, the writers found that over 90 per cent had been school failures. When the IQ was constant between 90 and 110, there was a mean difference of five years between the life-age and the reading status. The amount of school experience and rating in other subjects such as arithmetic was not reported.

Helen Robinson

Stulken (1937), who secured much information concerning his cases, found that about 20 per cent of the boys who were serious behaviour problems also had severe reading disabilities. He reported that about 66 per cent were retarded in reading one or more years below the level of their mental ages. After citing more statistical data, he concluded that this evidence indicated that reading disability was an important factor in producing school maladjustment. He added further:

In approximately 40 per cent of the cases the important factor in reading disability seemed to be related to personality factors such as emotional instability. . . .

In describing remedial treatment, he stated:

More important, however, than the progress in reading, is the changed attitude of the problem boy toward school when he realizes that he is learning to read. He ceases to play truant and instead becomes interested in his school work. Furthermore, when the problem boy gets a feeling of satisfaction from his school work he is less liable to go outside of school to win his success in antisocial and often delinquent behaviour.

Summary
Some evidence has been presented to indicate that reading disability and delinquency are coincidental in some cases; however, no causal relationship has been established. A great deal more should be known about other operative causes before one can be isolated and labelled as the cause of delinquency. Further studies should be made to throw light on the interrelationship.

References

BENNETT, CHESTER C. (1938) An inquiry into the genesis of poor reading *Teachers' College Contributions to Education* no. 755 New York: Teachers' College, Columbia University
BIRD, GRACE E. (1927) Personality factors in learning *Personnel Journal* 6, June, pp. 56–9
BLANCHARD, PHYLLIS (1928) Reading disability in relation to maladjustment *Mental Hygiene* 12, October, 772–88
BLANCHARD, PHYLLIS (1936) Reading disabilities in relation to difficulties of personality and emotional development *Mental Hygiene* 20, 410
CARTER, HAROLD D. (1936) Emotional correlates of errors in learning *Journal of Educational Psychology* 27, 55–67
CASTNER, B. M. (1935) Prediction of reading disability prior to first grade entrance *American Journal of Orthopsychiatry* 5, 379
DAMEREAU, RUTH (1934) Influence of treatment on the reading ability

and behavior disorders of reading disability cases *Smith College Studies in Social Work* 5, 182

DOLCH, EDWARD W. (1931) *The Psychology and Teaching of Reading* Boston: Ginn and Company

DURRELL, DONALD (1932) Confusions in learning *Education* 52, 330–1

FENDRICK, PAUL and BOND, GUY (1936) Delinquency and reading *Pedagogical Seminary and Journal of Genetic Psychology* 48, 236–43

*FERNALD, GRACE (1943) *Remedial Techniques in Basic School Subjects* New York: McGraw-Hill

GATES, ARTHUR I. (1936) (with assistance of Guy L. Bond) Failure in reading and social maladjustment *National Education Association Journal* 25, 205–6

GATES, ARTHUR I. (1941) The role of personality maladjustment in reading disability *Journal of Genetic Psychology* 59, 77–83

GILCHRIST, E. P. (1916) The extent to which praise and blame affect a pupil's work *School and Society* 4, 872–4

HARDWICK, ROSE S. (1932) Types of reading disability *Childhood Education* 8, 425

HOLLINGWORTH, LETA S. (1923) *Special Talents and Defects* New York: Macmillan

JAMESON, AUGUSTA (1939) Methods and devices for remedial reading in William S. Gray (ed) *Recent Trends in Reading* Supplementary Educational Monographs no. 49 Chicago: University of Chicago Press

KENDREW, E. N. (1935) A note on the persistence of moods *British Journal of Psychology* 26, 165–73

KIRK, SAMUEL A. (1934) The effects of remedial reading on the educational progress and personality adjustment of high-grade mentally deficient children *Journal of Juvenile Research* 18, 140–62

MONROE, MARION (1932) *Children Who Cannot Read* Chicago: University of Chicago Press

MONROE, MARION and BACKUS, BERTIE (1937) *Remedial Reading: A Monograph in Character Education* Boston, Massachusetts: Houghton Mifflin

NEWELL, NANCY (1931) For non-readers in distress *Elementary School Journal* 32, 183–95

*ORTON, S. T. (1937) *Reading, Writing and Speech Problems in Children* London: Chapman and Hall

PRESCOTT, DANIEL A. (1938) *Emotion and the Educative Process* Washington: American Council on Education

PRESTON, MARY I. (1939) The reaction of parents to reading failures *Child Development* 10, 3, 179

PRESTON, MARY I. (1940) Reading failure and the child's security *American Journal of Orthopsychiatry* 10, 240

RIDENOUR, NINA (1935) The treatment of reading disability *Mental Hygiene* 19, 387

SANOHARA, T. (1934) A psychological study of the feeling of shame *Japanese Journal of Psychology* 9, 847–90

Helen Robinson

SAUNDERS, MARY JANE (1931) The short auditory span disability *Childhood Education* 8, 59–65

SHERMAN, MANDEL (1939) Emotional disturbances and reading disability in William S. Gray (ed) *Recent Trends in Reading* Supplementary Educational Monographs no. 49 Chicago: University of Chicago Press

STULKEN, EDWARD H. (1937) Retardation in reading and the problem boy in school *Elementary English Review* 14, no. 5, 179–82

SULLIVAN, ELLEN B. (1927) Attitude in relation to learning *Psychological Monographs* 36, no. 169, 1–149

THORNDIKE, E. L. and WOODYARD, ELLA (1934) Influence of the relative frequency of successes and frustrations *Journal of Educational Psychology* 25, 241–50

TINKER, MILES A. (1934) Remedial methods for nonreaders *School and Society* 40, 526

TULCHIN, SIMON H. (1935) Emotional factors in reading disabilities in school children *Journal of Educational Psychology* 26, 446

WELLS, F. L. (1935) A glossary of needless reading errors *Journal of Experimental Education* 4, 35

WITTY, PAUL A. and SKINNER, CHARLES E. (1939) *Mental Hygiene in Modern Education* New York: Farrar and Rinehart

WOOLLEY, HELEN THOMPSON and FERRIS, ELIZABETH (1923) *Diagnosis and Treatment of Young School Failures* Bureau of Education Bulletin 1, Washington DC: Bureau of Education

3 Developmental aspects of reading difficulty

Introduction

The controversy over the existence of specific constitutional impediments to the learning of reading and writing is by now widely recognized. Resolution of the problems presented has been hampered partly by the fact that research in this area has to be interdisciplinary, and that the proper degree of collaboration between medical and psychological workers has seldom been achieved (Money 1962). Partly, too, difficulties reside in the nature of the conceptual basis of hypotheses about 'dyslexia', in the misunderstanding of terms and assumptions, and in the heterogeneity of evidence collected from case histories and larger studies.

In addition the topic has generated such a degree of disturbance that much of the discussion—oral and written—has been polemical and has not consisted of dispassionate assessment of the evidence. The matter has been further complicated by the fact that it has frequently been possible to postulate some other cause for failure, and in many discussions there has been a marked desire to settle for any explanation in preference to the notion of 'dyslexia'.

Alternative explanations for a severe degree of reading failure not explicable in social or cultural terms may retain some part of the conceptual framework of 'dyslexia' (Rutter *et al* 1970) or they may reject it entirely. For instance Merritt (1972) whose paper appears in this section (page 186) puts forward an explanation in terms of learning theory and neurotic reaction. There is no *a priori* reason why explanations of different kinds should be logically incompatible, that is to say why each should not sometimes be true; also a condition such as reading failure can be 'overdetermined'—i.e. there might be more than one set of associated circumstances which could account for the facts of any particular case.

The recently published *Tizard Report* (HMSO 1972, page 127) has recommended the substitution of the phrase 'specific reading difficulties' for the controversial term 'dyslexia'. The paragraphs in which this recommendation is made are reprinted at the beginning of this section. However, the comment in paragraph 10 that as part of the remedial process assessment must be made of 'the functions that underlie' reading skills, and that 'the identification of predisposing factors' may be important in taking preventive measures, suggests that the notion of developmental anomalies of different kinds is not being completely dismissed.

The papers which follow present a variety of views on the relationship of severe reading delay to aspects of development and learning, and include three examples of experimental work. They have been chosen not because

Developmental aspects

of the use they may make of any given term such as 'dyslexia' but because they illustrate an area of work and concern which merits serious consideration, and in which prejudice has no place.

References

*MONEY, J. (1962) (ed) *Reading Disability* Baltimore: Johns Hopkins Press
RUTTER, M., TIZARD, J. and WHITMORE, K. (1970) *Education, Health and Behaviour* London: Longman

3.1 Children with specific reading difficulties

TIZARD REPORT
Advisory Committee on Handicapped Children

Reprinted from Department of Education and Science (1972)
Children with Specific Reading Difficulties HMSO, paras 2–10

Introduction

2 Learning to read is part of the wider development of communication skills. Reading is a complex cognitive process requiring visual, auditory and motor skills to enable a child to recognize words and symbols, to associate them with the appropriate sounds and to invest them with meaning derived from previous experience. It is when a child has for some reason not fully developed one or more of these abilities that he is likely to be unusually slow in learning to read. Such delay is often accompanied by some degree of emotional disturbance.

3 Consideration of the proper educational needs of children with severe reading difficulties has been beset by conflicting descriptions and definitions of their condition. The term 'dyslexia' was originally used—and is still applied—by neurologists to describe severe difficulty in reading after a localized injury to the brain of an adult who was previously a competent reader. The same term was later applied to children with severe reading retardation who had never been competent readers. It is with these children that we are here concerned. However, much recent publicity has concerned a condition called by certain neurologists 'specific developmental dyslexia' which allegedly affects a minority of children with severe reading retardation, and it is this group which, it is claimed, require special recognition and special treatment. The validity of this more narrow view is open to question both on scientific and on practical (remedial) grounds. The position was further confused by Section 27 of the Chronically Sick and Disabled Persons Act, 1970, which used the unhelpful term 'acute dyslexia': the reading difficulties to which the Act intended to refer are not acute in the medical sense of coming sharply to a crisis; if, on the other hand, 'acute' is meant in the lay sense of severe, the Act omits to define the degree of severity.

Specific developmental dyslexia

4   The main controversy over 'specific developmental dyslexia' has centred on its etiology, or underlying cause. Some neurologists (including Dr MacDonald Critchley) and a few psychologists have postulated a syndrome of 'developmental dyslexia' with a specific underlying cause and specific symptoms, which may be found in children of normal or superior intelligence. It is said to be usually the consequence of a neurological delay in development which is of constitutional origin. It was defined in 1968 by a Research Group formed by Dr Critchley (as President of the World Federation of Neurology) and meeting in Texas as: 'A disorder manifested by difficulty in learning to read despite conventional instruction, adequate intelligence and sociocultural opportunity . . . [and] dependent upon fundamental cognitive disabilities which are frequently of constitutional origin.'

5   According to this view the 'disorder' is basically one of dysfunction in the synthesis and interpretation of information coming into the brain through and by the eyes and ears, the cause of which is specific and essentially neurological. This primarily neurological dysfunction is stated to be commonly associated with other disabilities such as clumsiness and difficulty in telling right from left. The dysfunction leads to characteristic difficulties in reading involving, for example, reversal of letters ('d' instead of 'b') and their transposition ('saw' instead of 'was'). If educational measures designed to overcome the reading difficulty fail, the 'localized constitutional immaturity of brain function' may be expected in most cases 'eventually to right itself'.

6   This view of 'specific developmental dyslexia' and its cause is by no means universally accepted by paediatric neurologists. Most educational psychologists also consider that the evidence on which it is based is unsatisfactory. The Education and Child Psychology Division of the British Psychological Society said in a letter to the Secretary of State that the clinical descriptions of the condition led to the conclusion that children with quite differing kinds of problems are being described. They seriously questioned the use of the term 'dyslexia' as a clinical entity, unless it is so carefully defined as to circumscribe its application to a very small proportion of poor readers indeed.

7   Among children with the most severe reading difficulties, a number of associated difficulties mentioned by Dr Critchley and others are indeed often found, but investigations such as that by Margaret Clark in Scotland and the Isle of Wight Study have shown that they are not all found in any one child, and the very varied combinations of difficulties do not fit easily into specific syndromes. As Margaret Clark said, 'The striking finding was the diversity of disabilities, and not an underlying pattern common to the group.' Furthermore, many children who display features said to be characteristic of 'dyslexia' can in fact read well; others who read badly display few if any of the classical diagnostic signs.

8   We take the view that, as these considerations suggest, there is really a continuum spanning the whole range of reading abilities from those of the most fluent readers to those with the most severe difficulties. In addition to children whose reading abilities are significantly below the standards which their general abilities in other spheres would lead one to expect, the continuum includes those children whose reading backwardness is only one aspect of their general retardation. It does of course also include children whose reading abilities are significantly *above* the standards which their general abilities would lead one to expect. Unless a 'specific developmental dyslexia' group could be positively and very precisely differentiated, there is a danger that attention would focus on the group assessed as 'dyslexic' to the disadvantage of those with perhaps equally severe difficulties but who happened not to be so assessed.

9   While we acknowledge that it is possible to separate a minority of children with severe reading difficulty (and often spelling, writing and number problems) who fulfil some of the criteria of 'specific developmental dyslexia', we are highly sceptical of the view that a syndrome of 'developmental dyslexia' with a specific underlying cause and specific symptoms has been identified. Since the term 'dyslexia' has recently been used so very loosely and misleadingly in the various ways described in paragraph 3, we think it would be better to adopt a more usefully descriptive term, 'specific reading difficulties', to describe the problems of the small group of children whose reading (and perhaps writing, spelling and number) abilities are significantly below the standards which their abilities in other spheres would lead one to expect.

10   There is general agreement among teachers, psychologists and neurologists—whatever their views on etiology—that the best way of dealing with specific reading difficulties is through appropriate remedial education. It is of course always necessary, as part of the remedial process, to make an assessment of a pupil's reading skills and an examination of the functions that underlie them—visual and auditory perception, association processes, language development and visuomotor skills such as handwriting; but we do not believe that the question of etiology has any great significance for the educationist, though the identification of predisposing factors may well have importance from the point of future prevention. The needs of children with specific reading difficulties are, in our view, most profitably considered as part of the wider problem of reading backwardness of all kinds, and it is to this wider problem that we therefore address ourselves in the remaining sections of this report.

3.2 Dyslexia: a problem of communication

Centre for Research in Educational Sciences,
University of Edinburgh

Reprinted from *Educational Research* (1969) 10, 2, pp. 126–33

In her paper to the Education Section of the British Psychological Society in 1964 (Vernon 1964) Professor Vernon referred to the continuing controversy between those who maintained that all reading delay was environmentally caused, and those who believed that in some cases a 'more fundamental constitutional condition' was involved.

In the following year, in the autumn issue of the AEP newsletter, there appeared a group of articles on dyslexia, contributed respectively by a neurologist (Reinhold 1965), an educational psychologist (Bannatyne 1965) and a college lecturer (Walbridge 1965), all of whom accepted that the term 'dyslexia' has some meaning. The issue for March 1966 contained in answer to these an article by Burt (Burt 1965) headed 'Counterblast to dyslexia', in which arguments about intelligence, motivation, emotional disturbance and suitable instruction were advanced.

In the latter part of the same year, two substantial works on reading were published in the United States and Britain. *The Disabled Reader: Education of the Dyslexic Child*, edited by Money and Schiffman in America, can be regarded as a sequel to the research symposium edited by Money which appeared some five years ago (Money 1962a). It contains sections on phenomenology and theory, teaching methods and programme organization, case studies illustrating different types of difficulty, and a final summing up, with a glossary, a bibliography of some 300 references and a bibliography of tests.

There are seventeen contributors, some of them British. Money's preface makes it clear that the terms 'dyslexic' child, or 'disabled' reader cover many types of disability, but indicates that the word 'disability' implies failure to learn in circumstances where learning might have been expected, and that it particularly excludes failure attributable to 'educational neglect or inadequate instruction'.

Standards and Progress in Reading (Morris 1966) contains the results of a detailed longitudinal survey of children in Kent. It is mainly concerned with the school conditions in which two selected groups, a group of 'good' readers and a group of 'poor' readers were taught, but pays attention also to domestic, social and personal characteristics. In the concluding chapter of *The Disabled Reader*, Edwards says: 'Unquestionably, there are special types of genuine learning disability.' In the concluding chapter of *Standards and Progress in Reading*, Morris says:

> It was concluded . . . that the study as a whole lends little support to the idea that 'specific developmental dyslexia' is an identifiable syndrome distinct from 'reading backwardness'.

This article has been written in an attempt to clarify some of the issues involved in these conflicts of judgment. It is not a comprehensive review, even of recent literature, but is selective in an effort to make certain points clear and is perhaps less about dyslexia than about attitudes to it. For comprehensive bibliographies and reviews the reader is referred to Benton (1962), Vernon (1964), Critchley (1964), Kinsbourne and Warrington (1966) and to the symposia in which the first and last of these references appear.

The conflict exemplified above is not new, nor are the origins of it easy to trace or explain in purely rational terms. But some explanation has to be found for the fact that side by side with the increasing recognition of backwardness and retardation, the development of more child-centred methods of teaching, the growing body of knowledge about the effect on learning of emotional stresses and cultural deprivation, the development of the Child Guidance Services, and the enormous expansion of special provision for the handicapped, there has persisted among administrators, psychologists and teachers a resistance to the notion that a condition describable as 'specific reading disability' exists. Most have wanted to regard all retardation (i.e. a state in which a child's reading ability was demonstrably below some level regarded as his 'potential') in terms of other causative factors. But some have tried to explain retardation away as largely a statistical artefact (Vernon 1956), and to deny that any 'expectation' of achievement other than a statistical one, based on observed correlations, is justifiable.

The assertion that the condition does exist (that is, that 'dyslexia' is a name for something more than the behavioural state of 'retardation in reading', in the same way that 'measles' means more than 'the state of being covered with a blotchy red rash') has come mainly from people in the medical profession; the history of medical interest in the topic is outlined by Critchley (1964). The resistance amounts, therefore, to an unwillingness among certain educators to accept medical opinion on an educational matter. To try to trace in detail the origins of the conflict of opinion would be a historical exercise outside the scope of this article. It is important, however, to look further at some of the things that have been said on both sides, not only as illustrations of the amount of feeling the topic has generated, but as clues to the possible resolution of what is, after all, a rather unproductive state of controversy.

On page 9 of his book on developmental dyslexia, Critchley (1964) accuses sociologists and educational psychologists of having 'invaded . . . what had hitherto been a medical province or responsibility'. 'Invaded' is an emotive term, and a derogatory one, and the passage from which this quotation is taken seems to imply clearly that sociologists and psychologists, by trying to relate a child's educational history to a whole network of genetic, economic, social, cultural, emotional and pedagogic influences, were arrogating to themselves the right to pronounce on what was, in fact, a medical condition; that they had succeeded in casting doubt on reputable evidence, and that they had obscured a distinction of great educational importance.

It is not hard to find equally harsh words uttered from the other side. For instance Wall (1961) speaking at the Nottingham refresher course held by the English Division of Professional Psychologists, had this to say:

> The word 'dyslexia' seems to be a jargon at its worst. . . . It means bad reading, and nothing is added but its Greek form. . . .

Going on to point out that reading is a culturally-determined activity, he asserted that

> Pseudo-medical terms seem to be not merely out of place but dangerously so. . . . Let us call our examinations and tests examinations and tests and not diagnoses.

Words such as these coming from the Director of the National Foundation for Educational Research make it hard not to conclude that the source of the 'resistance' has been the feeling that from the educationist's standpoint it was the medical specialists who had 'invaded' an educational domain and that the disagreement constitutes a battle for professional possession. But the skilled collaboration of doctors in the ascertainment and treatment of mental subnormality, severe emotional disturbance and infantile autism, all of which are in part cultural problems, has become accepted practice. What is different in the situation under review here? For one thing, the fact that neurologists and ophthalmologists have taken a keen interest in the particular difficulties and errors exhibited by children referred to them for reading and writing failure, and that they have often conducted psychological and educational examinations without calling on the help of a psychologist, may have put them in a special position. It is also, unfortunately, true that the descriptions given, and the labels and explanations proposed, have produced a multiplicity of obscure terms, and a great deal of conceptual confusion.

That medical men should have shown interest in the particular mani-

Dyslexia: a problem of communication

festations of reading/writing difficulty is completely understandable if we remember that the earliest thinking on the subject (Morgan 1896, Hinshelwood 1917) was in terms of analogy with acquired aphasia (i.e. that resulting from 'damage' by injury, vascular disease or tumours) and that the study of aphasic disorders in relation to brain function was in the early part of this century an immensely exciting new discipline in which it was believed that the key to understanding lay in trying to list, classify and systematize the varieties of receptive and expressive disorders displayed by patients with known cortical lesions. It is now fairly generally acknowledged that the analogy is unsound and misleading, and that a diagnosis of 'developmental dyslexia' does not imply cortical 'damage' (i.e. the disruption of a previous state of normality) and may indeed exclude it.

The nature of the terminology evolved (such as Orton's 'strephosymbolia', or Critchley's 'dyssymbolia', or Claparède's 'bradylexia'), is a result of standard medical practice in naming 'conditions'. The variety arises from the fact that attempts to identify what the children are suffering from have not led to uniform conclusions. All children have not exhibited identical abnormalities, samples of clinic cases have varied, and— more seriously—the same behaviour can be attributed theoretically to a variety of 'causes' or categorized in a variety of ways. This is, of course, a very general problem in the study of behaviour. But the profusion of terms, such as those exemplified above, has produced considerable bewilderment. There has also been serious confusion of a different kind over the exact meaning of the qualifying words 'specific', 'developmental' and 'congenital', and over the terms 'word blind' and 'syndrome'. I will consider these later.

The discussions reported in the Invalid Children's Aid Association symposium (Franklin 1962) testify further to the fact that many non-medical participants (though not the parents of nonreading children) found the concept of 'specific dyslexia' difficult—or else provocative of hostile feelings. Several speakers appeared to dismiss the clinical procedures used in identification of cases as 'unsound', while others who would admit to the existence in retarded readers of particular difficulties with orientation or space perception simply saw (to quote one speaker) 'no theoretical or practical use for the concept'. The claim was made that the description 'reading retardation' was quite adequate as a basis for remedial tuition. This is substantially what Wall (1961), Malmquist (1958) and Morris (1966) also claimed. The objection is to the notion that 'a condition' or 'a clinical entity' is involved—something to which the terms 'specific' or 'syndrome' are applicable.

At one point in the ICAA discussion Meredith remarked that he would very much like to know what underlay this 'resistance to the idea of something specific', and asked a very pertinent question: namely, whether a remedial worker would attempt to differentiate between different causes of retardation, and what action he would take if told that, of two retarded

Jessie F. Reid

readers, one had many associated spatial and motor difficulties while the other had not. No clear answer appears to have been given to this very important question. Daniels, however, gave his own personal objections to the notion of specific dyslexia. These rested largely, it seemed, on his own experimental evidence about the effect on a 'hard core' of nonreaders of intensive phonic training, which left only one child out of ten still unable to read. To have labelled these children 'dyslexic' (or even worse 'word blind') would, he claimed, have been to discourage at the outset all attempts to teach them. That is to say, he admitted that they had some special difficulty which caused them to need tuition which their classmates did not, and even said at one point that their 'disability' was 'akin to tone-deafness', but he rejected the *labels* because they carried the connotation of an incurable condition. Daniels, in other words, views the concept of 'dyslexia' not as useless, or bewildering, but as dangerous.

In his review of the literature, and of the history of attitudes towards the belief in specific dyslexia, Critchley (1964) obviously with this sort of pronouncement in mind, says that neurologists have been to blame for 'allowing psychologists to assert that neurologists believed the condition irremediable'. He cites Burt as one originator of this erroneous idea. Burt, writing in *The Backward Child* (1950), did indeed talk of 'so-called "word blind" children . . . who have made rapid and remarkable progress after a few weeks' intensive training at the hands of a psychological specialist', and Critchley points out that the adjective 'so-called' is objectionable, and that the claim about 'a few weeks' training' is doubtfully true. Burt's remarks do exemplify a view which not only calls the concept in question but almost holds it up to ridicule. But it must be asked whether the underlying attitude here is simply one of rational disbelief, or whether it is one of justifiable fear of what the term 'word blind' may become in the minds of the inexperienced or unreflecting teacher or parent.

In their contribution to *The Disabled Reader* Kinsbourne and Warrington make a similar point. They refer to the 'naïve notion' that 'impairment due to disease states is necessarily total and irremediable' and to the equally mistaken idea that thinking of reading disability as representing one extreme of a normal continuum of competence will dispose of these unfortunate connotations. They imply that such connotations do not need to be disposed of because they are not carried by the terms in question, namely 'congenital' and 'specific'.

The force of the term 'congenital' is to make a distinction between a condition acquired through disease or injury and one existing from birth. But again, doctors should remember that to the layman the term is known principally through its attachment to states that may be distressing and in many cases in fact irremediable, such as mental deficiency, or spina bifida, or syphilis, and that it functions in their minds almost as a 'pathic sign'. It is therefore understandable that there should have been resistance to the apparent finality of the term, and of the companion term 'word blind'. But it would appear that a failure of communication has existed in this area for many years, and it can only be a matter for regret if educators have spent time and energy strenuously opposing neurologists over something they did not say.

Critchley, besides describing psychologists as having been on occasion 'muddled and opinionated', criticizes them for having been 'more concerned with etiology than with cure'. This is a puzzling charge, but one which touches on a crucial issue. Concern with etiology has been the principal feature of medical intervention in the problem of the retarded reader—indeed it might be said to be in some cases the sole reason for that intervention. And, as we have seen, certain features of the way in which medical opinions have been expressed have probably helped to arouse resistance. It cannot be that etiology is here being set aside as of lesser importance than cure. What must be meant is that matters of etiology and diagnosis are a medical concern, while cure is the business of the psychologist and the remedial teacher. A view which might be thought to be similar is put forward by Reinhold (1965) who states that 'the final diagnosis of this condition should, of course, be left to the neurologist, as there are many conditions of organic brain damage whose symptoms mimic those of congenital dyslexia'. But there is a vast difference, if not a complete contrast, between feeling the need to call in the opinion of a medical specialist to assist in a differential diagnosis, and abandoning all interest in the origins of an educational difficulty. A remedial worker who did not retain a lively speculative interest in etiology would be reduced to the level of a technician, carrying out remedial exercises to someone else's specification. Moreover, the remedial worker has to deal with the emotional reactions of the child and of his parents, and an understanding of causes is a necessary part of the process of relieving anxiety. It might even be more true to say that educators have not concerned themselves sufficiently with etiology, in that they have sometimes put together for remedial purposes children who were retarded for a variety of reasons and who perhaps required very different sorts of help. It is possible that important distinctions have thereby been obscured. Edwards (1966) suggests also that educators have been slow to develop adventurous therapeutic techniques based in any scientific way on their findings. But such an undertaking is inseparable from an interest in causation and indeed presupposes it, so that Critchley's criticism seems here not only unjust, but misguided.

In his own contribution to the 1962 Symposium on Dyslexia, Money (1962b) remarks on the slowness which medicine and pedagogy have shown in coming together in joint study of problems of mutual interest, and on the desirability of greater collaboration. It is true, as any survey of the literature will show, that interdisciplinary studies have been very few in number. This fact has, no doubt, been part cause and part effect of the lack of understanding and trust between the disciplines concerned. The last twenty years have seen some improvement in this state of affairs,

Jessie F. Reid

together with a move away from the more anecdotal method of recording case studies to the collation and systematic analysis of test results, and from boldly speculative theorizing to more cautious and tentative explanatory attempts. But a study of these discussions (Money 1962a, Shankweiler 1964, Ingram 1965, Williams 1965, Money and Schiffman 1966) reveals how much methodological and theoretical difficulty still exists, and the extent to which attempts at rigorous study are beset by problems of identification and classification, and by the danger of circularity in reasoning.

Those who publish clinical studies of dyslexic children, who attempt theoretical systematizations, and who argue for the early recognition and special treatment of these cases, assume (a) that the category exists and (b) that members of it can be identified. To assert (a) without (b) would, of course, be not a scientific statement but an expression of faith. But how in fact do they claim to identify these children?

In the ICAA Symposium those in clinical practice frequently asserted that they could recognize a case of specific dyslexia almost unerringly by a number of signs and symptoms. However, they also admitted that no one of these signs was, by itself, definitive: any one might appear either in a retarded reader not suffering from dyslexia or, in passing, in a normal reader. The signs formed a 'variable syndrome', the uniquely distinguishing mark being the clustering—the coincidence of several signs together. Money (1962b) defends this as a respectable concept.

> It is not at all rare in psychological medicine, nor in other branches of medicine, that a disease should have no unique identifying sign, that uniqueness being in the pattern of signs that appear in contiguity.

But it is difficult to see how, unless certain of the signs are regarded as necessary, and perhaps even if they are so regarded, the identification can ever, on this basis alone, be more than a probabilistic one, with the probability increasing as the number of signs—or the severity of those present—increases.

A study of the writings of different neurologists will further show that they do not agree on the criteria by which they diagnose.

Critchley bases his belief in the existence of the condition on four crucial criteria: persistence into adulthood; the peculiar and specific nature of the errors in reading and writing; the familial incidence of the defect; and the frequent association with other symbol defects. But the first of these is diagnostic only in retrospect and the fourth leaves room for considerable variation. Other workers (e.g. Reinhold 1965, and see Vernon 1964) select other criteria, too numerous to list here, with the distinction between 'necessary' and 'sufficient' not always clear. It is probably these uncertainties, together with the need to show that alternative hypotheses about causation will not suffice, that has led to the practice of identification by elimination, resulting in some such statement as this:

This child is a very retarded reader of good intelligence. He has had an enlightened home and normal schooling. His vision and hearing are intact, and he has no overt neurological damage. He has no history of emotional upset prior to going to school and starting to learn to read. He wants to learn, but has failed. He must be dyslexic.

The important point to note about this mode of identification is that it is negative not positive, and that it does no more than place the residual cases in a category which medically is termed 'idiopathic'—that is, of unknown origin (Money 1962b). This is also a perfectly respectable notion, representing a state of knowledge in which one can recognize a condition operationally or behaviourally but give no explanation of its etiology. Eisenberg (1962) states exactly this position with regard to 'dyslexic' cases when he writes:

> The adjective 'specific' calls attention both to the circumscribed nature of the disability and to our ignorance of its cause. Operationally specific reading disability may be defined as the failure to learn to read with normal proficiency despite conventional instruction, a culturally adequate home, proper motivation, intact senses, normal intelligence and freedom from gross neurological defect.

There is, however, one totally unsatisfactory feature about this mode of definition, namely that it appears to imply that 'specific dyslexia' *as a condition* will exist only if all these other conditions obtain, i.e. that it will not occur in a child with defective eyesight or hearing, or in a child whose life is culturally deprived or whose school attendance has been disrupted, or who does not want to learn! One has only to write this to see that it makes nonsense of the notion of a 'congenital' or 'developmental' condition. What is being said is that the condition can *be identified with certainty* only if it exists in isolation; otherwise it will be impossible to disentangle it completely from other possible 'causes' of retardation. In the earlier Johns Hopkins Symposium (Money 1962a), Rabinovitch shows awareness of this difficulty, noting that very often he and his co-workers find themselves making a 'double-barrelled diagnosis'—secondary reading difficulty with a touch of primary disability. But it will be immediately obvious that this 'double-barrelled' diagnosis must be made by the use of positive clinical signs on the probabilistic basis indicated above, and that the point at which 'significance' is reached may well be somewhat arbitrary. Moreover, it is here that supporters of the doctrine of the parsimony of hypotheses find grounds for criticism. Why, they ask, invoke a cause which you cannot demonstrate when other perfectly feasible explanations are present?

The somewhat perplexing status of the individual 'clinical signs' which collectively add support to the diagnosis of dyslexia has also not been clarified by their heterogeneity. A rough four-fold classification of them might be made on the following basis:

1 Signs of perceptual difficulties of a more general kind ('spatial' difficulties, 'visuomotor' difficulties, and so on). Statements about these are normally inferences from results on performance tests, although they may also be based on observation of other behaviour (for instance, drawing) or on reports.

2 Signs of anomalies in development (of laterality, of speech, of motor control). Again, test results, observations and history-taking are the sources.

3 Circumstantial evidence (such as familial incidence of similar educational difficulties to those of the patient, handedness in the families etc).

4 The precise nature and severity of the difficulties themselves (e.g. the kind of errors made in spelling, the movements of the hand in writing, the speech rhythm in reading).

It is not always clear from discussions of the first three kinds of sign whether they are being regarded as clues to a cause, or whether they are merely being regarded as 'associated' difficulties, the cause remaining unknown. Especially has this been true of the discussions of the importance of laterality characteristics which, once noticed, invited much speculation about corresponding anomalies of cerebral dominance. But Zangwill (1962) makes it very clear that inferences about cerebral dominance from observations of laterality in hand, eye and foot are unjustified in the present state of knowledge.

Doubt has also been cast on the validity of the 'signs' in the great numbers of group studies which have investigated the correlation between ability in reading and other 'abilities' inferred from test results. Most of these studies have been done on heterogeneous groups of backward or retarded readers, and the effect has been to produce results that are inconclusive, or which contradict one another, and frequently appear to cast doubt on the notion that groups of associated difficulties exist. This point is made by Eisenberg (1966) and also by Vernon (1960, 1961, 1962), whose remarks are especially interesting, following as they do so soon after her comprehensive review of such studies (Vernon 1957). In a recent investigation, Belmont and Birch (1965) found no difference in laterality characteristics between backward readers and controls. But evidence of this kind does nothing to refute the claims of those who believe that 'dyslexia' exists. No one claims that *all* backward readers will show anomalies of laterality, and the same argument holds for any other characteristic investigated in this way. Likewise, Morris's correlational studies were bound to obscure rather than to highlight the few cases that might have an etiology which differed from the majority. This is not a criticism of her studies, but it is a criticism of the implication in her conclusion (quoted at the beginning of this article) that her studies cast doubt on the existence of dyslexia as a variety of reading disability.

What seems to emerge from the foregoing review is an overwhelming need for rigorous study in this area, study which would be undertaken at an interdisciplinary level and which would courageously submit the contentions of those who believe in dyslexia and those who do not to the most searching reappraisal and testing that can be devised. Since one of the standard scientific methods of demonstrating that a difference exists between two events or states of being is to make predictions the outcome of which will be different for the two events or states in question, it seems reasonable to suggest the setting up of a controlled experiment involving remedial methods. (This was in fact adumbrated by Vernon in 1962.) Two matched groups of 'dyslexic' children and two matched groups of retarded readers who are thought not to be 'dyslexic' could be selected. Within each pair one would receive tuition from teachers who 'believed in' dyslexia based, in the case of the dyslexic children, on a close diagnosis of the variety of disorder they were suffering from, while the other group would receive tuition of equal duration from teachers who did not believe in dyslexia but worked presumably at a phenomenological level. An analysis of variance design would be appropriate and would show whether (a) the 'dyslexics' as a whole made slower progress than the others, (b) whether 'dyslexics' taught on the basis of a diagnosis of dyslexia got on better than those who were not and (c) whether there was any overall difference between the results of the two groups of teachers.

An experiment of a different sort might pair children diagnosed as dyslexic by one specialist, with children whose retardation, equally severe, was of a different origin, and then set another specialist the task of picking the 'dyslexic' child from each pair. This may sound a slightly frivolous suggestion, but it is prompted by a consciousness of the confusing variety of criteria used, by the conviction that the notion of dyslexia would become more respectable if a greater degree of unanimity could be reached, and by the thought that such an exercise might help those taking part to analyse their dependence on scientific analysis and on intuition and clinical awareness of subtle kinds.

A third type of experiment might investigate, with suitable controls, the effect of training in the more general perceptual skills thought to be deficient, in an effort to see whether (a) improvement occurred in the skill in question (e.g. retention of shapes), and (b) whether any transfer took place to reading and writing. All investigations carry the limitation, of course, that it is not possible to discover whether 'dyslexics' are or are not characterized by x, unless x is *not* one of the criteria by which they have been initially identified.

The mention once more of variety in criteria leads to a further final point with which this discussion has not concerned itself so far. Current opinion seems to be moving in the direction of recognizing 'subtypes' of dyslexic disorder, thereby further complicating the notion of 'variable

Jessie F. Reid

syndrome'. Some writers have suggested that the postulating of an entity—
a 'condition'—is thereby rendered meaningless. But if all these subtypes
should prove to have in common a basis in some developmental anomaly
or delay, then it would seem that the use of one term to classify them
would still, both theoretically and practically, make sense.

References

BANNATYNE, A. D. (1965) The word blind centre for dyslexic children
  AEP Newsletter, no. 4, 17–9
BELMONT, L. and BIRCH, H. G. (1965) Lateral dominance, lateral aware-
  ness and reading disability *Child Development* 34, 257–70
BENTON, A. (1962) Dyslexia in relation to form perception and directional
  sense in J. Money (ed) *Reading Disability* Baltimore: Johns Hopkins
  Press
*BURT, C. (1950) *The Backward Child* Edinburgh: Oliver and Boyd
BURT, C. (1966) Counterblast to dyslexia *AEP Newsletter* no. 5, 2–6
CRITCHLEY, M. (1964) *Developmental Dyslexia* London: Heinemann
  Medical
EDWARDS, T. J. (1966) Teaching reading: a critique in J. Money and
  G. Schiffman (eds) *The Disabled Reader* Baltimore: Johns Hopkins
  Press
EISENBERG, L. (1962) Introduction to J. Money (ed) *Reading Disability*
  Baltimore: Johns Hopkins Press
FRANKLIN, W. (ed) (1962) *Word Blindness or Specific Developmental Dyslexia*
  London: Pitman Medical
HINSHELWOOD, J. (1917) *Congenital Word Blindness* London: H. K. Lewis
INGRAM, T. T. S. (1965) Specific learning difficulties in childhood *Public
  Health*, LXXIX, 2, January, 70–80
KINSBOURNE, M. and WARRINGTON, E. K. (1966) Developmental factors
  in reading and writing backwardness in J. Money and G. Schiffman
  (eds) *The Disabled Reader* Baltimore: Johns Hopkins Press
MALMQUIST, E. (1958) *Factors related to Reading Disabilities in the First
  Grade of the Elementary School* Stockholm: Almqvist and Wiksell
*MONEY, J. (ed) (1962a) *Reading Disability* Baltimore: Johns Hopkins
  Press
MONEY, J. (1962b) Dyslexia: a postconference review in J. Money (ed)
  Reading Disability Baltimore: Johns Hopkins Press
*MONEY, J. and SCHIFFMAN, G. (eds) (1966) *The Disabled Reader* Baltimore:
  Johns Hopkins Press
MORGAN, W. P. (1896) A case of congenital word blindness *British Medical
  Journal* 2, 1378
*MORRIS, J. M. (1966) *Standards and Progress in Reading* Slough: National
  Foundation for Educational Research
RABINOVITCH, R. (1962) Dyslexia: psychiatric considerations in J. Money
  (ed) *Reading Disability* Baltimore: Johns Hopkins Press

REINHOLD, M. (1965) Congenital dyslexia, *AEP Newsletter* no. 4, 13–7

SHANKWEILER, D. (1964) A study of developmental dyslexia *Neuropsychologia* I, 267–86

VERNON, M. D. (1957) *Backwardness in Reading* Cambridge: Cambridge University Press

VERNON, M. D. (1960) The investigation of reading problems today *British Journal of Educational Psychology* 30, 146–54

VERNON, M. D. (1961) Dyslexia and remedial education in *Proceedings of a Refresher Course on Dyslexia and Remedial Education* British Psychological Society: English Division of Professional Psychologists (In cyclostyle)

*VERNON, M. D. (1962) Specific dyslexia *British Journal of Educational Psychology* 32, 143–50

VERNON, P. E. (1956) Dullness and its causes, *Times Educational Supplement* 26th October

WALBRIDGE, A. (1965) A view of dyslexia by an educational psychologist *AEP Newsletter* no. 4

WALL, W. D. (1961) Recent research into dyslexia and remedial education in *Proceedings of a Refresher Course on Dyslexia and Remedial Education* British Psychological Society: English Division of Professional Psychologists (In cyclostyle)

WILLIAMS, D. J. (1965) A five-year followup study of fifteen children assessed as possibly dyslexic in 1960 Unpublished dissertation presented for Diploma in Education of Backward Children, University College, Swansea

ZANGWILL, O. L. (1962) Dyslexia in relation to cerebral dominance in J. Money (ed) *Reading Disability* Baltimore: Johns Hopkins Press

3.3 Severe reading disability— some important correlates

GILBERT R. GREDLER

Professor of Educational Psychology,
Temple University, Philadelphia

Reprinted from J. E. Merritt (1971) (ed) *Reading and the curriculum*
Ward Lock Educational, pp. 188, 191–211

Reading problems in children continue to be of concern to many different groups of individuals: school personnel, parents and researchers. Of particular concern to all is the child who shows extreme difficulty in learning how to read and with whom the usual remedial methods have been unsuccessful.

The intent of this paper is to review the problem of severe reading disability and to look at important correlates of this condition in order to arrive at some valid conclusions concerning causal factors and remedial programmes.

Any discussion of reading disability must deal with the factors of socioeconomic class, ethnic group membership and sex grouping. Too often studies of reading disability cases fail to take into account these sociological factors. By carefully considering possible etiological factors, we can gain much useful knowledge about reading disability. Eisenberg states that we must know the source of a fever in a population in order to gain valid information as to the epidemiology of infections. The same logic applies to the study of reading disability. To say that perceptual lags, emotional maladjustment and handedness problems are major determiners of the 57 per cent reading disability rate in the inner city school system, is to ignore the several other factors which play an important part. Poor teaching is more likely to be prevalent in the inner city school (Eisenberg 1966). A recent study (Beez 1968) indicates that lowered expectation on the part of teachers actually leads the teacher not only to expect less from such a child but not to attempt to teach the child the same number of learning exercises in comparison with a child who is perceived more positively.

Other factors that are important can be categorized as deficiencies in cognitive stimulation and deficiency in motivation, which can in turn be linked to social pathology as well as psychopathology (Eisenberg 1966).

In studying what I am calling severe reading disability, we are concerned with children whose reading shows a significant discrepancy below their age and ability level and is also not in accord with the child's cultural and educational experience (Harris 1970).

Factors involved in reading disability: Some important studies

The major thrust of this paper is a consideration of concomitants of specific reading disability. We are concerned with the children who fail to learn to read, despite adequate classroom instruction, and where cultural adequacy of the home environment, degree of motivation, sensory mechanism, and level of intelligence are not *major* determiners of the disability (Eisenberg 1966).

Too often severe reading disability is still seen as being linked to one factor rather than to a host of causative factors. The writer is impressed with the regularity of the classroom teacher's comment that a child has reading problems due to reversals (e.g. was for saw). What is often forgotten is that the normal child in learning to read manifests the same errors; the important variable for the severe disability case is the *frequency* and *persistence* of these errors (Eisenberg 1966). For example, Schonell (1942) found that by the age of eight to nine, 60 per cent of all children backward in reading were still showing reversals of such letters as b, d, p, q, w and m, while only 12 per cent of a sample of normal children did so.

Resistance to a careful consideration of the many-faceted problem of severe reading disability is commonplace. Spache (1969) writes satirically on the various diagnostic and remedial absurdities he finds in the field. Abrams (1969) is concerned lest we forget that in reality emotional considerations ('disturbances in ego functioning') must still be foremost in any discussion of severe reading disability.

Isom (1969) offers us important information in his study of children's referral for reading retardation. He states his findings thus:

> It was found that almost all poor readers were deficient in the ability to process sequentially presented material, particularly via the auditory as opposed to the visual channel. This deficit is expressed in developmental terms. The poor readers lagged behind the average readers with regard to the age at which they could state their complete birthdate, the months of the year or days of the week. They also lagged in the acquisition of ability to write, with correct spelling, their name, residential address, phone number, and the letters of the alphabet. These are behaviours or tasks that are learned by most children without formal instruction or with very limited instruction. The poor readers were universally unable to acquire these skills at the same age as children with normal reading ability.

Isom gives us a more sophisticated approach in looking at reading retardation, saying in effect that the syndrome also includes deficiencies as regards the concept of time, quantity and number, as well as a memory factor.

Anthony (1968) also helps us to see the interrelationship of several

Gilbert R. Gredler

factors in his study of cerebral dominance and reading disability. Looking at dyslexics (children with reading scores a minimum of one standard deviation below the mean at the pupils' grade level) and nondyslexics (children with reading scores from grade level to one standard deviation above the mean) Anthony divided these pupils into mixed-dominant and dominant categories, based on their performance on the Harris Tests of Laterality. Then he studied the importance of such factors as perceptual-motor level, directionality, as well as sensory integration in these two groups. Anthony's subjects were composed of sixty children with a mean chronological age of 8 years 6 months and of normal intelligence. The basic hypothesis of this study was that children who are dyslexic and mixed-dominant will also show below average perceptual development, will show more indications of neurological impairment, will perform more poorly on a measure of directional differentiation, as well as having more difficulty with tasks of auditory–visual integration.

What Anthony is saying is that a severely retarded reader of normal intelligence will manifest disturbances on a number of important dimensions. When such disturbances are found in conjunction with a child of mixed dominance, it will invariably mean the child is a poor reader.

The results from Anthony's study would indicate that mixed dominance *by itself* does not predict a child's reading performance. This study also has important implications for the school psychologist. The results indicate more precisely the kind of diagnostic information needed in order to come to meaningful conclusions concerning the nature of the child's learning disabilities.

Anthony favours a maturational lag theory saying that such a lag is a global stress factor in that it limits the subject's coping capacity and thus serves to make the subject more vulnerable to environmental pressure.

The importance of directionality and laterality

Such findings also show the need for us to understand the conceptual importance of the development of directionality in the child. Jastak (1965) states that the letters a child is required to perceive can only be processed accurately if attention is given to their space or directional value. He holds that children with severe reading disability have failed to develop the proper directional clues which are necessary in learning to read. Thus, 'when the development of directional differentiation is blocked, reading disability results'. Jastak speculates that 'children with reading disability may be normal in all respects except to the acquisition of symbols based on directional clues'.

Basic to the development of directionality in the child is the establishment of laterality. Laterality is conceived as the awareness *within* the body of left and right. Directionality is considered to be the projection of laterality on to external objects; it would deal with left and right differentiation of external objects in space (Anthony 1968).

The laterality status of the child in turn is supposedly reflective of lack of dominance in hemisphere development. Zangwill (1962) states the problem thus:

On balance, the evidence suggests that an appreciable proportion of dyslexic children show poorly developed laterality. . . . If poorly developed laterality can be linked with incomplete cerebral dominance, it might be said that these patterns of disability reflect faulty establishment of assymmetrical (i.e. normally lateralized) functions in two hemispheres . . . but we have also to consider why all ill-lateralized children do not exhibit backwardness in reading.

A number of studies do indicate that many retarded readers show lack of lateralization of function or inconsistency of preference of hand, foot and eye functions (Monroe 1932, Vernon 1957). Other investigations indicate that problems of measurement affect the result obtained. Silver (1963) questions whether peripheral dominance (i.e. eye, hand, foot, preference) reflects true cerebral dominance. Stephens et al (1967) in looking at eye/hand preferences and reading readiness of first grade children, question the importance of such preferences. They found no relationship between mixed eye/hand preferences, reading readiness and performance on visual-motor tests.

They also state that their negative results indicate that neurological impairment or minimal brain dysfunction is not a factor in reading performance of first grade children. However one would question applying a label of neurological impairment to children showing only a mixed hand/eye performance pattern. Bond and Tinker (1967) cite a number of studies which indicate that there is no relationship between laterality and reading disability. In one such study (Tinker 1965) no such relationship was found in a group of pupils from grades two, four and six. Here is where the difficulty arises, for the study is then quoted as further valid evidence that we should expect no relationship. The conclusion would be better stated that no relationship was found in children of superior ability, for only children whose mean IQ ranged from 126 to 131 were studied. Koos (1964) found a relationship between reading ability and mixed dominance but only for children below the median IQ of her sample. Similarly Trieschman (1968) found no relationship between mixed dominance and reading ability. In her sample only those children whose IQ was below 125 showed a reading retardation which was linked with mixed dominance of the subject.

In addition to raising questions about the influence of ability level, we need to question once again the attempt to find one causal factor which will explain the severity of the reading disability. Trieschman also makes the important point that differences in outcomes of studies as to important factors linked with reading disability are partially a function of how the sample of children is chosen. Children retarded in reading and chosen randomly from a school population such as Tinker's might show fewer

Gilbert R. Gredler

disabling facets of their disability than children referred to some type of clinic for diagnosis and treatment.

Anthony's study mentioned previously is also important because it attempts to show how *one* factor such as mixed dominance *cannot* be utilized to explain all reading disability cases. But it does show very adequately how a number of factors taken together (i.e. mixed dominance status, poor perceptual development, below average directionality, inadequate intersensory performance) can all combine to limit the child's ability to learn to read.

The importance of perceptual factors in severe reading disability

A number of authorities have emphasized the importance of perceptual processes in learning to read. De Hirsch (1957) states how adequate perceptual development is necessary or letters and words will remain undifferentiated and diffuse. Adequate development of spatial relationships is important or the child cannot cope with a pattern (i.e. words) which is laid out in space. Figure/ground relationships are important or the child will not be able to differentiate letters (figures) from the page (background). There must be adequate awareness of a L/R direction or the child cannot proceed with correctly understanding the symbol sequence of words.

Thus we might expect disturbance of the perceptual function to be one facet of a reading disability syndrome. And this often proves to be the case. In the study previously mentioned (Trieschman 1968) boys between seven and nine were studied to determine various factors which were present in those who were severely disabled readers. Children were presented with symbol material which reflected in part some of the features found in letters of the alphabet (i.e. straight lines, curved lines, angles etc). Results indicate that poor readers made many more perceptual errors than normal readers.

In this study perceptual competency was measured by the child's ability to match the standard stimulus with comparison stimuli. The results reinforce Jastak's (1965) ideas wherein he emphasizes that accurate performance in the reading process involves attention to the space and directional aspect of the letters. Thus children who have severe reading problems frequently will have failed to develop the proper directional clues which are necessary in learning to read. Adequate directional differentiation can be measured in part by performance on perceptual tasks such as those used by Trieschman.

In another study which dealt with boys aged 8 years 10 months to 10 years 11 months, and who were all two to three years below expected grade level, the subjects were consistently below age expectations on a test of visual-motor performance. Yet all these children showed additional dysfunctions, i.e. performance scale in excess of verbal on an ability scale; conceptual difficulties in space, time and directional areas, and articulatory difficulties (Haworth 1970).

Gredler (1969) cites the importance of visual perception in reading disability. He stresses, as does Benton (1962), that the development of visual perceptual abilities is of special importance when the young child is learning to read. Here is where adequate perceptual abilities will aid the child in perceiving the similarities and differences of letters and words. Adequate development of spatial relationships will aid the child to successfully perceive the pattern of letters which are laid out in space. Adequate visual perceptual development will result in the child being able to note the differences in two dimensional visual symbols (Gofman 1966). Lovell's (1964) work can also be cited wherein he found perceptual dysfunction in a group of backward readers. It was Lovell's thesis that some cortical or subcortical dysfunction disturbs visual perception and in turn results in limited progress in reading.

Gibson (1966) emphasizes that learning to differentiate the graphic symbols is *one* important element in learning to read. She adds that there are several different aspects of the reading process which are important: receiving communication, decoding graphic symbols and relating them to speech and getting meaning from the printed word. Gibson states that once the child progresses from spoken language to written language there are three stages of learning tasks which must be looked at: (a) learning to perceive differences in graphic symbols; (b) learning to associate letters with sounds; (c) learning to use progressively more complicated units of structure as typified by spelling patterns. It is therefore logical to expect some disturbance of the visual perceptual process in disabled readers if we concede that learning to perceive differences in graphic symbols is one important aspect of the reading process.

In one study, Gibson (1963) investigated the perception of graphic symbols which were similar to letters. The task involved perceiving differences between the standard stimulus and transformation of that stimulus. The subject was required to match the standard stimulus with an identical form. Gibson found a decrease in number of errors made from age four to eight years and also found a high relationship between such errors and errors made with transformation of real letters.

Some of this material was used in Trieschman's work which has been previously cited. In another study Gibson and Gibson (1955) investigated the relationship between a standard stimulus figure and variants of that standard stimulus. Their rationale was that perceptual development will reflect increase in specificity of response. Drawings similar to scribbles were used as standard stimuli. Other cards were presented which differed from the original drawing on three dimensions: (a) the number of coils present; (b) the degree of compression or stretching; (c) the orientation of the figure (two kinds). In addition other cards were made up which contained stimuli quite different from the standard stimulus cards and thus were easily distinguishable. Results indicated that the younger the child the less the specificity reacted to by the subject.

In one of the few experiments done using the Gibson material, Whipple and Kodman (1969) investigated perceptual learning of fourth and fifth graders of normal intelligence and whose reading level ranged from eight to twenty-four months below their grade placement level. The results indicate that the perceptual level abilities of the child retarded in reading were distinctively inferior to those of the normal reader with the same IQ. Checking the norms of this task it was found that the perceptual ability of the ten year olds was similar to the perceptual ability level of the normal six to eight year olds used in the Gibson and Gibson study.

Gibson states that perceptual development reflects both maturation and learning. She contends that performance on the perceptual level tasks mentioned above reflects both the influence of age and changes which occur as the results of practice. For her the child's perceptual development (or his reduction in stimulus dependency) is tied in with attentional ability (Gibson 1963). With an adequate attentional level the child has learned to select the critical aspects of the stimuli presented to him. Vernon (1970) puts the issue somewhat differently:

. . . it would seem that any increase in the extent and accuracy of form perception through learning is doubtful. Where there is some improvement, it probably results from improvement in the capacity to direct attention towards particular aspects or details of the forms presented which facilitates their discrimination and identification.

How improvement in perceptual development can come about and can be planned for cannot be considered in detail at this time. But we can state briefly the important features of perceptual development. Gibson says that criteria of perceptual learning include an increase in specificity of discrimination which is also called an increase in correspondence with the stimulus offered. In perceptual learning the capacity of ascertaining the distinctive features of objects and learning invariant relationships is acquired. For Gibson adequate spatial orientation would mean that an object in space is seen the same regardless of how it is oriented. However a child learning to read must supplant the law of object constancy (Money 1966) as defined above with the law of directional constancy wherein an alphabetic letter cannot change its position without changing its name or meaning (e.g. h and y). In addition the law of form constancy (Money 1966) means that a letter can be changed only within certain limits before it is considered a different letter (e.g. c and e). But other differences are tolerated and the letter will be the same regardless of these differences (e.g. g and G). Money also adds that there can be difficulty with conceptual discrimination in such words as their—there, to—too.

Goins (1958) investigated the role of visual perception in the reading achievement of young children. Her work indicates the importance of being able to hold a gestalt in mind against distraction. Obviously competence in this task involves being able to note details of the perceptual figure. For Goins a successful performance on a perceptual test requires manipulating parts of the whole with the whole pattern acting as a distractor. On a perceptual test of reversals, successful performance requires ability to keep in mind a figure against the distraction and confusion of figure and ground (i.e. the reversed and nonreversed figures). Success on these tasks indicates that the child shows adequate strength of closure.

Of course strength of closure reflects ability to deal with the specificity of the stimulus figure as outlined by Gibson. For Vernon (1970) adequate performance on such perceptual tasks as incomplete patterns and reversal figures would also reflect successful scanning and search efforts on the part of the child.

The controversy concerning the role of visual perception

It would seem from the foregoing discussion that there would be some consensus as to the importance of visual perception in the development of reading and in reading disability, but Vernon (1957) states:

It seems possible that the childish tendency to overlook the orientation and order of shapes and letters is prolonged in the backward reader, partly as the result of continued immaturity, but partly also because of his general cognitive confusion.

Vernon also emphasizes that the children may show poor visual memory. She continues:

It appears that some cases of severe reading retardation, but not all, do show a poor ability to relate shapes and details of shapes and to reason about them. We cannot assume, however, that the inability to read is due to this deficiency. It is possible . . . that it is a sign of lack of maturation. The normal reader may grow out of this immature type of behaviour. But backward readers may fail to do so because they have not developed habits of orderly and systematic analysis of shapes into their essential constituents. This deficiency then is the result rather than the cause of the reading disability; or both may be produced by some other defect.

Thus for Vernon, the emphasis on defects in visual perceptual development have been overstressed. She would emphasize the failure of the disabled reader in analysing, abstraction and generalization, all of which can be subsumed under the overall label of cognitive difficulties.

Wolf (1968) is also quite concerned lest we overemphasize visual perception as an important factor in reading disability. He states:

One variable that has received considerable attention in the literature as related to specific dyslexia is visual perception. With the exception of the suggested difficulties in visual imagery and visual memory, controlled studies have failed to substantiate that visual imperception is relevant to specific dyslexia.

Benton (1962) also inveighs against assigning too much influence to the role of visual perception in reading disability. He states:

My conclusion is that deficiency in visual form perception is not an important correlate of developmental dyslexia.

However Benton states that a certain level of visual perceptive development is obviously necessary in learning how to read. He mentions that retardation in this area will affect the child's progress in acquiring reading skills.

But this factor accounts . . . for only a very small proportion of cases of developmental dyslexia in older school children (i.e. above the age of ten).

Critchley (1970) concurs with Benton's approach to the problem. Much of the controversy as to the relative influence of visual perception in reading disability is reminiscent of the argument concerning the role of eye movements in reading disability. Faulty eye movements were once held responsible for poor reading (Hildreth 1936). However Critchley maintains, as do other authorities, that faulty eye movements may be better considered as an outcome of difficulty in reading. This is the same thesis used in arguing against the primacy of visual perceptual development. Instead the child with poor development in visual perception is seen as showing an 'immature' type of behaviour due to lack of development of habits of systematic analysis of shapes. For Vernon the defect in visual perception is a result rather than a cause of reading disability.

However, if we follow Gibson's thesis we would need to consider seriously the idea that a child with severe reading disability is often an individual whose perceptual learning has not kept pace with other children. Thus special attention would need to be given to this area.

For Vernon it is 'cognitive incapacity' of some kind or other that needs to be ascertained. Discussion of cause and effect here is important for the programming implications involved. In the USA much importance is attached today to visual perceptive training. Frostig (1963), in contrast to Benton and Vernon, places major emphasis on perceptual development:

The development of visual perceptive processes is the major function of the growing child between the ages of three and seven and . . . at this age level perceptual development becomes a most sensitive indicator of the developmental status of the child as a whole.

Kessler (1970) reacts somewhat negatively to the emphasis on visual perception:

On the face of it, it seems reasonable to say that a child does not 'perceive' the 'gestalt' of letters or words and cannot read, but there is a danger of circular reasoning, that is, giving the phenomenon of failure to read another fancier name.

Kessler feels the perceptual proponents have not precisely stated their theoretical assumptions:

The explanation as to why a given child should have the perceptual deficit is vaguely given as a function left behind in successive waves of maturation.

Kessler (1970) also questions Frostig's emphasis on the development of perceptual processes in the child of five to seven and suggests that cognitive development within that age period might influence perceptual development.

Perhaps some of the difficulties of ferreting out the exact role of visual perception in the reading process is that researchers tend to be victims of a stereotypy of thinking that a factor must have an all or none influence. We must be prepared to understand that cognitive variables, as well as perceptual and personality variables, may also be specifically involved in severe reading disability. To say that one particular factor *must* predominate is to underestimate the complexity of psychological processes which operate within any individual. It would appear that there is no one persuasive factor which can be held accountable for severe reading disability whether it be perceptual, cognitive or motivational in nature.

An example of two factors (perceptual and cognitive) which combine to affect performance is seen on the letter recognition test. In this test a child is exposed to a line of letters and asked to find and circle a certain letter. Many of the letters used are those commonly confused by children with severe reading disability. The score is the number of seconds required for the child to locate all the letters. Dyslexic children do quite poorly on this kind of test (Wolf 1968). We would postulate that this would be so if we follow perceptual theories of directional and form constancy (Money 1962). However Wolf points out that the identity of a letter is more than a perceptual act; it also involves cognition. Vernon would probably emphasize that performance on the letter recognition test reflects the degree of competency of search procedures on the part of the child.

In this study of dyslexic readers at the third and fourth grade level Wolf categorized the children into subgroups based on variables with the highest factor loadings. He found three different syndrome patterns containing fourteen variables which differentiated three groups of dyslexics from each other and from normal reading groups. It is interesting to note that one dyslexic subgroup was quite low in the letter recognition subtest, one performed at an average level and one above average. Yet the subgroup that performed best on the letter recognition test performed most poorly on the verbal scale of the IQ test, and the subgroup that performed best on the verbal scale performed most poorly on the letter recognition subtest.

If, as has been suggested, the letter recognition test is perceptual-conceptual in nature then we might have expected, based on prior reasoning, that those children with the higher verbal IQ might have done better. That they did not suggests the need for measures such as the letter recognition test in order to tease out all the specific processes involved in the dyslexic's difficulties.

Also popular as a measure of perceptual development is the Bender–Gestalt. Results of several studies have shown its sensitivity to perceptual development in retarded and normal readers. Bean (1967) found a significant difference in performance on the Bender with retarded and normal readers from grades seven, eight and nine. Connor's (1968) study of Bender performance of good and poor readers however, indicates some of the pitfalls of interpretation in trying to assess the importance of the perceptual performance in reading.

Connor (1968) investigated perceptual test performance in good and poor reading groups at the first grade level. He found, as was to be expected, that poor readers make more errors on the Bender–Gestalt. Numbers of distortion errors were also found significantly more often in the poor reading group. Connor went one step further and asked if significant group differences also meant that we could predict reading performance of individuals from their Bender scores.

When comparing Bender scores of good and poor readers, he found no difference as to number above or below the mean Bender scores for the chronological age of the group. Connor concludes that 'such test performance should be used with extreme caution in predicting or diagnosing poor reading performance'.

Perhaps it would be more accurate to state that when significant differences are found between groups on any test, such differences will not necessarily mean that the test can be used to predict accurately the performance of specific individuals.

Connor defined his sample by taking the upper and lower 27 per cent of the second group population as representatives of good and poor readers. Poor readers thus defined would probably have different characteristics than a sample drawn from a clinic population.

In a monumental study by Doehring (1968), patterns of impairments in severe reading disabilities were also investigated. Results indicated that a wide variety of skills were impaired and that retarded readers had the most difficulty with visual or verbal tasks which required sequential processing of material. Doehring rejects the theory that immaturity of gestalt functioning as reported on perceptual tests was of primary importance. However, most of his perceptual measures were measures of perceptual speed which would be only one aspect of visual perceptual development. On one perceptual test (Thurstone Reversals) retarded readers performed significantly more poorly. Doehring considers such a test more of a measure of directionality, while other investigators (Goins 1958) have cited it as one important aspect of overall perceptual development. It is important to note that while Doehring found sequential processing skills poorly developed in his retarded readers aged ten to fourteen, Weiner (1970) found no difference in the sequential processing skill of her sample of good and poor readers of fourth grade level. Weiner makes the same statement that Benton makes about the role of visual perception in reading, namely that serial-order ability may be a more important variable in the reading performance of young children.

Recent research on visual perception

The importance of visual perception in the academic process is seen in a study of first graders matched as to IQ but separated into high and low groups on the basis of a perceptual measure (Ferguson 1967).

Results indicated that those children with perceptual quotients of below 90 on the Frostig will be below grade level in reading and arithmetic at the end of first grade. In a followup study of these children it was found that the differences between the high and low perceptual groups persisted up to and throughout the second grade (Fullwood 1968). While such studies dramatically illustrate the importance of the visual perceptive factor we must express caution in drawing conclusions.

While the groups were equated on the major variable of intelligence through the use of the Stanford–Binet, we must ask if there were not other factors of major importance which could help to account for the differences at the end of the first grade and second grade. To explain adequately the differential functioning of these two groups, specific study of such processes as directionality, intersensory integration and personality functioning should be directly assessed. For example, 14 per cent of the high perceptual group did not achieve up to the level predicted at the end of the second grade, which suggests that other factors were operating which need to be investigated.

It is our thesis that a number of factors are involved in the successful accomplishment of the act of reading. The principles of perceptual learning are indeed specific enough, so that when these principles are inadequately incorporated into the repertoire of the developing child he will have difficulty in learning to read. For the older child with severe reading disability, there is sufficient perceptual disability found that for many of such children inadequate progress in the perceptual area would be a major contributor to the reading disability.

Because successful academic achievement involves a level of maturity of several cognitive processes, auditory and visual perceptual maturity, adequate motivational level and a certain minimum level of emotional adjustment, attention must also be given to these factors in any study of reading disability.

Gilbert R. Gredler

A study by Lovell and Gorton (1968) provides us with further insight into factors involved in severe reading disability. Fifty backward readers, nine to ten in chronological age and with normal intelligence, were studied in an effort to ascertain the various psychological factors involved in the syndrome. A control group of fifty normal readers was also utilized.

Six components were extracted in the factor analysis; these components accounted for 86 per cent of the variance of the scores in the retarded group and 77 per cent of the variance in the normal group. Most important of the factors extracted was one labelled by Lovell and Gorton as reflecting a neurological integrity-impairment syndrome which accounted for 48 per cent of the variance. Included in this component were measures of auditory–visual integration, figure rotation, spatial orientation, left/right discrimination, and motor performance.

This investigation can be considered a more sophisticated approach to ascertaining important attributes of reading disability. The authors have recognized that a number of factors have to be considered as being involved with the poor reading performance of children.

Theories of causation

The label given to a specific condition often determines future attitudes about the individual involved. Educators often inveigh against the use of the word dyslexia because they feel it implies that little can be done to help the child. Bender (1958) postulates that maturational lag in gestalt formation or an undifferentiated abstractedness is the prime factor involved in language and reading difficulties. But Vernon (1958) gets quite upset when such theories are expounded saying:

> All theories which attribute reading disability to some general lack of maturation are unsatisfactory in that they give no explanation as to why reading alone should be affected, and no other cognitive activities.

If we will concede that the term 'maturational lag' is but an indication of cortical immaturity or degree of neurological integration, then we can perhaps consider it to have a primary role in reading disability. The results of Lovell and Gorton's study certainly indicate that there is a neurological component which is important in reading achievement. Impairment in this area will result in reading retardation.

However, the term 'immaturity' is to be avoided at all costs. This word has such negative connotations that little will be done for a child so labelled. A typical American response to a young child who is doing poorly in reading is to say that he is 'immature' and that he should have stayed at home another year or repeated kindergarten so that he would then be mature enough to start the reading process. A study by Gold (1966) indicates that the favourite term to diagnose reading difficulties of children referred to a dyslexic centre was that they were 'immature'.

It is also important to avoid this term because it tends to absolve school personnel of any responsibility to help the child. The term 'immaturity' is so nonspecific and nebulous in scope that it offers no real clue as to what is wrong with the child, and why he cannot cope with the reading process successfully.

Ascribing reading difficulty to a developmental lag or to cortical immaturity is but a small step for many teachers to an acceptance of a generalized concept of overall immaturity as *the* reason for poor reading. In all time-oriented systems, a time for starting school must be selected (Cohen 1970). American children start to go to school between 5 years 9 months and 6 years 5 months old; British children start school a year before. Yet many teachers in both systems ascribe a child's failure to the fact that he is 'immature' and needs another year to grow up and then all will be well. The importance of being more precise is self-evident. How we can effectively programme for the child is the important question.

Theoretical positions on reading disability: A summary

It is evident that a number of researchers can be identified as having a particular bias concerning causal factors which will 'explain' disability in reading. Unfortunately, many investigations of severe reading retardation are nothing more than a thinly disguised treatise in championing a particular viewpoint. Modern statistical techniques are used to 'prove' conclusively that such and such a factor is important. While there is no substitute for sound research and statistical design, there *is* a great need for an objective appraisal of the point we have reached in our total understanding of the severely disabled reader.

We know that there still exists a school of thought which emphasizes that reading retardation is primarily tied in with the neurotic defences of the individual. While definite attention has to be given to the status of ego controls of the reader, we also agree with Clements that too many reading cases have been dismissed as reflective only of neurotic symptoms. Others have been guilty in overvaluing the importance of a single index such as mental ability, forgetting that wide differences in reading performance are found in children of the same ability level.

Then there is a school of thought which has emphasized the neurological component in the child's reading difficulty. This school has progressed from being concerned only with organic brain damage to a consideration of minimal brain dysfunction to the current emphasis on central processing dysfunctions as the important factor in reading disability. Also included in this neurological school are those who think that ascertaining cerebral dominance or laterality in the child is a sufficient explanatory concept of reading disability. At present there are those who champion the perceptual factor as being *the* most important.

The concept of 'maturational lag' or immaturity of a specific function is preferable to an overall indictment of the child as 'immature'. For

Gilbert R. Gredler

Money (1966) rotation errors are indicative of 'developmental dyslexia with arrest at an immature level'. He talks of maturational lag showing itself in a variety of ways—by slow language development or delayed maturation of intersensory transfer. He also mentions that such lag may be due to neurological deficits. This latter concept is similar to Rabino-vitch's (1962) delineation of primary reading retardation in which there is a 'disturbed pattern of neurologic organization'.

Bender (1966) speaks of maturational lag as 'slow differentiation in an established pattern'. For Bender, children with dyslexia show

> neurologic patterns (which) remain immature and poorly differen-tiated and the longitudinal course shows lag in maturation. Global primitiveness and plasticity in all the perceptual experiences with immature perceptual motor gestalten involve the child's own self-awareness, body image, identification, time, and space orientation and object and interpersonal relationships. . . .

Bender poses an interesting point when she questions whether a child who is of borderline impairment as regards congenital immaturities and motivational problems may 'compensate and never manifest a clinical problem in the absence of exogenous strains'.

Two recent studies help to further clarify the concept of 'immaturity'. Hyatt (1968) found that first grade children referred as 'immature' by their teachers showed deficits in several areas of psycholinguistic function-ing and remained at these deficit levels up to and including their second year at school. Those children who had deficits in visual-motor sequencing and auditory–vocal sequencing Hyatt called poor in 'active listening and seeing'. She states:

> The child must be able to think and interpret as he listens and sees and maintain this activity over long periods of time to keep up with ongoing developments in the classroom.

Hyatt suggests that the children found to be seriously deficient in the above sequencing skills be placed with highly trained specialists who would follow a very carefully worked out programme with them. Her proposals are important to note for this marks the appearance of an attempt to redefine the reading difficulties and resultant school failure of the young child on grounds other than overall emotional immaturity or being 'too young'.

Others also argue for redirection of our work with children who have learning disabilities. Santostefano (1969) suggests that the dyslexic child may scan printed material in a passive manner and take in only small bits of information at a time. He, therefore, would attempt to programme for the child in order to increase the amount and rate of information with which he can deal. His interest is in rehabilitating the cognitive controls the child is utilizing.

While we may rightly be concerned with the mechanistic aspects of the behaviour modification school and of the central processing deficit model, nevertheless proponents of these approaches are attempting to pinpoint factors important in the child's learning problems. This approach is to be preferred to categorizing a child as emotionally immature or ascribing his difficulties to the fact that he came to school too young. Currently popular among some researchers is the 'expectation bias' phenomenon (Beez 1968) as an explanatory concept of why some children do not do well in learning tasks. This school of thought is a reflection of the importance of the attitudinal structure when attempting to explain lack of learning.

A school psychologist or educational psychologist called upon to diagnose the reading problems of an elementary school child will certainly need to understand as fully as possible the various theoretical positions on severe reading disability. For each such case he will want to look at the following:

1 Personality structure so as to be able to make valid statements about the child's motivation.
2 The cognitive structure of the child.
3 The central processing mechanisms and their level of operation.
4 The environment of the school which means not only the quality of the interaction going on in the classroom, but the quality of the teaching.

References

ABRAMS, J. C. (1969) Further considerations of the ego-functioning of the dyslexic child—a psychiatric viewpoint in G. D. Spache (ed) *Reading Disability and Perception* Newark, Delaware: International Reading Association

ANTHONY, G. (1968) *Cerebral dominance as an etiological factor in dyslexia* Unpublished doctoral dissertation, New York University

BEAN, W. J. (1967) *The isolation of some psychometric indices of severe reading disabilities* Unpublished doctoral dissertation, Texas Technological College

BEEZ, W. V. (1968) *Influence of biased psychological reports on teacher behavior and pupil performance* Proceedings, 76th Annual Convention American Psychological Association, 605–6

BENDER, L. (1968) Neuropsychiatric disturbances in A. H. Keeney and V. T. Keeney (eds) *Dyslexia: Diagnosis and Treatment of Reading Disorders* St Louis: C. V. Mosby

BENTON, A. L. (1962) Dyslexia in relation to form perception and directional sense in J. Money (ed) *Reading Disability: Progress and Research Needs in Dyslexia* Baltimore: Johns Hopkins Press

BOND, G. L. and TINKER, M. A. (1967) *Reading Difficulties: Their Diagnosis and Correction* New York: Appleton-Century-Crofts

Gilbert R. Gredler

CLEMENTS, S. and PETERS, S. J. (1962) Minimal brain dysfunction in the
school age child *Archives of General Psychiatry* 6, 185–97
COHEN, R. (1970) The role of immaturity in reading disabilities *Journal
of Learning Disabilities* 3, no. 2, 73–4
CONNOR, J. P. (1966) The relationship of Bender visual motor gestalt test
performance to differential reading performance of second grade
children Unpublished doctoral dissertation, Kent State University
CRITCHLEY, M. (1964) *Developmental Dyslexia* London: Heinemann
CRITCHLEY, M. (1970) *The Dyslexic Child* London: Heinemann
*DE HIRSCH, K. (1957) Tests designed to discover potential reading diffi-
culties at the six year old level *American Journal of Orthopsychology* 27,
566–76
*DOEHRING, D. G. (1968) *Patterns of Impairment in Specific Reading Disability*
Bloomington: Indiana University Press
EISENBERG, L. (1966) The epidemiology of reading retardation and a
program for preventive intervention in J. Money (ed) *The Disabled
Reader* Baltimore: Johns Hopkins Press
FERGUSON, N. U. (1967) The Frostig—an instrument for predicting total
academic readiness and reading and arithmetical achievement in the
first grade Unpublished doctoral dissertation, University of Oklahoma
FULLWOOD, H. L. (1968) A followup study of children selected by the
Frostig developmental test of visual perception in relation to their
success or failure in reading and arithmetic at the end of second grade
Unpublished doctoral dissertation, University of Oklahoma
GIBSON, J. J. and GIBSON, E. G. (1955) Perceptual learning: differentiation
or enrichment *Psychological Review* 62, 33–40
GIBSON, E. J. (1963) Perceptual development in H. W. Stevenson (ed)
62nd Yearbook of the National Society for the Study of Education Chicago:
University of Chicago Press
*GIBSON, E. J. (1966) Experimental psychology of learning and reading in
J. Money (ed) *The Disabled Reader* Baltimore: Johns Hopkins Press
GIBSON, E. J. (1968) *Trends in perceptual development* Paper presented at
meeting of Eastern Psychological Association, Washington DC
GOFMAN, H. T. (1966) The training of the physician in evaluation and
management of the educationally handicapped child in J. Hellmuth
(ed) *Educational Therapy* volume 1 Seattle: Special Child Publications
GOINS, J. T. (1958) Visual perceptual abilities and early reading progress
Supplementary Educational Monograph no. 87 Chicago: University of
Chicago Press
GOLD, L., HEUBNER, F. M. and BICE, M. O. (1968) Characteristics of
pupils who attend a regional learning center for treatment of developmental dyslexia data cited in A. J. Harris (1970) *How to Increase Reading
Ability* New York: David McKay
GREDLER, G. R. (1968) Performance on a perceptual test with children
from a culturally deprived background in H. K. Smith (ed) *Perception
and Reading* Newark, Delaware: International Reading Association

GREDLER, G. R. (1969) A study of factors in childhood dyslexia in J. I. Arena (ed) *Selected Papers On Learning Disabilities* Pittsburgh Association for Children with Learning Disabilities

GREDLER, G. R. (1969) Factors in severe reading disability: the psychological test correlates in *Selected Convention Papers* Washington DC Council for Exceptional Children

HAWORTH, M. R. (1970) *The Primary Visual Motor Test* New York: Grune and Stratton

HILDRETH, G. (1936) *Learning the Three Rs* Minneapolis: Minneapolis Education Publications

HILDRETH, G. (1950) Development and training of hand dominance: IV Developmental problems associated with handedness in *Journal of Genetic Psychology* 76, 39–100

HYATT, G. (1968) Some psycholinguistic characteristics of first graders who have reading problems at the end of second grade Unpublished doctoral dissertation, University of Oregon

JASTAK, J. and JASTAK, S. (1965) *Wide Range Achievement Manual* Wilmington: Delaware Guidance Associates

ISOM, J. B. (1969) An interpretation of dyslexia: A medical viewpoint in G. D. Spache (ed) *Reading Disability and Perception* Newark, Delaware: International Reading Association

KESSLER, J. (1970) Contributions of the mentally retarded toward a theory of cognitive development in J. Hellmuth (ed) *Cognitive Studies* 1 New York: Brunner/Mazel

KOOS, E. (1964) Manifestations of cerebral dominance and reading retardation in primary grade children in *Journal of Genetic Psychology* 104, 155–65

LOVELL, K. (1964) A study of some cognitive and other disabilities in backward readers of average intelligence as assessed by a nonverbal test *British Journal of Educational Psychology* 34, 58–64

*LOVELL, K. and GORTON, A. (1968) A study of some differences between backward readers of average intelligence as assessed by a nonverbal test *British Journal of Educational Psychology* 38, 240–8

MONEY, J. (1962) Dyslexia: a postconference review in J. Money (ed) *Reading Disability: Progress and Research Needs in Dyslexia* Baltimore: Johns Hopkins Press

MONEY, J. (1966) On learning and not learning to read in J. Money (ed) *The Disabled Reader* Baltimore: Johns Hopkins Press

RUBIN, E. Z. (1964) *Secondary emotional disorders in children with perceptual motor dysfunction* Paper presented at annual meeting, American Orthopsychiatric Association, Chicago, Illinois

SANTOSTEFANO, S. (1969) Cognitive controls vs. cognitive styles: An approach to diagnosing and treating cognitive disability in children *Seminars in Psychiatry* 1, no. 3, 291–317

SILVER, A. A. (1963) Diagnostic considerations in children with reading disability *Bulletin of the Orton Society*, 13

Gilbert R. Gredler

SPACHE, G. D. (1969) Diagnosis and remediation in 1980 in G. D. Spache (ed) *Reading Disability and Perception* Newark, Delaware: International Reading Association

STEPHENS, W. E., CUNNINGHAM, E. S. and STIGLER, B. J. (1967) Reading readiness and eye/hand reference patterns in first grade children *Exceptional Children* 33, 7, 441-576

STILLWELL, R. J., ARTUSO, A. A., HEWETT, F. M. and TAYLOR, F. D. (1970) An educational solution *Focus on Children* 2, no. 1, 1-15

TINKER, K. J. (1965) The role of laterality in reading disability in J. A. Figurel (ed) *Reading and Enquiry* Newark, Delaware: International Reading Association

TRIESCHMAN, R. B. (1968) Undifferentiated handedness and perceptual development in children with reading problems *Perceptual and Motor Skills* 27, 1123-34

VINOGRADOFF, V. (1969) *The role and function of the diagnostic teacher* Paper presented at annual meeting of Council for Exceptional Children, Denver, Colorado

VERNON, M. D. (1957) *Backwardness in Reading* Cambridge: Cambridge University Press

VERNON, M. D. (1970) *Perception Through Experience* London: Methuen

WEINER, J., BARNSLEY, R. H. and RABINOVITCH, M. S. (1970) Serial order ability in good and poor readers *Canadian Journal of Behavioral Science* 2, 116-23

WHIPPLE, C. I. and KODMAN, F. Jr (1969) A study of discrimination and perceptual learning with retarded readers *Journal of Educational Psychology* 60, no. 1, 1-5

WOLF, C. W. (1969) Psychoneurological and educational characteristics of specific dyslexia in D. Knowlton and B. Kratoville (eds) *Ideas for Action* Proceedings of the 14th convention of the Texas Association for Children with Learning Disabilities Houston, Texas: ACLD

ZANGWILL, O. L. (1962) Dyslexia in relation to cerebral dominance in J. Money (ed) *Reading Disability: Progress and Research Needs in Dyslexia* Baltimore: Johns Hopkins Press

3.4 Specific developmental dyslexia

SANDHYA NAIDOO
National Children's Bureau

Reprinted from *British Journal of Educational Psychology* (1971)
41, 1, pp. 19–22

In 1963, the Invalid Children's Aid Association established the Word Blind Centre for Dyslexic Children in London. The Centre's aims were primarily to provide facilities for the investigation and teaching of intelligent children who experienced considerable difficulty in learning to read and to research into the nature and causes of specific dyslexia.

Two basic concepts are implicit in the term 'specific dyslexia': (a) the reading disability is specific and (b) it stems from anomalies of maturation or development which are primarily constitutionally determined. Although some definitions seem to suggest that the condition is found only in children of at least average intelligence, it is recognized that it may be found in the dull as well as in the bright child.

There is little doubt about the existence of specific reading disabilities. It is the second concept which is controversial. From studies of children with specific reading difficulties comes evidence of developmental delays and dysfunctions. Frequently reported are a history of late speech development (Ingram and Mason 1965, Rutter, Tizard and Whitmore 1970), defects of articulation (Schachter 1967, Doehring 1968), disorders of language (Johnson and Myklebust 1967, Mason 1967), difficulties in retaining and reproducing a sequence of sounds (Johnson and Myklebust 1962, Belmont and Birch 1966, Doehring 1968), poor sound discrimination (Wepman 1960, Clark 1970), difficulties in the discrimination of shapes varying in orientation (Galifret-Granjon 1952, Lyle 1969), constructional apraxia (Zangwill 1960, Kinsbourne and Warrington 1963), specific deficits of visual recall (Lyle 1969), visuomotor impairment (Brenner and Gillman 1966), difficulties in the integration of auditory, visual and tactile sensory patterns (Birch and Belmont 1964, Beery 1967, Clark 1970) and right/left confusion (Hermann 1959, Belmont and Birch 1965). A history of lateness in sitting and in walking unaided and findings of poor motor coordination and of marked motor impersistence are reported in the Isle of Wight Survey (Rutter, Tizard and Whitmore 1970).

Sandhya Naidoo

Minor deviant neurological responses have been found, these being remarkably persistent over a number of years (Cohn 1961, Silver and Hagin 1960, 1964). These are disorders and delays in functions whose development depend as much upon neurological integrity, organization and maturation as upon opportunities for learning.

Four major hypotheses, not necessarily mutually exclusive, have been proposed to account for the constitutional basis of specific reading disabilities associated with these developmental anomalies and delays.

First is the genetic hypothesis based on the frequency with which reading disorders are found in other members of a child's family (Hallgren 1950, McGlannan 1968, Rutter *et al* 1970). While family histories may be cautiously interpreted, more convincing evidence comes from three studies of uniovular and binovular twins (Hermann 1959).

The second hypothesis postulates that cerebral dominance is late in becoming established or does not become fully established, thus affecting the acquisition of both speech and reading (Orton 1937, Ettlinger and Jackson 1955, Zangwill 1960). An explanation of the apparently contradictory findings relating laterality to reading and language disorders is offered by Annett (1964).

The third hypothesis explains the isolated developmental delays as simply reflecting unusual but essentially normal variations in the maturation of a part of the brain (Rutter *et al* 1970). Delayed maturation implies that, given the opportunity for learning, a normal level of function will ultimately be achieved and this seems to occur in some children (Critchley 1964).

Lastly, some specific reading disorders are thought to have arisen from organic brain dysfunction, particularly when there is also evidence of neurological disorders and of predisposing factors such as abnormal perinatal conditions (Kinsbourne and Warrington 1963, Boshes and Myklebust 1964).

The presence of associated delays and disorders in children with specific reading difficulties has been well established. Many of these, as well as the reading difficulty, may result from adverse environmental conditions or be aggravated by them. There are many children, however, whose difficulties cannot be so explained. At the Centre we have, for example, examined many verbally uninhibited children from homes where standards of spoken English are high, but who show defective patterns of speech. Each of the disorders listed above has been found, despite more than adequate levels of intelligence and more than adequate opportunities to develop particular skills, and these strongly suggest constitutional delays or dysfunctions.

The diversity of associated features and the difficulties in acquiring just some of the skills essential in reading, writing and spelling, have led to attempts to distinguish subgroups or types of specific dyslexia. Kinsbourne and Warrington (1963), Ingram (1964) and Johnson and Myklebust (1967) have described two types, each with a characteristic cluster of signs. The clusters are not identical but they are broadly similar. Thus Ingram's audio-phonic group, Kinsbourne and Warrington's language retarded group and Johnson and Myklebust's auditory dyslexics are characterized by speech and language delays and disorders. Likewise there are similarities between the visuo-spatial group (Ingram), the developmental Gerstmann syndrome (Kinsbourne and Warrington) and the visual dyslexic (Johnson and Myklebust), visuo-spatial disorders and frequently clumsiness being found. Ingram identifies a third group with both audiophonic and visuo-spatial disorders and our experience at the Centre supports the existence of such a group. Very recently Lyle (1970) has produced some evidence which suggests relationships between birth variables and perceptual and perceptual-motor distortions and between developmental variables, particularly speech delay, and formal learning difficulties mostly verbal in nature.

The attempt to identify subgroups seems to me to be theoretically sound. At the Centre, we have found thinking in such terms most valuable in planning remedial programmes. The principles upon which we have worked and the methods used are described in *The Assessment and Teaching of Dyslexic Children* (Franklin and Naidoo 1970). We suspect that prognosis is related not only to the severity of the disorder but also to the type of the disorder but this requires substantiation by formal investigation.

Whether specific dyslexia exists as a clinical entity has been, in my opinion, confused by a demand for unequivocal evidence of a single disorder of single identifiable etiology. Such insistence would disqualify the use of 'cerebral palsy', for example, as a meaningful clinical term. The etiological factors in cerebral palsy vary and sometimes cannot be identified. The types of motor disorder are varied and are accompanied by sensory, intellectual, perceptual, speech and language disorders which vary from child to child. Different descriptive terms and different sub-classifications are used by different authors. Nonetheless, 'cerebral palsy' has meaning in distinguishing a particular group of handicapped children. I would suggest that 'specific dyslexia' and its alternative terms, are similarly useful to distinguish children whose specific reading disability is associated with developmental delays, minor neurological dysfunctions or isolated maturational lags which are indicative of inherent developmental anomaly. It is important that such distinction be made in order to provide appropriate facilities for assessment and teaching. Such provision has become more urgent since the Chronically Sick and Disabled Persons Bill, including a clause relating to dyslexic children, was passed.

Controlled experiments are needed to compare the response to teaching of dyslexic children and those whose reading disorders are not so classifiable. Many of the children taught at the Centre have had considerable prior remedial tuition with little success. Our teachers have commented on qualitative differences of response between dyslexic children, slow learners and children whose retardation is associated primarily with sociocultural and emotional factors. The dyslexic child, even when bright, appears to learn to read and to spell more slowly. Such observations need to be formally explored. The Centre's research has been concerned with the identification of features characteristic of specific dyslexia and an attempt is made by cluster analysis to distinguish subgroups or types. The subjects are 98 boys selected on criteria which meet the requirements of many definitions of specific dyslexia. They are matched for age and type of school with 98 boys unselected for reading ability and of comparable socioeconomic status. The data relate to developmental history, perinatal history, physical and neurological status, motor coordination, right/left discrimination, finger localization, laterality, intelligence, speech, visual recall, auditory discrimination, behaviour, home and school factors and the presence of familial reading, spelling and speech difficulties and left-handedness. A report of the research will be published in due course. (Now published—Naidoo 1972 [ed].)

References

ANNETT, M. E. (1964) A model of the inheritance of handedness and cerebral dominance *Nature* 204, 4953-9

BEERY, J. W. (1967) Matching of auditory and visual stimuli in average and retarded readers *Child Development* 38, 867

BELMONT, L. and BIRCH, H. G. (1965) Lateral dominance, lateral awareness and reading disability *Child Development* 36, 57

BELMONT, L. and BIRCH, H. G. (1966) The intellectual profile of retarded readers *Perceptual and Motor Skills* 22, 787

BIRCH, H. G. and BELMONT, L. (1964) Auditory–visual integration in normal and retarded readers *American Journal of Orthopsychiatry* 34, 852

BOSHES, B. and MYKLEBUST, H. R. (1964) A neurological and behavioral study of children with learning disorders *Neurology* 14, 1, 7

BRENNER, M. W. and GILLMAN, S. (1966) Visuomotor ability in school children—a survey *Developmental Medicine and Child Neurology* 8, 686

*CLARK, M. M. (1970) *Reading Difficulties in Schools* Harmondsworth: Penguin

COHN, R. (1961) Delayed acquisition of reading and writing studies: a neurological study *Archives of Neurology* 4, 153

CRITCHLEY, M. (1964) *Developmental Dyslexia* London: Heinemann

*DOEHRING, D. G. (1968) *Patterns of Impairment in Specific Reading Disability* Indiana: Indiana University Press

ETTLINGER, G. and JACKSON, C. V. (1955) Organic factors in developmental dyslexia *Proceedings of the Royal Society of Medicine* 48, 998

FRANKLIN, A. W. and NAIDOO, S. (eds) (1970) *The Assessment and Teaching of Dyslexic Children* London: Invalid Children's Aid Association

GALIFRET-GRANJON, N. (1952) Le problème de l'organisation spatiale dans les dyslexies d'évolution in *L'Apprentissage de la Lecture et ses Troubles* Paris: Presses Universelles France

HALLGREN, B. (1950) Specific Dyslexia *Acta Psychiatrica et Neurologica* Suppl. 65

HERMANN, K. (1959) *Reading Disability* Copenhagen: Munksgaard

INGRAM, T. T. S. (1964) The dyslexic child *Word Blind Bulletin* 1, 4, 1

INGRAM, T. T. S. and MASON, A. W. (1965) Reading and writing difficulties in childhood *British Medical Journal* 2, 463

*JOHNSON, D. J. and MYKLEBUST, H. R. (1967) *Learning Disabilities: Educational Principles and Practice* New York: Grune and Stratton

KINSBOURNE, M. and WARRINGTON, E. K. (1963) Developmental factors in reading and writing backwardness *British Journal of Psychology* 54, 145

LYLE, J. G. (1969) Reading retardation and reversal tendency: a factorial study *Child Development* 40, 833

LYLE, J. G. (1970) Certain antenatal, perinatal and developmental variables and reading retardation in middle class boys *Child Development* 41, 481

McGLANNAN, F. K. (1968) Familial characteristics of genetic dyslexia: preliminary report from a pilot study *Journal of Learning Disabilities* 1, 3, 185

MASON, A. W. (1967) Specific (developmental) dyslexia *Developmental Medicine and Child Neurology* 9, 183

MYKLEBUST, H. R. and JOHNSON, D. J. (1962) Dyslexia in children *Exceptional Children* 29, 1, 14

NAIDOO, S. (1972) *Specific Dyslexia The Research Report of the ICCA Word Blind Centre for Dyslexic Children* London: Pitman

*ORTON, S. T. (1937) *Reading, Writing and Speech Problems* London: Chapman and Hall

RUTTER, M., TIZARD, J. and WHITMORE, K. (1970) (eds) *Education, Health and Behaviour* London: Longman

SCHACHTER, M. (1967) La dyslexie-dysorthographie chez des ecoliers avec un Q.I. d'au moins 0–80 au test de Binet-Simon: À propos de 87 observations *Rivista di Psichicatria* 2 (4), 271

SILVER, A. A. and HAGIN, R. A. (1960) Specific reading disability: Delineation of the syndrome and relationship to cerebral dominance *Comprehensive Psychiatry* 1, 126

SILVER, A. A. and HAGIN, R. A. (1964) Specific reading disability: Followup studies *American Journal of Orthopsychiatry* 34, 95

WEPMAN, J. M. (1960) Auditory discrimination, speech and reading *Elementary School Journal* 60, 325

ZANGWILL, O. L. (1960) *Cerebral Dominance and its Relation to Psychological Function* Edinburgh: Oliver and Boyd

3.5 Backward readers—research on auditory–visual integration

ASHER CASHDAN
Faculty of Educational Studies, Open University

Reprinted from W. K. Gardner (1970) (ed) *Reading Skills: Theory and Practice* Ward Lock Educational, pp. 99–106

Teaching backward readers

The number of children in our junior schools who do not reach a satisfactory standard in reading is still distressingly large. One cannot measure this purely in terms of how much their reading ages lag behind their chronological age. For one thing, two years of retardation is clearly more significant in an eight year old than in an eleven year old. For another, the important issue is not the normative one—how children compare with each other or with the average for a particular age—but rather the effective level of literacy they eventually reach. Nevertheless, as Joyce Morris's researches have shown, children who fall seriously behind at primary school level do not often become competent readers later on. So, to use reading age terminology, if a reading level of eleven years is considered a minimum for anything approaching real literacy in adult life, then we must be quite concerned about any child who leaves the junior school with a reading age of less than nine. And far too many still do so—in fact the educational standards attained by at least 10 per cent of schoolchildren are sufficiently low to give us good cause for concern.

The organizational problems of remedial provision are outside the scope of this paper. But it is important to note that followup studies of the more typical arrangements have tended to produce discouraging results: in the long run much of our effort seems to prove abortive. It seems timely, therefore, to look at the main orientations in remedial work and to see what suggestions can be made.

It has long seemed to me that there are two main approaches to helping the child who has reading difficulties. Some teachers concentrate on seeing the child in his total context. Thus they focus their attention on his emotional and social life, his interests and his motivational problems. Very often they will spend some time working with the child semitherapeutically or providing him with general cultural enrichment and language practice before doing any work in reading at all. And their reading work, too, tends to be informal, to focus on interests and meaning rather than upon specific skills. Other teachers approach the whole task from the point of view of the 'learning programmer'. They work systematically through the basic reading skills, with the expressed aim of progressively advancing the pupil's mastery of the elements involved in translating the spoken into the written code, followed by their integration into the complex skills of efficient reading.

Of course, most backward children need both kinds of help, but not many teachers function equally well in both spheres. Hopefully, the child who gets personal and background help will soon have the confidence and motivation to teach himself; while the experience of success in mastering some of the technical skills will help the general adjustment of those children who encounter the other type of teacher. My concern is not to support the one or the other approach. Clearly the ideal is a real synthesis of both of them. At the same time I cannot help feeling that the cognitive analysis—exploring what it is that the poor reader cannot do— is one that needs particular attention. And it is with one small aspect of this that this paper will now be concerned.

Intersensory skills in reading

Birch and Lefford (1963) suggest that one of the major ways in which human beings are superior to lower animals is in their ability to translate incoming messages in one sensory channel into those presented through another. For example, if you put your hand behind your back and I put a pencil into it you will know what it is immediately, although you normally recognize such an object visually. In other words, you can integrate tactile with visual information. Birch and Lefford have studied the development of such skills in primary age children using simple geometrical forms and the three modes of vision, touch and kinaesthesis (moving the hand round the object). They show that infants have not yet acquired the ability to perform such tasks competently and that it is only in the later junior school years that children can manage such tasks with ease. They go further and suggest that 'the development of intersensory functioning follows a general law of growth' and that 'the emergence of such functioning is developmental'. In other words, they are implying that, like the components of Piaget's stages, this type of skill develops relatively independently of specific environmental factors, that it unfolds as it were naturally and that it would not be easy to hasten artificially. We shall return to this argument later.

Birch has applied this work in various fields. In particular (Birch and Belmont 1964) he has shown that backward readers perform less well than comparable normal children at an intersensory task. In fact, learning to read obviously draws heavily on such skills. The child has to learn to integrate auditory and visual messages. He has to appreciate how a *heard* sequence of sounds is represented by a *seen* sequence of symbols. Birch and Belmont's auditory–visual integration task consists of sets of rhythmic taps which the child listens to and then has to identify from a choice of visual patterns. A typical item is as follows:

auditory taps   visual stimuli

.. ..

The child hears the auditory taps and then has to say which of the three visual stimuli (shown to him on a card) is the same as what he heard. It is quite a reasonable inference that if backward readers have particular difficulty with this task by comparison with those who are good readers, this is in part what is holding them up; though in such matters it is never easy to say with certainty which difficulty is the chicken and which the egg! Birch clearly thinks that the retarded reader will often be suffering from a developmental lag in this type of skill, even if his general intelligence is relatively good.

The nature of this deficiency does, however, bear further consideration. Blank and Bridger (1966) think that the important problem may lie not in the 'cross-sensory' integration, but rather in the backward readers' reluctance to use verbal coding. What happens is that the child fails to translate the stimuli because he falls down in the mediating aspect. If he said to himself, in effect, 'That was two and then a pause and then another two' the problem is solved. By using flashing lights instead of auditory stimuli, Blank and Bridger were able to show that the difficulty still existed, although the whole task was now in a single mode (that is, both parts were visual). Furthermore, children who were good at 'verbal labelling'—that is, naming the stimuli in the way just suggested—found the task much easier than those who did not seem to do this, even though both groups of children clearly had the requisite vocabulary at their command. One way of putting this, as these researchers say, is by suggesting that the backward readers do not attend as well and fail to adopt strategies that would help them.

Whether one adopts the Birch analysis or that of Blank does make a practical difference. In the one case, one might be inclined to spend time helping the child to translate messages from one mode to another, perhaps devising special exercises to facilitate this. In the other, the focus would need to be on language and on isolating the features to which attention must be paid. Furthermore the Birch approach with its stress on 'developmental emergence' is less encouraging to the teacher than one which points to a more obviously remediable deficit.

The investigation

One of my advanced students (Fearn 1968) has recently carried out a small investigation which we hope makes the position a fraction clearer.

Our aim was twofold: to confirm the Birch and Belmont findings in a group of retarded readers; and then to see how far the difference between our normal and retarded readers could be lessened by a modification in the test procedure. As this modification consisted of offering the children language labels, we hoped at the same time to be able to support Blank's suggestion that this is where the main difficulty lies.

We took a group of twenty-two nine year olds, whose average Burt reading ages were 6.5 years and matched them for age, sex, socioeconomic group and nonverbal intelligence (Raven's Matrices) with a similar number of good readers—Burt mean 10 years. Each group was subdivided at random into two subgroups of eleven children. In each group one subgroup was given the 'instructed' version of the test, and the other the 'uninstructed' version (Table 1).

TABLE 1   *The groups*

	Good readers (N)	*Backward readers* (R)
UNINSTRUCTED (U)	Group UN (7 boys, 4 girls)	Group UR (7 boys, 4 girls)
INSTRUCTED (I)	Group IN (7 boys, 4 girls)	Group IR (7 boys, 4 girls)

In both versions the identical test material was used. After three demonstration examples each child was given a twenty item auditory–visual test of the type explained above. After items 5, 10 and 15 an extra example was given—different each time. Whenever any example was given the experimenter pointed to the correct selection and said, irrespective of the child's choice, 'It is this one.' In the 'instructed' version the same tasks were presented in the same way except that with every example the examiner gave a verbal description of the taps made, before he exposed the visual pattern. For instance with the example given earlier he would have said, 'That was two taps and then two taps'—that is, he indicated the number and position of taps and pauses.

The purpose of the 'instructed' condition was to see if the retarded group would show better performance when the idea of verbal labelling was presented to them than when they were left to devise their own strategies (if any). The intervention was a mild one in that no suggestion was made to the child that he should code in this way—he was simply exposed to the fact that the experimenter did this with the examples. In the case of the normal children, no differences were expected between the instructed and the uninstructed groups, on the grounds that these children would probably spontaneously be making use of verbal labels.

As a further check, each child was then given a second task. He was presented with twenty further items but this time he was merely required, after listening, to explain verbally what he had heard.

Results

After appropriate analysis of variance and 't' tests had been applied, it was seen that the experimental hypotheses were amply confirmed. Both groups of good readers scored better than the backward ones. The instructed retarded readers performed better than the uninstructed group, but there were no differences between the two groups of good readers. The findings were virtually identical for both tasks. Mean scores are given in Table 2.

TABLE 2   *Task scores (maximum 20)*

Group	Mean number correct	
	Task 1	Task 2
UN	16.0	15.17
UR	9.82	5.64
IN	16.45	15.27
IR	13.51	9.73

Comments on the results

Looking first at the uninstructed or natural condition it seems clear that the good readers can manage an auditory–visual task better than backward readers, even when they are of similar nonverbal intelligence. On reflection, we should probably have matched them on verbal ability too, but this would have been harder to do and it seems fairly safe to say that the verbal abilities of the poor readers were well up to the demands of the task—their inferiority was more in their ability to use a verbal strategy without it being suggested to them.

In the instructed condition Group IR scored significantly better than the other poor readers (Group UR) though they were still significantly poorer than the good readers. But they had closed the gap somewhat (in Task 1 Group UN performed significantly better than Group UR at the .001 level, whereas the difference between Groups IN and IR was only significant at the .05 level). These results seem to suggest that although auditory–visual integration tasks are not performed as well by backward readers as by more competent ones, the differences lie more in their willingness to attend and plan and to label spontaneously, rather than in a major and relatively irremediable failure in international ability, whether due to maturational lag or minor neuropathology. If such a study were repeated with the addition of a deliberate training programme, I would expect to see the poor readers close the gap entirely.

In the same vein, another of my students (Mrs O. S. Gregory) looked at the possibility of training backward children to perform the kind of word analysis skills which Bruce (1964) found quite difficult for normal children before the middle of the junior school age range. In essence, the experimenter presents the child with a word such as *table* or *pin* and asks him what would remain if the sound t or p respectively were removed. Mrs Gregory found that after a relatively short training period her group of eight year old retarded readers could perform this task quite well. Again, an apparently 'developmental' function begins to look relatively teachable.

Some conclusions

In the light of these admittedly rather small studies what kind of conclusions can we reasonably draw? Clearly, we need to decide to what extent specific skills such as the ability to integrate auditory and visual 'messages' are crucial in learning to read and how far we can help children who are slow to acquire them. We must admit that we are not yet in a position to give definitive answers; but we have confirmed that retarded readers are poor at this kind of task, and reading does involve, at least in part, the ability to translate heard sequences of phonemes into a visual code (and vice versa). But Blank's work, as well as our own, certainly suggests that strengthening children's verbal labelling skills gives them specific help in this kind of task and quite possibly in the reading situation also. The more general question of the validity of Birch's analysis is one that will have to wait on much further study. It would be interesting to know at how young an age one could train children to perform well on intersensory tasks—and it may well be that what proves relatively easy to do with a retarded nine year old may be well beyond the powers of a normal five year old.

Finally, what is the relevance of this kind of research for the practising teacher—particularly in remedial work? Three points seem to be worth making. First, the value of relatively abstract research must seem problematical at times to those who are engaged wholly in the day to day work of the classroom. But there is enormous potential in such studies, even when there is no immediate pay-off. With but a little imagination we can see the investment value of any hard work that we put into understanding the development of children's skills—and their deficiencies—even when we are working at one remove from the classroom. As in the physical sciences, all fundamental study proves of value in the end—some immediately and some in the longer term. We do pitifully little basic research in child development in this country and we need both the courage and the support to do far more.

My second and third points are more immediate. The one is that we must continue to take the mystique out of learning difficulties. If as some neurologists have seemed to argue (Critchley 1964), we were to stop at the point where all our tests yield negative results and say simply that the child has a 'maturational lag' and cannot yet manage complex higher order skills, such as reading, we would be doing a pretty incomplete job. What we must do is to find out what it is that the child cannot do which makes reading progress difficult for him—in other words we need to continue to work towards a satisfactory model of both the components and the totality of reading ability.

The remaining point is simply that even in our present state of knowledge in this field we can certainly draw out some useful guide lines for the remedial practitioner. We can suggest that the child might usefully be briefed on the nature of the auditory–visual translations he is being asked to accomplish. Rather than assuming that the child has the mental sets of the established reader we must help him to achieve these, quite often by offering him appropriate vocabulary. J. F. Reid (1967) has pointed out how often normal five year olds are unaware of the precise significance of terms such as *letter* or *word*, as well as how quickly they can learn these. Further analysis of the kind I have been discussing in this paper could provide us with a better appreciation of how reading skills develop in normal children as well as with ideas about what we might already do for those who show difficulties.

References

BIRCH, H. G. and BELMONT, L. (1964) Auditory–visual integration in normal and retarded readers *American Journal of Orthopsychiatry* 34, 825–61

BIRCH, H. G. and LEFFORD, A. (1963) Intersensory development in children *Monograph of the Society for Research in Child Development* 28, no. 5

BLANK, M. and BRIDGER, W. H. (1966) Deficiencies in verbal labelling in retarded readers *American Journal of Orthopsychiatry* 36, 840–7

BRUCE, D. J. (1964) The analysis of word sounds by young children *British Journal of Educational Psychology* 34, 157–70

CRITCHLEY, M. (1964) *Developmental Dyslexia* London: Heinemann

FEARN, D. (1968) Do children differ in auditory–visual integration tasks even when given verbal labels? Dissertation: Manchester University

GREGORY, O. S. (1968) Phonic analysis in young children Dissertation: Manchester University

REID, J. F. (1967) Talking, thinking and learning *Reading* 1, no. 1, 5–9

3.6 A retrospective study of 82 children with reading disability

T. T. S. INGRAM, A. W. MASON and
I. BLACKBURN
Department of Child Life and Health,
University of Edinburgh

Reprinted from *Developmental medicine and child neurology* (1970)
12, 3, pp. 271–81

This investigation of 82 dyslexic patients was designed to throw light on the controversial condition of specific reading disability, especially in its relationship to underlying brain function.

Selection of patients

Between 1962 and 1968, 206 children (156 boys and 50 girls) were referred to the authors with alleged reading difficulties, mostly from the neurological and speech clinics of the Royal Hospital for Sick Children, but others by family doctors, school medical officers or psychologists. All the patients had a careful history taken as well as neurological and psychological examinations.

Thirty were excluded from further consideration because they were under seven years of age, when the assessment of educational attainments is unreliable, 90 because their educational difficulties were explicable on the grounds of low intelligence (IQ under 80), unfavourable home environment, interrupted schooling, inadequate teaching or poor motivation, and a further four because their testing could not be completed. The final series comprised 82 highly preselected patients, 66 boys and 16 girls.

By this careful selection of patients it was hoped to eliminate from the series any contaminating environmental, intellectual or emotional variables known to adversely affect the learning of reading. Unfavourable conditions which were not excluded were neurological dysfunction, a history of slow speech development or a family history of reading or speech difficulties. All 82 children were considered to show mild, moderate or severe underachievement in reading or spelling. Mild underachievement was defined as an attainment quotient (as measured by the Schonell Tests R1 and S1) of 10 to 14 points below the IQ assessed on the Stanford–Binet Intelligence Scale 1960 Revision (Form L-M). Underachievement was defined as moderate where a disparity of 15 to 29 points existed between the two quotients and as severe where the disparity was 30 or more points.

Considered as a group, these children were reading at an average of more than two years below their chronological age, despite the fact that all but six of the group were of average or higher intelligence. Only three children, all of superior intelligence, were reading at the level of their chronological age but even they were more than three years below the level of their mental age. Sixty-two of the group fulfilled an operational definition of children suffering from 'specific dyslexia'—i.e. children who, in the absence of low intelligence, emotional disturbance or adverse environmental (especially educational) factors, experience difficulty in learning to read and spell, although they perform satisfactorily in school subjects independent of reading—particularly in mechanical arithmetic.

Investigations

Medical
Detailed history-taking elicited information about any family history of speech, reading or spelling difficulties, about sinistrality or ambidexterity or about the presence of any neurological or psychiatric disorders. It also elicited details of the mother's health during pregnancy and of the labour and delivery which resulted in the birth of the child. Parents' accounts were supplemented by notes from maternity hospitals in the majority of cases. Full histories of each child's development in infancy and earlier childhood were taken from parents and guardians and, whenever possible, additional information was obtained from nurseries, nursery schools and schools. Questions were asked about the child's health and details of any serious illnesses were sought from attending doctors and hospitals. Parents were asked detailed questions as to any symptoms of emotional disturbance in the child, such as temper tantrums, excessive withdrawal, bed-wetting, nail-biting, truancy or delinquency.

Patients were subjected to a physical examination, including a detailed neurological assessment. Simple tests for eye, hand and foot dominance were given. Tests of visual fields were not employed. The tests for hand dominance consisted of asking the child to use a top which was driven by one hand, to throw a ball one-handed and to break a stick using both hands (in this test it is found that the dominant hand is operative in performing the breaking action). Eye dominance was tested by asking the child to look through a hole in a piece of paper held in front of his face by the examiner, then while holding it himself with his preferred hand and then while holding it with his nondominant hand. The only test of foot dominance was to ask the child to kick a ball placed centrally about one foot in front of him, on three different occasions. Electroencephalograms were obtained in 38 patients. Air-encephalography was felt to be unjustified.

An attempt was made to classify children according to the likelihood of their suffering from 'brain damage' by taking their histories into account and by indications of brain dysfunction ascertained in the course of neurological examinations and electroencephalography.

Birth histories were judged arbitrarily in the same way as were those of patients suffering from cerebral palsy in a previous study (Ingram 1964). They were scored for the possible traumatic, hypoxic and toxic insults that the fetus might have suffered. Mild or moderately severe pre-eclampsia was scored as one hypoxic insult; severe pre-eclampsia or antepartum haemorrhage or prolapse of the cord as two. Mid-cavity forceps delivery was counted as one traumatic insult, but labour prolonged beyond 36 hours in a first gestation or beyond 24 hours in a second gestation, breech extraction and high forceps delivery counted as two. Apnoea up to five minutes was considered as one hypoxic insult; more prolonged apnoea or cyanosis for more than an hour counted as two. Patients born after uncomplicated pregnancies, labours and deliveries who were normal in the neonatal period were placed in category 0, those with one or two insults in category 1, those with three or four in category 2, those with five or more insults in category 3.

A history of clumsiness or slow motor milestones sufficiently severe to make the parents seek medical advice placed the child in category 1. A history of convulsions with fever, strabismus or other conditions frequently associated with chronic brain disease placed the child in category 2. A history of definite head injury, meningitis or encephalitis, or of persistent neurological impairment such as ataxia or neglect of a hand, placed patients in category 3.

Patients were also classified according to the findings of neurological examination. Those with no abnormal neurological signs were placed in category 0 and those with minimal incoordination or a mild excess of contralateral associated movement (for example on the Fog test) were placed in category 1. Category 2 covered those with more evidence of motor impairment, particularly those showing the choreoid syndrome or mild asymmetries in the reflexes without definite paresis. Patients with definite cerebral palsy or epilepsy were placed in category 3.

The electroencephalograms of patients were also classified into four categories. Normal records for age were in category 0; records in which there was a mild excess of slow activity or minor asymmetries but no paroxysmal activity were placed in category 1; records in which there was a definite excess of slow activity which might be paroxysmal were placed in category 2; records with focal spike activity, spike wave activity or other evidence of epilepsy were placed in category 3.

Psychological

All patients were given the Stanford–Binet Intelligence Scale 1960 Revision (Form L-M). They were also given standardized tests in reading (Schonell Test R1), spelling (Schonell Test S1) and, except for six children for whom school reports were accepted, mechanical arithmetic (Schonell Forms A or B). The Goodenough Draw-a-Man Test was given to 49 children under the age of ten (the test does not measure the upper levels of ability after this age). Diagnostic reading tests (Schonell R5, 6 and 7) were administered as appropriate.

Children were placed in one of two categories. The first consisted of 62 children who were underachieving in reading and spelling only and who thus fulfilled the operational definition of specific dyslexia—for the sake of brevity this group will be referred to as the 'specifics'. The second group of 20 children had general learning difficulties in that as well as underachieving in reading and spelling they also performed below expectation in arithmetic (the criterion being an arithmetic quotient 15 or more points below intelligence quotient). This group will be referred to as the 'generals'.

An attempt was made to assess the importance of audio-phonic difficulties and visuo-spatial difficulties in the processes of reading and spelling.

Audio-phonic difficulties are shown in (i) inability to synthesize letters correctly sounded individually into the appropriate words (*b u n* sounded and the word uttered as *but*); (ii) confusion of vowel sounds in recognition of words (bed read as bad); (iii) poor phonic knowledge (lack of acquaintance with the sound of diphthongs); (iv) general inability to analyse words into their natural auditory units.

Visuo-spatial difficulties are manifest in (i) confusion of letters of the same shape but different orientation (b, d, p); (ii) slow recognition of even simple words; (iii) poor visual discrimination of words closely similar in shape (*road* and *read*); (iv) directional errors (*saw* read as *was*), although this type of error may also occur as a result of an audio-phonic difficulty described under (i) above.

Findings

General variables (Table 1)
The two subgroups of specifics and generals are similar in age, social class and intelligence. The specifics show a higher percentage of boys than do the generals, although the difference between the two groups is not significant. However, when the χ^2 test of significance is applied to the intra-

TABLE 1 *General variables*

	No.	Intelligence			Age in years			% Girls	% Social Classes I and II†
		Mean	Range	S.D.*	Average	Range	S.D.*		
SPECIFICS	62	108	81–165	16	$9\frac{10}{12}$	7–$15\frac{7}{12}$	$2\frac{1}{12}$	18	68
GENERALS	20	107	81–131	13	$10\frac{4}{12}$	$7\frac{1}{12}$–$15\frac{11}{12}$	$2\frac{5}{12}$	25	70

*S.D. = Standard Deviation   †Registrar General's classification

group differences between the numbers of boys and girls constituting the groups, it is found that for the specifics the difference is significant at the .01 level, while for the generals it is not significant.

History variables (Table 2)
When the family histories of reading and spelling difficulties were taken, only siblings, parents and uncles and aunts of patients were taken into consideration. Forty per cent of the specific group and 25 per cent of the general had a positive family history. Although this difference is not statistically significant, it lies in the expected direction according to other studies. There was also a higher incidence of family speech difficulties in the specific than in the general group, but the difference was not significant.

The figures in this table may be compared with those obtained from a group of 30 children of equivalent intelligence and social class who read normally, only 9 per cent of whom had a history of reading difficulties in the family. The difference between this normal group and the specifics is significant at the .01 level.

The possibility that a genetic factor may exist in reading disability has emerged from the work of Hallgren (1950) and Hermann and Norrie (1958).

TABLE 2   *History variables*

	No.	*Personal speech difficulties* (%)	*No.*	*Family speech difficulties* (%)	*Family reading difficulties* (%)
SPECIFICS	62	56	60	30	40
GENERALS	20	50	20	20	25

* The statistical significance of differences between percentages in the two groups has been assessed by the standard error formulae

Neurological aspects (Table 3)
This analysis shows the distribution of specifics and generals by the likelihood of their having evidence of brain damage or cerebral dysfunction, as assessed by birth history, developmental history, clinical examination and electroencephalography. The findings are remarkably consistent. The specific group have less evidence of brain damage or dysfunction than the generals, whether this is assessed by birth and developmental history, clinical examination or electroencephalography. Neurological examination and EEG findings (the two criteria of cerebral function on which most reliance was placed, since they did not rely upon retrospective examination) show these contrasts very clearly. For 68 per cent of the specifics there were no positive neurological findings, in comparison with only 35 per cent of the generals, whereas there were positive neurological findings (categories 2 and 3 combined) for 60 per cent of the generals,

T. T. S. Ingram, A. W. Mason and I. Blackburn

TABLE 3   *Neurological aspects*

	No.	Categories (%)			
		0	1	2	3
BIRTH HISTORY					
Specifics	60	65 *	15	18	2
Generals	20	30	40	20	10
DEVELOPMENTAL HISTORY					
Specifics	62	72 *	13	12	3 *
Generals	20	20	25	30	25
CLINICAL EXAMINATION					
Specifics	62	68 *	10	17	5 *
Generals	20	35	5	25	35
EEG RESULTS					
Specifics	26	66 *	15	12	7
Generals	12	16	9	50	25

* Differences significant at the .01 level

but for only 22 per cent of the specifics. Again, 66 per cent of the specifics had normal EEGs, compared with only 16 per cent of the generals. All these differences are significant at the .01 level.

Nature of reading difficulties (Table 4)
In the early stages of reading, pupils must learn to recognize the written symbol (letter, syllable or word), to associate it with the corresponding auditory images and then to synthesize these into words. At a later stage, visual recognition of words becomes the rule; the child finally learns to read by making a series of rapid hypotheses, often on slight contextual clues, inappropriate responses being inhibited as he proceeds (Luria 1966).

Whereas the specific group made primitive errors involving confusion even of letters or auditory–phonic synthesis, these were much less frequent in the general group. For example, while 77 per cent of all specifics made mistakes of audio-phonic origin, only 11 per cent of the generals did. Only 2 per cent of the specifics were free of primitive errors as against 40 per cent of the generals. Both these differences were significant at the .01 level.

Audio-phonic difficulties were not the major cause of reading failure in all the specific patients. For example, one eight year old boy with entirely normal development and of very high intelligence, whose auditory–phonic capacities seemed well-developed in all aspects, could not recognize simple words like *dog*, *man* or *my* in print. In such cases, some inadequacy in visual recognition must be postulated.

TABLE 4   *Nature of reading difficulties*

	No.	Word discrimination and recognition %	Audio-phonic %	Mixed %	Neither %
SPECIFICS	62	87	77 *	66	2 *
GENERALS	20	60	11	55	40

		Word recognition and discrimination only %	Audio-phonic only %
SPECIFICS	62	21	11
GENERALS	20	5	0

* Significant at the .01 level

Goodenough and Stanford–Binet IQ comparisons
The 49 scores obtained from the Goodenough Test are compared with the Stanford–Binet scores in Table 5. Both groups of children showed marked depression of Goodenough scores, but the more spectacular discrepancies occurred in the specific group. There were no obvious correlations between the likelihood of brain damage and scores on the Goodenough test.

TABLE 5   *Goodenough and Stanford–Binet IQ comparisons*

	No.	S.B. = Goodenough to within 15 points %	S.B. > Goodenough by 15 to 19 points %	S.B. > Goodenough by 30+ points %
SPECIFICS	35	23	37	40
GENERALS	14	43	28.5	28.5

Severity of underachievement (Table 6)
When degree of failure is examined, the two groups differ only slightly in the direction of more severe failure in the specific group.

TABLE 6 *Severity of reading underachievement*

	No.	$RQ < IQ$ *by 10 to 14* *points* %	$RQ < IQ$ *by 15 to 29* *points* %	$RQ < IQ$ *by 30+ points* %
SPECIFICS	62	0	35	65
GENERALS	20	10	30	60

Discussion

The definition of dyslexia
The word 'dyslexia' has been and is being used in a number of different ways. It can be useful when it is used as a short term to denote difficulty in learning to read and, inevitably, the associated difficulty in learning to spell. The definition is then an operational one and can be arbitrarily defined in terms of the difference between the child's achievements on tests of intelligence and on tests of reading and spelling. There may or may not be difficulties in other school subjects.

The terms 'specific dyslexia' or 'specific developmental dyslexia' are susceptible of operational definition. Neither term should be used to imply any particular causation, such as genetic defect or brain damage.

Confusion has arisen for several reasons. Authors have described series of children with very varied clinical and psychological findings; mass surveys of populations of schoolchildren are liable to produce reading failures too heterogeneous in their origins and manifestations to allow for satisfactory groupings; and adequate combined neurological and psychological assessments have been lacking.

Retarded speech development and dyslexia
Since a proportion of the patients were referred from a speech clinic, the preponderance (more than 50 per cent) with a history of deviant speech development was to be expected. However, it is interesting that Ingram and Reid (1956) found almost as high a proportion of such children in a group with specific dyslexia diagnosed in a Department of Child Psychiatry where no such selecting factor would, apparently, be operating. The relationship between slow speech development and later difficulties in learning to read and spell is being further explored by the authors in a longitudinal investigation (Mason 1967 and 1969).

In some patients in the present series, the retardation of speech development was severe and children of seven or eight years of age were found to be making the articulatory errors characteristic of three year olds.

Difficulties

The most marked difference between the two groups is in the high incidence of audio-phonic difficulties among the 'specifics' despite a similar proportion of children with a history of speech difficulties in each group. It appears to reflect the greater severity of reading failure in the 'specifics', for audio-phonic skills are the most basic for reading. Soviet psychologists (Levina *et al* 1965) are convinced that audio-phonic difficulties associated with speech difficulties (especially when evidenced by phonemic substitutions) underlie all reading difficulties. In France, Tomatis (1967) has expounded a similar view.

The evidence from this study of visual–perceptual and auditory-phonic inadequacy in reading disability, deduced from errors, supports the findings of a number of experimental investigations made of the association between children's reading ability and their visual–perceptual development (Maslow *et al* 1964, Lyle and Goyen 1968), their auditory-perceptual organization (Wepman 1962) and the integration of the modalities (Birch 1962, Birch and Belmont 1965, De Hirsch *et al* 1966, Lovell and Gorton 1968). Vernon (1962) used Piagetian theory to postulate an immaturity in dyslexic children in the ability to make the coordination of visual and auditory perception necessary for the reversible operations basic to reading. Davol and Hastings (1967) have recently demonstrated the close relationship between reading ability and the mastery of visual–spatial relations. Current research at Cornell University into the learning of reading, based on a study of the phonemic, semantic and syntactic constraints utilized by a reader according to modern linguistics also supports the view that visual factors play a vital part especially in the improvement in visual discrimination between the ages of four and eight years (Gibson 1968).

Dyslexia and indications of brain damage
The pioneer work of Lord (1937), Dunsdon (1952) and Taylor (1959) indicated clearly that perceptual difficulties, in addition to mental and physical handicaps, impaired the early educational progress of many children who suffered from cerebral palsy. On the other hand, the reported incidence of neurological evidence of 'brain damage' varied greatly in different series of children diagnosed as having specific dyslexia (Hallgren 1950, Drew 1956, Hermann 1959, Ingram 1959). Such discrepancies stemmed partly from differences in the selection of patients and partly from differences in the techniques and interpretations of neurological examination. Authors have referred to the 'clumsiness' of many of their patients, and 'developmental dyspraxia' has been described as a common concomitant of 'dyslexia' (McCready 1910, Orton 1937, Eustis 1947). Rabinovitch *et al* (1954) describe 'a nonspecific awkwardness and clumsiness in motor function'. In a group of backward readers studied by Lovell and Gorton (1968), 12 per cent showed the symptoms described by

Prechtl and Stemmer (1962) but none of the control groups of normal readers did.

In the present series, the proportion of the 'generals' with abnormal neurological signs is significantly higher than that of the 'specifics' (significant at the 0.01 level).

In spite of the fact that evidence of brain damage was more often, though not exclusively, associated with general learning difficulties, it was not associated with a greater degree of difficulty in learning to read (see Table 6). In fact the reverse was the case. Of the 'generals' 70 per cent in category 0 (no clinical evidence of brain abnormality) showed severe reading failure, against only 57 per cent of those in category 3 (definite evidence of brain damage). In the 'specific' group, 60 per cent in neurological category 0 were severe reading failures, compared with only 33⅓ per cent in category 3.

These conclusions establish that severe specific reading disability can be present without any clinical evidence of brain abnormality and that the latter is more likely to be accompanied by general educational difficulties than by a specific reading disability.

The 'specifics' with no positive neurological signs whose reading has been followed up all showed a good initial spurt on the commencement of remedial tuition but have remained severe failures.

All these findings show that the assumption that specific dyslexia must be associated with organic brain defect is unfounded (Morris 1966).

Interpretations of depressed Goodenough scores
There are indications that it may be permissible to interpret the depressed Goodenough scores in both groups of children as coming from the authors' longitudinal study of the relationship between retarded speech development and reading disability (Mason 1969). All the evidence so far suggests that depressed Goodenough scores, in relation to Stanford–Binet IQs of children in the speech-retarded group who are also failing in reading, are explicable in terms of a maturational lag in those aspects of intelligence that are measured by the Goodenough test, especially visuo-perceptual and motor development (see also Abercrombie and Tyson 1966). Maslow *et al* (1964), having established a positive correlation between it and the Frostig Visual Perceptual Test for young children, claim that the Goodenough test can be used as an indicator of perceptual development.

It appears likely then that the depressed Goodenough scores of the younger children in this study may also be interpreted in terms of maturational lag, especially as a high proportion of these children had a history of retarded speech development and as there was nothing bizarre about their drawings.

Difficulty in learning to read viewed as a result of failure of maturation
Harris (1963) quotes studies which have demonstrated the influence of the acquisition of language on drawing (Stotijn-Egge 1952) and the im-

portance of visual, auditory and kinaesthetic perceptual experience in improving the quality of the drawing of the human figure (Mott 1945). Soviet psychologists (Luria and Yudovich 1959, Luria 1961) underline the importance of language in the development of perceptual as well as conceptual processes.

Fry (1966) describes the basic motor, auditory, kinaesthetic and visual skills (best seen in the language learning of partially deaf children) which enter into early language learning. Mastery of oral language itself underlies the acquisition of reading, which in turn requires the integration of visual–perceptual, auditory and kinaesthetic processes (Birch 1962).

Lovell and Gorton (1968), using factor analysis, have demonstrated a clear link between reading skills, auditory–visual integration and motor performance in a group of backward readers aged 9–10 years randomly selected from a total age group of 697 pupils.

In view of these mutually compatible arguments from many sources, it does not seem unreasonable to suppose that an immaturity in even one of the basic perceptual or motor functions will have repercussions on one or all of the development of language, the readiness to learn reading or the ability to draw.

References

ABERCROMBIE, M. L. J. and TYSON, M. C. (1966) Body image and draw-a-man test in cerebral palsy *Developmental Medicine and Child Neurology* 8, 9

BIRCH, H. G. (1962) Dyslexia and the maturation of visual function in J. Money (ed) *Reading Disability: Progress and Research Needs in Dyslexia* Baltimore: Johns Hopkins Press

BIRCH, H. G. and BELMONT, L. (1965) Auditory visual integration, intelligence and reading ability in school children *Perceptual and Motor Skills* 20, 295

DAVOL, S. H. and HASTINGS, M. L. (1967) Effects of sex, age, reading ability, socioeconomic level and display position on a measure of spatial relations in children *Perceptual and Motor Skills* 24, 375

*DE HIRSCH, K. JANSKY, J. J. and LANGFORD, W. S. (1966) *Predicting Reading Failure* New York: Harper and Row

DREW, A. L. (1956) A neurological appraisal of familial congenital word blindness *Brain* 79, 440

DUNSDON, M. I. (1952) *The Educability of the Cerebral Palsied Child* London: Newnes

FUSTIS, R. S. (1947) The primary etiology of the specific language disabilities *Journal of Pediatrics* 31, 448

FRY, D. B. (1966) The development of the phonological system in the normal and deaf child in F. Smith and G. A. Miller (eds) *The Genesis of Language* Cambridge, Massachusetts: MIT Press

GIBSON, E. J. (1968) Learning to read in N. S. Endler and coworkers *Contemporary Issues in Developmental Psychology* New York: Holt, Rinehart and Winston

GOODENOUGH, F. L. (1926) *Measurement of Intelligence by Drawings* New York: World Books

HALLGREN, B. (1950) Specific dyslexia *Acta Psychiatrica Scandinavica* suppl. 65

HARRIS, D. B. (1963) *Children's Drawings as Measures of Intellectual Maturity* New York: Harcourt, Brace and World

HERMANN, K. (1959) *Reading Disability* Copenhagen: Munksgaard

HERMANN, K. and NORRIE, E. (1958) Is congenital word blindness an hereditary type of Gertsmann's syndrome? *Psychiatrica et Neurologica* 136, 59

INGRAM, T. T. S. (1959) Specific developmental disorders of speech in childhood *Brain* 82, 450

INGRAM, T. T. S. (1964) *Paediatric Aspects of Cerebral Palsy* Edinburgh: E. and S. Livingstone

INGRAM, T. T. S. and REID, J. F. (1956) Developmental asphasia observed in a department of child psychiatry *Archives of Diseases in Childhood* 31, 161

LEVINA, R. and coworkers (1965) Nyedoststatki Ryechi u Uchashchichsya Moscow: Isdatelstvo Procveshcheniye

LORD, S. E. (1937) *Children Handicapped by Cerebral Palsy* London: Commonwealth Fund

LOVELL, K. and GORTON A. (1968) Some differences between backward and normal readers of average intelligence *British Journal of Educational Psychology* 38, 240

LURIA, A. R. (1961) *The Role of Speech in the Regulation of Normal and Abnormal Behaviour* London: Pergamon

LURIA, A. R. (1966) *Higher Cortical Functions in Man* London: Tavistock Publications

*LURIA, A. R. and YUDOVICH, F. I. (1959) *Speech and the Development of Mental Processes in the Child* London: Staples Press

LYLE, J. G. and GOVEN, J. (1968) Visual recognition, developmental lag and stephosymbolia in reading retardation *Journal of Abnormal Psychology* 73, 25

McCREADY, E. B. (1910) Biological variations in the higher cerebral centers causing retardation *Archives of Pediatrics* 27, 506

MASLOW, P., FROSTIG, M., LEFEVER, D. and WHITTLESEY, J. R. B. (1964) The Marianne Frostig developmental test of visual perception, 1963 *Perceptual and Motor Skills* 19, 463

MASON, A. W. (1967) Specific (developmental) dyslexia *Developmental Medicine and Child Neurology* 9, 183

MASON, A. W. (1970) Followup of educational attainments in a group of children with retarded speech development and in a control group in M. M. Clark and S. M. Maxwell (eds) *Reading: Influences on Progress* UKRA

Study of children with reading disability

* MORRIS, J. (1966) *Standards and Progress in Reading* Slough: National Foundation for Educational Research

MOTT, S. M. (1945) Muscular activity as an aid to concept formation *Child Development* 16, 97

* ORTON, S. T. (1937) *Reading, Writing and Speech Problems in Children* London: Chapman and Hall

PRECHTL, H. F. R. and STEMMER, C. J. (1962) The choreiform syndrome in children *Developmental Medicine and Child Neurology* 4, 119

RABINOVITCH, R. D., DREW, A. L., DEJONG, R. N., INGRAM, W. and WITHEY, L. (1954) A research approach to reading retardation *Research Publication of the Association for Nervous and Mental Disorders* 34, 363

SCHONELL, F. J. (1942) *Backwardness in the Basic Subjects* Edinburgh: Oliver and Boyd

SCHONELL, F. J. and SCHONELL, F. E. (1950) *Diagnostic and Attainment Testing* Edinburgh: Oliver and Boyd

STOTIJN-EGGE, S. (1952) *Investigation of the Drawing Ability of Low-grade Oligophrenics* Leiden: Luctor et Emergo

TAYLOR, E. M. (1959) *Psychological Appraisal of Children with Cerebral Defects* Cambridge, Massachusetts: Harvard University Press

TOMATIS, A. (1967) *La Dyslexie* Paris: Centre du Language

*VERNON, M. D. (1962) Specific dyslexia *British Journal of Educational Psychology* 32, 143

WEPMAN, J. M. (1962) Dyslexia: its relationship to language acquisition and concept formation in J. Money (ed) *Reading Disability: Progress and Research Needs in Dyslexia* Baltimore: Johns Hopkins Press

3.7 Reading failure: a reexamination

JOHN E. MERRITT
Professor of Educational Studies, Open University

Reprinted from Vera Southgate (1972) (ed) *Literacy at all levels*
Ward Lock Educational, pp. 175–84

Introduction

There have been many studies over the years which have shown a relationship between some neurological, perceptual, emotional, sociological or other factors and reading disability. An admirable review of studies of this kind is to be found in Gredler (1971). There is, however, a major problem in interpreting studies of the kind he describes: *in the case of every factor that is supposed to contribute to reading disability we can find a child who should be at risk who can read perfectly well.* In other words, it is no great problem to find a child who is emotionally disturbed, ESN, perceptually impaired or socially disadvantaged who can read tolerably well, even though children in these categories tend to be below average readers or even severely backward. How then do these various influences tend to affect some children, but not others?

I would like to discuss two concepts which, in my view, may be rather important in helping us to understand how this comes about. The two concepts to which I refer are *error factors* and *reading neurosis*.

Error factors

Error factor theory was developed by Harlow (1959) to account for the way in which human beings and animals learn to make discriminations and also how they 'learn to learn'. In initial learning to read, it is necessary for children to discriminate between the sounds of speech, and to discriminate letters and words. It is also necessary for them to learn how to learn new words which they encounter in print. What light may error factor theory throw on this?

First, what is error factor theory? According to this theory, a particular discrimination can only be learned if the correct general response is already in the response repertoire. Obviously, a child cannot discriminate red if he is colour-blind. Similarly, he cannot respond to length if he cannot judge size and distance, or to position if he cannot perceive body–object relationships, and so on. So much is obvious.

The critical point that Harlow emphasized, however, is that in learning to make a new discrimination in a particular situation the child, or animal, must *select* from his repertoire of responses that response which is *appropriate* in the new situation.

An important element in the child's selection is the preference he has for the various responses already in his repertoire. If, for example, you want a child to respond to 'twoness' the child may have a preference for 'redness'. Your verbal prompting may, for a variety of reasons, go over his head. And if you want him to attend to volume, as in a Piaget-type experiment, the child may prefer to respond to length.

The examples, of course, are endless, so we must group them in some way if we are going to talk about them sensibly.

Harlow suggested that four error factors were of particular importance: stimulus perseveration; differential cues; response shift; and position preference.

Stimulus perseveration
This refers to a tendency to persist in those responses to a stimulus which are based on preferences as in the examples given above. The preferences may be innate, as in the rat's preference for darkness; on the other hand, they may be the result of previous learning, as when a child taught to read by sounding separate letters says 'wu-a-su' for 'was' or 'tu-hu-e' for 'the'.

If opportunities for learning the correct response are plentiful such errors tend gradually to disappear. Sometimes they persist. This depends to some extent on the treatment the child receives each time he makes a response and we can see how in considering the next error factor.

Differential cue
We can easily make it quite clear to a child that he is correct in making a particular response. For example, we can show our approval when he says the word on the card we show him. But it is less easy to make sure that the child is responding to the relevant features of the printed word. If, for example, he is responding to a flash card, he may be responding to any one of a number of cues when giving the right word. He might be responding simply to word length, or to a dirty mark, or a tear on the card. He might be responding to the relative size of the word against the area of the background. If there are a number of words he might be responding to the position of the word in relation to other words. Some children will do almost anything rather than read!

The influence of this differential cue factor has been found to be a highly persistent source of errors. We can easily see why if we look at the effects of rewarding a correct response in a rather erratic fashion—a procedure known as 'intermittent reinforcement'. If we are constant in rewarding or reinforcing a correct response, the incorrect responses soon drop out and learning is fairly rapid. If on the other hand we are rather erratic in reinforcing a response, that response tends to become relatively fixated and highly resistant to change. Now, if the child is responding to a stimulus for the wrong reason, then in terms of *his* perception he will be receiving intermittent reinforcement.

Consider, for example, the case where a child is required to learn a fairly small number of words. They may occur as the first sentence in a reading scheme, as a set of words on a flash card, or as a block of words on a chart. Let us suppose that the child responds to position. He may possibly think that he is correct when he gives a particular word because it is the first word on the line, the third word shown to him, or the word in the top left-hand corner. He is bound to be right occasionally by chance alone. If he adds another cue, i.e. word length, he will be wrong less often. In terms of *his* perception he is then receiving intermittent reinforcement for responding to position and word length instead of shape. He will, therefore, become even more strongly fixated in responding to a cue that is either wrong, or inadequate. Many children confuse 'here', 'there', 'this' and so on—typical first words in sentences in reading primers. And many children confuse words like 'on', 'do', 'to', 'is' and so on—typical flash card or lotto words. Much of this may well be accounted for in terms of the intermittent reinforcement of differential cues—the classic route to error fixation.

Response shift

Children, like animals, tend to be unpredictable, even when there seem to be good grounds for us to expect them to be consistent. Even when they have achieved a high level of performance on a task, making no mistakes, they will often shift quite unexpectedly and make a 'foolish' error. Harlow (1959) explains this in terms of an exploratory drive, and reports that it seems difficult to suppress.

But when a child produces a response shift of this kind and makes a 'silly' mistake, what is the typical response of the teacher of an over-large class at the end of a tiring day? Hopefully, one may say that the teacher is usually tolerant. But it is hard to be tolerant when tired—particularly when faced with behaviour that seems to be at the least perverse and at the worst provocative.

It would be some help, at least, if the teacher knew that such behaviour is not necessarily blameworthy—that it is in some cases beyond the child's control. If we don't feel that a child is necessarily blameworthy, we often find it easier to deal with his behaviour with wisdom and good nature instead of inadvisedly and with impatience.

Position preferences

This is a special case of stimulus preservation. The source of position preference is often 'handedness', something that occurs in animals as well as man. But these are relatively unimportant sources of error in man, and the notion that handedness itself is an important factor in reading failure seems to be largely discredited (Clark 1970).

A complication: the suppression of a suppression
In general, Harlow's position is that one does not positively learn a 'new' response. What happens, rather, is that a number of responses that already existed are suppressed. Thus, in learning to recognize a letter we may learn, for example, not to attend to colour, line thickness, position, background detail or figure–ground relationships. We may then respond primarily to shape—a response tendency we possessed in the first place.

But let us consider the response to orientation—a very important factor in reading. For the first five years of our lives we have been learning to treat orientation as an error factor in identifying objects (Vernon 1957, Merritt 1970a). But nearly half the letters of the alphabet can only be distinguished from other letters by responding to their orientation. In the case of the following letters we must decide what they are by noting whether they are placed facing left or right, or one way up or the other: b-d-p-q; u-n; h-y; f-t.

The same argument applies to sequence. For example a child does not think of his train as being different merely because he switches the position of a couple of the carriages, or if he runs his train across from right to left instead of from left to right. It is still the same train. However a response to sequence is certainly in his repertoire in some circumstances. He soon learns that to be last in a queue is not very rewarding. What he does learn is to ignore sequence as a means of *recognizing* objects. That is to say, having learned to suppress his responses to orientation as an important factor in recognizing objects, he must now suppress that suppression. Little wonder that he is confused when he has to learn that 'was' is not 'saw', 'on' is not 'no', 'goal' is not 'gaol' and so on.

But there is worse to come. I have said that he has to suppress his suppression of response to sequence when looking at letters. He has got to do the same in order to learn to read sequences of words from left to right. But then he has to learn *not* to use a position response as a means of identifying words i.e. he must learn to recognize a whole word by its letters, not by its position in relation to other words.

If you find this confusing then what about the child? Just imagine trying to programme a computer to follow those instructions. And if you find this confusing you clearly do not understand an important element in the learning task. If *you* do not understand it then the child must be learning in spite of your teaching—not because of it. What a marvellous brain even the ESN child must have!

Let us return for a moment to the opening theme: if this orientation problem owes so much to learning, what do we gain by stressing the neurological aspect? If a child's difficulty with orientation does owe something to a neurological deficit of some kind we certainly cannot

John E. Merritt

operate on his brain. Whatever may have predisposed the child to experience difficulty, the remedial problem consists of developing the
appropriate learning sets. This is where more attention is really needed
both for practical and theoretical reasons.

Interaction of errors

Now let us consider the sum of all these factors. If we had 100 per cent
control over the learning situation for any child, we could, arguably, get
rid of the error factors fairly efficiently. But we do not have so much
control, nor anything like it. By chance alone some children will happen
to be exposed to a better array of learning situations than others.

Perhaps this point could be emphasized by means of an illustration.
During the last war, a 'buzz bomb' attack was launched on London and
certain districts were badly hit. In the second, third and subsequent
waves of bombing, certain districts which had already suffered severe
damage were hit again and again. It was then rumoured that the bombs
were being deliberately directed at certain targets.

A bit of careful analysis was enough to show that this was not the case.
If a limited number of bombs are directed in a certain general direction
then, by chance, they will tend to scatter and not all districts will be hit
in the first wave. In the next wave, each district already hit is just as
likely to be hit or missed as any other district. The same applies to subsequent waves. Until rather a large number of bombs have been launched,
therefore, there will be quite a number of districts which, by chance,
receive far more than their fair share. And, of course, some will receive
none.

Now let us relate this to the learning situation and consider the reinforcement of errors occurring in a similar way. It must be remembered
that we are talking about what *the child* perceives as reinforcement and
what *the child* perceives as the response that is being reinforced. As the
reinforcements don't occur very frequently, those that do occur will tend
to be spread rather unevenly between children and rather unevenly
within the total number of responses that any individual child makes.
Some will occur in such a way that learning is facilitated. Others will tend
to reinforce errors in the manner described above. Some children will be
very lucky. Some will be very fortunate. And many will be moderately
lucky and moderately unlucky. Hence, even if all children were equal
in all respects at the outset, their performances would tend to vary quite
appreciably over a period of time.

But of course all children are not identical at the outset. Some are
bright and others are less bright, some have minor perceptual lags and
others have some degree of emotional disturbance.

A child with one or more minor handicaps may be lucky. He may get
the reinforcements he needs just at the optimal moments. He may then
become quite a good reader. Another child may just happen to suffer
a pattern of reinforcements which fixates a number of errors in critical

areas. Being in any case at risk he suffers even more than the average child.

When a number of separate factors can all affect a situation, they usually interact. Thus, if we apply both water and fertilizer to soil, the water will influence growth, the fertilizer will influence growth, and some combinations of water and fertilizer will influence growth to a much greater extent than can be accounted for in terms of the separate effects. The interaction effects of all the factors affecting reading almost certainly operate in this way. The child with two defects is thus thrice handicapped.

Cumulative effects

In reading, as in mathematics, failure tends to be cumulative. If a child fails in certain elementary skills he will make little progress until the failure is remedial. If he is lucky, he may encounter a teacher with a good insight into the reading process who can help him. Or he may eventually realize how to help himself. Many children are not so fortunate and they build up a ballast of errors that sinks them as far as educational achievement is concerned. Again, there is this rather frightening element of sheer chance. And the consequences of being unlucky are disastrous.

Reading neurosis

I should like to draw your attention to a theory I presented at a UKRA Conference in Nottingham (Merritt 1970b). At that time I proposed that the term 'reading neurosis' should be used in a rather specific way. I made this proposal within the context of a different kind of debate and it got lost in the general furore that surrounded that particular issue. I should like, therefore, to restate the points I made.

The story really starts with Pavlov, or more strictly, with Shenger-Krestovnikova in 1914. A dog was trained to salivate when a luminous circle was projected on a screen. This was achieved by projecting the circle immediately prior to feeding. The circle, by the process known as 'conditioning', came to mean 'grub up'. Once this was achieved, an ellipse was occasionally presented but this was not followed by food. The dog then salivated when it saw the circle but did not salivate when it saw the ellipse. The shape of the ellipse was then changed by stages until it was almost that of a circle. There came a point at which discrimination ceased to improve and actually got worse over a period of three weeks. At this stage the dog clearly did not know whether it was on its head or its elbow—if we may paraphrase a colloquialism!

The whole behaviour of the dog underwent a sharp change. The dog, previously a docile animal, began to squeal in its stand, struggled in its harness, bit through some of the apparatus, and barked violently when taken into the experiment room. Later investigations reported signs of anxiety such as whining and trembling, a breakdown of the learning

John E. Merritt

already achieved, and a very much delayed response to the stimulus. A refusal to eat in the experiment room was reported by Dworkin and yawning and drowsiness were reported by Muncie and Gantt. Among the symptoms observed in a wide range of researches summarized by Hilgard and Marquis (1964) were the following:

1 hyperirritability
2 resistance to entering the learning situation
3 motor abnormalities, tics and tremors
4 changes in social behaviour, including refusal to join the flock, and symptoms of 'suspicion' and 'aggressiveness'
5 inability to resist making incorrect responses
6 loss of the ability to delay a response
7 autonomic symptoms including abnormalities of respiration, eliminative functions and heart action.

In a related set of experiments it is reported by Liddell (Hilgard and Marquis 1964) that experimental neurosis in sheep were very persistent, lasting for thirteen years or more.

Masserman (1950) reported the following symptoms which were observed in cats when they were punished for making a response which had previously been rewarded:

1 restlessness and agitation or, sometimes, passivity
2 fear responses—trembling, cowering, hiding, attempting to escape from the learning situation
3 'compulsively' stereotyped behaviour
4 regression to earlier patterns of behaviour.

I would add that experimental neurosis is often fairly specific, i.e. it is possible for it to be closely related to the task situation and for behaviour to be otherwise fairly normal.

The dominant element in these experiments appears to be the necessity of making an overly difficult discrimination. There is then a clash between a tendency to respond and a tendency not to respond. Sometimes the tendency not to respond arises because punishment is introduced. Sometimes it arises merely because the response is not rewarded—which is really rather extraordinary. Evidently, we do not need to punish children to induce stress—as the sensitive teacher well knows.

Let us consider the earlier analysis of learning in terms of error factors. The subject, according to Harlow, is required to suppress responses already in his repertoire—some of them the result of earlier learning. If the discriminations to be made are rather crude, or rather obvious, it would seem that the suppression of the wrong responses presents no great problem. Very often, however, the discrimination is neither crude nor obvious. For example, in the case of the development of number concepts, children with limited preparatory experience find the concepts difficult to attain. They do not appreciate which responses to suppress in order to respond to the very abstract numerical properties of the stimuli. Little wonder that so many develop 'number shock'. Indeed, there are very many otherwise normal adults who have the greatest difficulty in dealing with numbers, particularly under stress, as a consequence of early learning difficulties.

Does it not seem likely that there is a relationship between this sort of difficulty and the experimental neurosis induced in animals? In both cases there has been some initial learning and this has broken down when the discriminations have proved too difficult, too confusing. In both cases there is often a tendency to become anxious in the task situation. In both cases there is a strong tendency to avoid the situation altogether and to try to escape once it occurs—struggling, in the case of the animal, and making excuses for doing something else, being uncooperative, or being cooperative but engaging in distracting behaviour, in the case of the child. In both cases there may be a tendency to regress to earlier behaviour patterns. And in both cases there is often a breakdown of earlier learning. The child who seemed to have mastered a concept yesterday seems to have forgotten it today.

In both cases, stereotyped behaviour may occur. In maths, for example, the child may go through meaningless mechanical rituals without the slightest hope of solving the problem presented. Eliminative disorders, too, may occur in both situations. Bed-wetting and soiling are often equally likely to be due to other causes. However, they are a regressive type of behaviour and may well be precipitated by the stress of learning failure.

I have chosen the example of maths deliberately. From our point of view, in maths the material is quite clear and unambiguous. It is far from unambiguous to the child.

I need hardly add that reading presents much greater difficulties. The ambiguities are built-in. Letter orientation and letter sequence call for the suppression of well-established learning sets. For example, a response to single letters has to be suppressed in the case of digraphs. Another feature is that single letters can stand for many sounds—often sounds that are normally represented by digraphs, and so on. If asked deliberately to design a situation for trying to induce experimental neurosis, one could scarcely do better than use the beginning reading situation as a model. Indeed, the only consolation in all this is that the presence of a teacher who is warm in manner and methodical in approach makes an appreciable difference. This may be linked with the observation of Liddell (1954) that lambs are less likely to become neurotic in experimental situations when the ewe is present.

Of course it may possibly be the case that some cognitive disability, not reflected in IQ tests, accounts for the seemingly normal children who fail to make satisfactory progress, as Vernon (1957) suggests. As she says, a multitude of minor causes may hit such children particularly

John E. Merritt

badly. Such a disability would be hard to demonstrate, however, and the arguments based on the evidence presented here do seem rather impelling. They are impelling enough, in my view, to justify a considerable amount of attention by those who are actively engaged in research in this field.

Conclusions

I have argued that neurological hypotheses about causes of reading disability do not take us very far. Perhaps we might qualify this by adding 'except in very severe cases'. Such cases, I would suggest, are few. For most children who are diagnosed as 'dyslexic' or as having 'severe reading disability' we can find some children with similar disabilities who can read. What I have suggested, therefore, is that certain children may certainly be regarded as 'at risk' on the grounds of a variety of handicaps. But I have argued that it is a combination of circumstances in learning situations which may by chance act together to impair learning ability in ways indicated by error factor theory. The effects of these hazards are cumulative.

In addition I have suggested that they can occur in such a way as to induce a very persistent and severe learning disability—reading neurosis—a highly specific disability which may or may not transfer as a *neurotic* response to other learning situations. It does, of course, affect learning in other areas in which reading is required.

In my opinion these vagaries of the learning situation could well account for the 20 per cent or so of our children who are inadequate as readers. If this is the case we may regard beginning reading as a process akin to the slaughter of innocents rather than the exposure of the inadequates.

I am sure that teachers would appreciate more help in trying to understand the learning problems and possible modes of treatment of these unfortunates, and would prefer less emphasis on factors they could not conceivably control and which serve, largely, to justify our own failures.

References

*CLARK, M. M. (1970) *Reading difficulties in schools* Harmondsworth: Penguin
GREDLER, G. R. (1971) Severe reading disability—some important correlates in J. E. Merritt (ed) *Reading and the curriculum* London: Ward Lock Educational
HARLOW, H. F. (1959) Learning set and error factor theory in S. Koch (ed) *Psychology: A study of a science* vol. II New York: McGraw-Hill
HILGARD, E. R. and MARQUIS, D. G. (1961) *Conditioning and Learning* London: Methuen
LIDDELL, H. S. (1954) Conditioning and emotions in *Scientific American* 190, 48–57

MASSERMAN, J. H. (1950) Experimental neuroses in *Scientific American* March

MERRITT, J. E. (1970a) Reading skills re-examined in E. Stones (ed) *Readings in Educational Psychology—Learning and Teaching* London: Methuen

MERRITT, J. E. (1970b) An evaluation of the research report on the British experiment with ita in J. C. Daniels (ed) *Reading: Problems and Perspectives* United Kingdom Reading Association

VERNON, M. D. (1957) *Backwardness in Reading* Cambridge: Cambridge University Press

4 Diagnosis and treatment

Introduction

Permeating all thinking about correlates of reading failure is the question of how we make the inference from observed correlation to some kind of causal connection, and what kinds of conclusion about action we can then draw. In the Plowden Report (HMSO 1967) this problem is admirably summed up in the following terms:

> Association, though necessary, is not sufficient evidence of causality. For example, a factor loading—or a first order correlation coefficient—showing a positive relationship between size of class and school attainment does not justify the corollary that increasing class size will improve scholastic ability. A similar association with number of books in the home does not mean that if one made a present of a dozen books to a family, this would improve the child's school work. Winning the pools, and thus dramatically raising the family income, is unlikely to have any advantageous educational effect on the children, despite the correlation between income level and attainment. If the school nurse disinfests the hair of one or two children, this is irrelevant to the results on the next arithmetic test, in spite of the Manchester results on 'cleanliness'.

In short, positive correlation does not signify a direct causal link, and there is therefore no simple prescription to be derived from any such results. They can, however, suggest causes and means of improvement, and many of the papers in sections 2 and 3 have already included discussion in these areas.

In some cases, the direct causal connection between reading failure and other circumstances seems fairly plausible. Psychological diagnostic procedures usually take into account not only environmental correlates, but some assessment of the subject's perceptual, motor and psycholinguistic skills. Often, remedial work is based on these findings. In other cases the concomitants established must be seen as symptoms, or as consequences, of more fundamental disorders in our society and our institutions, and the ultimate remedies as lying in areas which may be quite remote from the immediacies of the classroom.

It is ideally desirable, in the interests of getting firmer evidence, to carry out some experimental manipulation of potential causes and observe the results. In many cases this cannot be done, either because ethical considerations preclude the kind of procedure that would be necessary, or because potential causes are not within anyone's direct control. So action has often to be taken on the basis of a hypothesis, if it seems to be both plausible and supported by correlational and followup evidence. Experimentation with potential causes is sometimes possible, however, and it is of course normally possible in studies of 'treatment variables'—methods and materials, the effect of the duration of remedial instruction, the size of remedial groups, the introduction of counselling. Studies of this latter kind are important, because the remedy for something that has gone wrong frequently consists not in removing the cause (which may be a series of events in the past and therefore irremovable) but in treating the resulting condition.

The papers which follow illustrate a variety of approaches to remedial work and to the problem of making it more effective. The procedures described are concerned with causes, and also directly with the resulting poor attainment—with attempting to specify the nature and extent of errors and to teach in ways which will put them right and thus extend the reader's independent skill.

The emphasis is on the successful fusion of diagnostic and teaching methods with a regard for the whole child as an emotional and social being.

Reference

DEPARTMENT OF EDUCATION AND SCIENCE (1967) *Children and their Primary Schools* (Plowden Report) London: HMSO

4.1 Diagnosing learning difficulties: a sequential strategy

K. WEDELL

School of Education, University of Birmingham

Reprinted from *Journal of Learning Disabilities* (1970), 3, 6, pp. 23–9

There has recently been considerable comment on the inadequacy of the psychological assessment of children with learning difficulties. It has been pointed out that the information yielded by these assessments is often neither sufficiently relevant nor sufficiently detailed to be of use to those concerned with the day to day management of children. A diagnostic strategy is proposed which may enable the psychologist better to use his time to obtain the information needed. Diagnosis is presented as an ongoing process of hypothesis verification. Some of the problems involved in this strategy are discussed.

Current practices in the diagnosis of individual children with learning difficulties have been widely criticized (Engelmann 1967, Gallagher 1966, Lovitt 1968). In general, these criticisms make the point that the diagnostic findings arrived at have little practical significance for those concerned in the day to day management of the child's difficulties.

For the educational psychologist, the problem often lies in obtaining information which has (a) practical relevance to the child's management and which (b) is sufficiently specific to indicate appropriate action. One of the main reasons for the psychologist's difficulty lies in his often self-imposed dependence on psychometric instruments. The psychologist may feel that his main contribution to diagnosis lies in his expertise in applying objective means of assessment, and thus may confine himself to using these, even in those cases where he knows that his findings will be of little help. The diagnostic strategy proposed in this paper is intended to redirect rather than to replace, the psychologist's use of psychometric instruments.

Diagnosis is, to a large extent, an attempt by systematic observation to arrive in a short period at information which could usually be obtained by informal observation over a longer period. In children, one of the main needs for diagnosis arises from the desire to prevent or reduce the potential effects of a disability. For this reason time becomes an important element in the choice of diagnostic procedure, if not for the more frequent reason

K. Wedell

of pressure of work. Any diagnostic strategy must take into account the psychologist's need to arrive at the relevant information as quickly as possible. How quick this may be depends, of course, on the complexity of the diagnostic problem, and on the size of error margin compatible with the decision the psychologist has to make. Frequently the available alternative courses of action open to the psychologist in making recommendations or provision for a child are relatively few, and several diagnostic outcomes would indicate the same action (Wedell 1966). In such a case, there may be little need for a high degree of specificity in diagnosis, and the relevant findings might be arrived at in a shorter time. An example of such a diagnostic problem would be the case of a three year old child whose language was delayed without evidence of hearing loss. Although ultimately there would be a need to distinguish the psychogenic and other etiological factors, the immediate recommendation of admission to a nursery programme would not depend on such a distinction. By contrast, a request for the diagnosis of a nine year old boy's specific reading failure would require correspondingly specific information to permit the recommendation of appropriate remedial action.

This paper is primarily directed at the application of a diagnostic strategy to the diagnosis of the cognitive and educational features of children's learning difficulties. Such an approach has of course to be based on certain assumptions about the nature of the relevant factors underlying educational attainment. Since the present paper is concerned with describing strategy rather than with the validity of these assumptions, they will be set out without further comment. In crude outline, it is assumed that a child's performance depends on:

1 the adequacy of his physical condition (e.g. sensori-motor function)
2 the development of basic cognitive skills (e.g. language, perceptuo-motor skills)
3 the acquisition of relevant concepts (cf. Piaget)
4 a knowledge of how to apply (2) and (3) to educational tasks
5 adequate motivation to make progress
6 opportunities for all the above to develop or be acquired.

Faced with the need to diagnose the cause of a child's failure in school, the psychologist will have to consider all these factors, or, if working in a diagnostic team, those factors not likely to be investigated by others. The diagnostic strategy proposed here calls for a sequential consideration of these factors at different degrees of specificity.

This strategy implies a further assumption, namely that most educational—and other tasks—depend for their successful completion on a number of component skills or processes. If a given task is successfully achieved, it is assumed that the component skills and processes subserving it are also functionally adequate. If the task is failed, on the other hand, the psychologist knows only that one or more of the component skills are

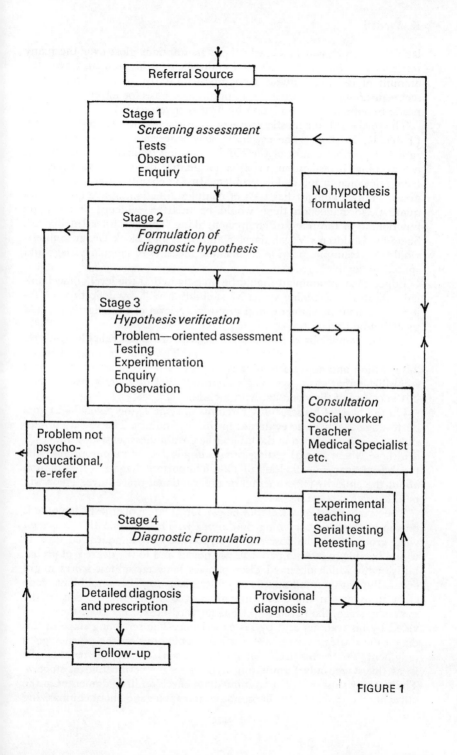

FIGURE 1

lacking, but not which. Clearly these assumptions gloss over the many intricacies of interaction between component skills, and also over the amount of ignorance about such interactions. In general, however, it seems justifiable to use such assumptions as a basis for formulating diagnostic hypotheses, for validation by further investigation.

The proposed diagnostic strategy consists of four successive stages (Table 1). In stage 1 the psychologist is concerned to cover the whole range of possible causes of the child's learning difficulty at the level of a 'screening' investigation, in order to identify those areas that seem to have relevance to the child's problem. In the cognitive and educational areas, the psychologist has tests of complex functioning available. Adequate performance on these would be used as evidence of adequate functioning of the relevant component skills. The Wechsler Intelligence Scale for Children's Vocabulary, Similarities and Block Design Subtests would, for example, provide a screening measure of language usage and spatial reasoning.

Educational attainment should be investigated at the level of mechanical skills at this screening stage. Most children will, by definition, be referred for poor attainment, and any higher level of investigation would probably be unrealistic.

Similar standardized screening measures are not available to assess motivational and other etiological factors. The items mentioned under 'observation and conversation' may appear rather comprehensive, but it seems likely that most psychologists normally tick off these items mentally in the course of their contact with a child.

On the basis of his screening attempts in stage 1, the psychologist goes on to stage 2, where he evaluates his initial findings. The variety of possible outcomes are listed in the table. The possibilities mentioned under (a) are those where formal testing proves impossible or inappropriate. The psychologist can, nonetheless, still obtain important diagnostic information about the child by experimental or observational procedures. These will be discussed in stage 3.

The psychologist may feel that he can formulate a diagnostic hypothesis on the basis of his 'screening' findings, (b). The question thus arises on what grounds does he base such a hypothesis? In standardized tests he would be able to refer to performance norms and to the degrees of probability, with which observed discrepancies between subtest scores might occur. But with a small sample of subtests such findings would have wide error margins. In the observational and conversational aspects of the screening stage, the psychologist has no yardsticks other than those provided by his training and by his experience. The screening stage of this diagnostic strategy thus places a considerable onus on the psychologist's judgment. This seems justifiable for two reasons. Firstly, the psychologist is, at this stage, only formulating hypotheses for verification in stage 3. The strategy thus builds in an immediate check on his judgment. On the other hand one should, perhaps, not be too apologetic about emphasizing

TABLE 1 *Outline sequential strategy*

Numbers to right of items indicate lines of further investigation if deficient performance is found. (+) indicates further investigation if no impairment found.

Stage 1 Screening assessment

A OBSERVATION AND CONVERSATION

Rapport, motivation and attention 44
Social adequacy and interests 37–39
Adjustment 35–38, 41, 42
History: personal 40, medical 42, educational 41
Sensori-motor state 24–27, 29–31, health 42
Speech 28

B TESTING

General abilities (abbreviated individual intelligence test.)
    verbal 10–13, 22, 23
    nonverbal 18–23
Educational achievement
    reading (word recognition) (+)1; 4–6
    spelling (word spelling) (+) 2; 4, 6, 7
    maths (oral problem with explanation of method) (+) 3; 8, 9

Stage 2 Evaluation of screening assessment

POSSIBLE OUTCOMES

(a) Rapport too poor for reliable evaluation
    (i) discontinue testing and observe 44
    (ii) build rapport for subsequent testing
(b) Formulate hypothesis
    (i) no problem: discontinue assessment
    (ii) problem not psychoeducational; rerefer
    (iii) screening indicates areas for further investigation (stage 3)
(c) No hypothesis possible

Stage 3 Hypothesis testing

A TESTING

EDUCATIONAL SKILLS (assessment leading to 44, 45 where required)

1 Adaptive skills: reading (comprehension) 10–13
2   spelling (composition) 10–13
3   maths (problems) 12–14. 1
4 Basic skills: reading: knowledge of letter sounds 14–16, 18, 19
5   blending 14, 18, 28
6   knowledge of spelling patterns 14–17 and rules 22

spelling: knowledge of letter sounds 14–16, 18, 19
  spelling patterns 14–17 and rules 22
7   handwriting 19, 20, 33
8   maths: written sums 20
9   basic operations 22, 31

COGNITIVE SKILLS (assessment leading to 44, 45 where required)

10 Language: expressive: vocabulary 14, 18, 26, 28
11   syntax 14, 15, 18
12   receptive: vocabulary 14, 15, 18
13   syntax 14, 15, 18
14 Memory: auditory: verbal 18
15   nonverbal, rhythm 18
16   visual: simple 19
17   sequential 19
18 Perception: auditory 26, 27
19   visual 24, 25, 31
20 Perceptuo-motor: pencil copying 19, 29, 31, 21
21   3-dimensional copying 19, 29, 31

CONCEPT DEVELOPMENT AND REASONING

22 e.g. Piagetian analysis (seriation, conservation and levels of reasoning) 12, 13, 19, 44
23 e.g. cognitive style (e.g. Kagan's reflexivity, impulsivity) 44

SENSORY SCREENING

24 Vision: acuity 42
25   eye-movement 42
26 Hearing: speech sounds 42
27   pure tone 42

MOTOR FUNCTION SCREENING

28 Articulation 43
29 Fine motor skills 39, 40–42
30 Gross motor skills 39, 40–42
31 Awareness of body coordinates 41

LATERAL PREFERENCE

32 Eye 40–42
33 Hand 40–42
34 Foot 40–42

ADJUSTMENT

35 Personality 40–42
36 Attitudes 40–42
37 Family relations 40

K. Wedell

TABLE 1   (*continued*)

---

38 Peer group relations	40, 41	instruction and rewards in free-field or
39 Social adequacy	40, 41	structured situations 45

B CONSULTATION

40 Family and personal history (psychiatric social worker, local authority
health and welfare workers)

41 School behaviour: peer and teacher–
pupil relations; study habits. (School
headmaster, class teacher, counsellor)

42 Medical information (e.g. paediatric,
psychiatric, ENT)

43 Speech (speech pathologist)

C EXPERIMENTAL INVESTIGATION (cognitive
and behavioural)

44 e.g. response to graded clues, brief

Stage 4   Diagnostic formulation

A PROVISIONAL DIAGNOSIS

45 (i) recommend

(a) experimental action (e.g. in
classroom)

(b) retesting

(c) serial testing

(ii) problem not primarily psychoeducational: transfer case as appropriate.

B Full diagnostic formulation and recommendation for action, including provision for report back on adequacy of
diagnosis.

---

the psychologist's judgment. In the last analysis, however objective the techniques he uses, his contribution in practical situations is based on the adequacy of his judgment, as is the case with the contributions of other clinicians.

Both hypotheses (i) and (ii) in alternative (b) will probably lead the psychologist on to some confirmatory investigation in section 3. It is probably only in rare instances, such as undiagnosed severe sensory loss or misreferral that he would terminate his assessment at this stage.

The psychologist may well judge that he is unable to formulate a hypothesis on the basis of his screening assessment. This situation is referred to in alternative (c), and would clearly lead him on to extend his screening investigations in each of the areas in his search for a hypothesis. He might, for example, go on to more subtests of an intelligence scale, further questioning, further tests of educational attainment or more formal assessment of personality or adjustment.

Stage 3 clearly forms the main part of the psychological investigation. The aim here is to continue the analysis of the component functions in those areas where the child fails, until the psychologist reaches the level where the child succeeds. This 'process of elimination' implies a knowledge of the relevant hierarchies of skills. While some research is available to indicate such hierarchies (Wedell and Horne 1969), in general the psychologist, like the teacher, has to rely on rule of thumb. This is an area for much needed research.

The sequence of this analysis of component skills and processes is indicated in the table. In the area of educational attainment, the sequence moves from mechanical skills to their components, then to cognitive skills, and finally to sensori-motor adequacy. Existing diagnostic tests such as the Illinois Test of Psycholinguistic Abilities (1968) and the Frostig Developmental Test of Perception (1966) fit in well as analyses at some of these levels. It is worth emphasizing, however, that the diagnostic sequence works from the target task (educational achievement in this case) downwards rather than the other way about. It was mentioned earlier that too little is yet known about the type and degree of component skills required in most educational tasks. While one may thus for example attribute known educational failure to specific cognitive defects, the present state of our knowledge makes an inference in the opposite direction very uncertain. The same can, of course, be said of emotional disturbance in relation to a child's earlier experiences. While in some cases one can ascribe maladjustment to specific aspects of a personal history, those same aspects in another child might have no effect.

Having formulated his hypothesis in stage 2, the psychologist may of course find it not substantiated by further investigation in stage 3. In this event, he would clearly have either to follow up a secondary hypothesis he might have formulated, or to widen his screening investigation in his search for one. In most cases, the etiology of learning difficulties is multiple, and several hypotheses from stage 2 would have to be followed up. More extensive intelligence testing might be indicated where the psychologist feels that a change in level of education may have to be recommended (e.g. EMR or ESN, provision). In such a case the normative level of the child's performance may clearly become more crucial, and so need to be based on a broader sample of his functioning.

There is one exception to the downward sequential analysis in stage 3. This refers to the investigation of what, by some, has been called the 'adaptive level' of educational proficiency. Clearly, failure may occur above the level of mechanical proficiency, for example in those children whose teaching has been too much in the form of drill, or who have achieved mechanical efficiency with such effort that they can hardly pay attention to applying these skills. This is often illustrated in the meagre compositions of children who have had difficulty in spelling and handwriting.

The investigation of sensory and motor function in stage 3 is seen here only as a more systematic screening procedure using tests such as the Reed Hearing Screening Tests (Reed 1960). Such testing would be aimed at a 'fail safe' level, leading to referral for specialist investigation in relevant cases (stage 3 B).

Assessment for lateral preference has been included for the sake of convention, rather than because of any conviction about its contribution to an understanding of learning difficulties. An exception to this would be unestablished or left-handedness, in its effect on the acquisition of handwriting.

It is difficult to spell out a sequential approach to the investigation of emotional adjustment, since this will vary so much with the individual psychologist's orientation. Presumably each psychologist will extend this section according to his own interests, competence and the availability of other professional help. If this area appears to be very relevant to a child's difficulties, the psychologist will wish to check his findings with those of the parents or the teachers. Findings on behaviour in a diagnostic setting may often be discrepant with findings in other settings. It may, for example, be important that the psychologist should establish more exactly the positive and negative motivational factors affecting the child's response in school, by consultation with his teachers.

Where facilities exist, the psychologist may seek amplification from psychiatrists and psychiatric social workers (stage 3 B), which may lead to a recommendation for onward referral at stage 4.

So far we have been concerned with the psychologist's application of his armamentarium of tests. The inclusion of stage 3 c emphasizes that the psychologist should apply his training in experimentation in the diagnostic setting. There are two main ways in which he may do this. The first involves the use of miniature learning situations. The psychologist may wish to discover how far a child is from attaining the next relevant level of skill above the one at which the child has been found competent. He may thus embark on a brief period of training during his diagnostic session. This would be exemplified by giving a child who has a knowledge of letter sounds a brief lesson in blending, to discover whether he has any idea of what is involved in this skill.

The other situation in which a psychologist may wish to use experimental techniques is the one referred to in stage 2, where the child does not respond to formal testing. Here, the psychologist may obtain considerable information of use to those responsible for the child, for example, by testing his response to specific stimuli (sound, light, people, objects etc), by testing his span of attention under various circumstances, and his response to different kinds of rewards (Lovitt 1968). The sequence of the psychologist's investigation may follow either his own formulation, or one implied by the referrer's statement of the problem.

More extended experimentation, involving either observation or teaching, may also form a recommendation at stage 4.

Stage 4 refers to the point at which the psychologist, or the team, conclude their initial investigation. The most common outcome will probably be a provisional diagnosis leading to some recommended action. Just as in stage 2 such a diagnosis is appropriately regarded as a hypothesis, validation for which is provided by the outcome of the recommended action. Even in those instances where a more definitive diagnosis is claimed, followup investigation should be instituted as a check on the validity of the diagnosis.

The psychologist or the diagnostic team may feel unable to arrive at a diagnosis after an initial assessment. Such a conclusion may lead to a variety of further strategies according to the nature of the case. The psychologist may feel the need to check the reliability of his findings with a retest after a period of time. He may be interested in evaluating the rate of a child's development, and so use his initial assessment as a base line against which to measure future progress.

Remedial action may be used in a more systematic experimental way as a test of a specific hypothesis. For example it is sometimes difficult to assess the extent to which a specific cognitive defect constitutes a handicap to a child who has very poor motivation to learn. Such an issue could be decided by exposing the child to a strongly motivating teacher regime (e.g. Hewett 1968) and observing its effect. This example also illustrates the way in which the psychologist and teacher can cooperate in diagnosis. A 'specialist' too often feels that his position obliges him to arrive at diagnostic conclusions on his own, wrongly supposing that his role is diminished by invoking the help of others—including the referrer.

Lastly, the psychologist may feel that his diagnostic assessment is at least sufficient to indicate that a child's problem is not primarily psychoeducational and requires investigation in another area of specialty. Psychiatric investigation and treatment is an obvious example of this.

It should, perhaps, be emphasized that the list of possible investigations mentioned in Table 1 is by no means allinclusive. It is offered only as an example. Psychologists will differ in their views of relevant functions, and each will tend to build up a list of his own.

Conclusion

The sequential strategy of diagnosis outlined here is aimed at enabling the psychologist to maximize the use of his time in arriving at findings which are both relevant and sufficiently specific to be of help to those concerned in the day to day management of the child. For many psychologists, this approach will not be new. Others may object that it forces the psychologist too much into areas such as skill analysis, about which too little is as yet known and which consequently leave the psychologist without any clearly defined means of formulating his diagnostic hypothesis. It may be argued that without a clear means of defining a discrepant function, too much is left to clinical judgment. To this objection, three points can be raised. Firstly, were it even possible to define discrepant function in probabilistic terms, a clinical judgment would have to be made about its relevance in an individual case. Secondly, this problem is common to diagnosis in all clinical disciplines. Thirdly, by exposing the problem, the strategy will hopefully draw attention to an area in which research is badly needed.

References

ENGELMANN, S. (1967) Relationship between psychological theories and the act of teaching *Journal of School Psychology* 2, 93–100

GALLAGHER, J. J. (1966) Children with developmental imbalances: a psychoeducational definition in W. M. Cruickshank (ed) *The Teacher of Brain-Injured Children* Syracuse: Syracuse University Press 1966

K. Wedell

HEWETT, F. M. (1968) *The Emotionally Disturbed Child in the Classroom* Rockleigh, New Jersey: Allyn and Bacon
LOVITT, T. C. (1968) Assessment of children with learning disabilities *Exceptional Children* 34, 233–9
WEDELL, K. (1966) Discussion in P. J. Mittler (ed) *Aspects of Autism* British Psychological Society
WEDELL, K. and HORNE, I. E. (1969) Some aspects of perceptuo-motor disability in 5½ year old children *British Journal of Educational Psychology* 39, 174–82

4.2 Basic principles of remedial instruction

G. L. BOND and M. A. TINKER
United States Office of Education;
University of Minnesota

Reprinted from G. L. Bond and M. A. Tinker (1957) *Reading Difficulties: Their Diagnosis and Correction* Appleton-Century-Crofts, pp. 241-66

The complexity of the reading act, the nature of reading difficulties, and the many characteristics of child growth and development that have a bearing on reading success make it clear that no two cases of disability are exactly alike. No two cases of reading disability result from the same set of circumstances, no two have exactly the same reading patterns, no two cases have the same instructional needs, and no two can be treated in exactly the same manner. Every child is different in many ways from every other child. Because a child's difficulties in reading stem from a wide variety of causes, the diagnosis of his case involves a study of the child to find out his instructional needs and everything else that may influence a remedial programme for him.

The remedial teacher studies the diagnostic findings and then arranges a learning situation that will enable the child henceforth to grow in reading at an accelerated rate. The remedial teacher's problem is to appraise materials and methods in order to select the combination that will best suit a given disabled reader. The many kinds of reading confusions children manifest indicate that no two disabilities will be corrected exactly the same way. Nonetheless, there are some basic principles underlying remedial instruction irrespective of the specific nature of a particular reading disability. There are certain common elements among corrective programmes, whether we are treating a comprehension case, a problem of word recognition, or an oral reading limitation.

Among the more important general categories of basic principles underlying treatment of disabled reading are the following:

1 Treatment must be based on an understanding of the child's instructional needs.
2 Remedial programmes must be highly individualized.
3 Remedial instruction must be organized instruction.
4 The reading processes must be made meaningful to the learner.

5 Consideration of the child's personal worth is necessary.
6 The reading programme must be encouraging to the child.
7 Materials and exercises must be suitable to the child's reading ability and instructional needs.
8 Sound teaching procedures must be employed.
9 A carefully designed followup programme is necessary.

Treatment must be based on an understanding of the child's instructional needs

The remedial programme must be designed to emphasize those phases of reading growth that will enable the disabled reader to grow rapidly and solidly. The programme designed for each child must be based on a diagnosis of his instructional needs. The purpose of the diagnosis is to obtain information about each child that is necessary in order to formulate a remedial programme suited to him. Watkins (1953) has shown that the child who is in trouble in reading often has an unequal profile showing an unfortunate pattern of reading skills and abilities. Some phases of reading will be well learned while other phases will be developed poorly. Still other phases may have been overemphasized to the point that they restrict the child's development in reading. The diagnosis must ferret out these inconsistencies in the child's attack on reading.

The child having difficulty in reading will show irregular performances. He may have a large sight vocabulary but he is unable to phrase well. He may be high in word recognition but low in comprehension. A reading diagnosis is designed to locate the inconsistencies that preclude rapid and effective growth in reading. The diagnosis is designed to locate essential areas of growth that have been neglected, those that have been faultily learned, or those that have been overemphasized. It is impractical to start a remedial programme in reading until the nature of the instruction needed by the disabled reader has been established. Otherwise, the programme may stress areas already overemphasized or omit areas needing attention or perhaps underemphasize such areas.

The remedial programme must be based on more than an understanding of the child's reading needs. It must also be based on the child's characteristics. The child who is hard of hearing needs a different approach to reading than does his counterpart with normal hearing. The child with poor vision needs marked adjustments in methods and, if his limitation is severe enough, in materials also. The child who is a slow learner needs modified methods and so does the child who is emotionally disturbed. The modifications of instruction for such children will be discussed in a later chapter.

As each case is different, there can be no 'bag of tricks' nor can there be a universal approach which will lead to the solution of disabled readers' problems. Many times, remedial training suited to one child would be detrimental to another. If, for example, a remedial programme has been planned to develop more adequate phrasing, the child might well be required to do considerable prepared oral reading in order to help him to read in thought units. The same recommendation would do serious harm to the youngster who is already overvocalizing in his silent reading. It would exaggerate the faulty habit he had acquired and increase his disability. To sum up, every remedial programme must be made on the basis of a thorough appraisal of the child's instructional needs, his strengths and weaknesses, and the environment in which correction is to take place.

Clearly formulate the remedial programme

After the diagnosis has shown the kind of instruction that is needed, the remedial programme should be carefully planned. This requires writing down what is to be done for each case. This must be done because it is too difficult to remember each child, his needs, the level of his attainments, and his limitations with the exactness that is necessary in order to conduct an effective corrective programme. The written case report should indicate the nature of the disability and the type of exercises recommended to correct the difficulty. It should identify the level of material that is to be used. The written report should state any physical or sensory characteristics of the child that need to be corrected or for which the programme needs to be modified. Any indication of faulty personal adjustment or unfortunate environmental conditions should be included. The child's interests, hobbies and attitudes should become part of the written record. Most important, it should include a description of the remedial programme recommended and the type of material and exercises to be used.

The remedial programme should be modified as needed

The original plan of remedial work is not to be considered a permanent scheme of instruction. It will need to be modified from time to time as the child progresses in reading. Often a child who is having difficulty in learning changes rapidly in respect to his instructional needs. The better the diagnosis and the more successful the remedial work, the more rapidly will the child's needs change. One disabled reader, for example, may have failed to build analytical word recognition techniques but is depending on sight vocabulary and context clues as his means of recognizing new words. He would be given remedial work designed to teach him the analytical techniques. After a time, he may develop considerable skill in word study, but he may not make a corresponding gain in rate of reading. His problem would no longer be one of developing word analysis. In fact, emphasis on this phase of the programme might become detrimental to his future reading growth. The use of larger word elements and other more rapid word-recognition techniques and further building of sight vocabulary would be advisable. As the problem changes, so must the programme of remediation be modified in order to meet the new reading needs of the child.

G. L. Bond and M. A. Tinker

Since the child's instructional needs change rapidly, it is unwise to set him into a remedial programme that resembles the production line in a factory. Such a programme assumes that once a given child's level of reading performance is identified, all that is needed is to put him through a set of exercises uniform for all children. There is no single method suited to all children even in the developmental reading programme. The disabled reader whose needs change rapidly as his limitations are corrected, is in dire need of a programme that readily adjusts to every change in his reading pattern. To achieve success, a remedial programme must be based upon a continuous diagnosis and it must be modified as the child's instructional needs change.

In some instances, the original programme for remediation does not result in improvement. When this occurs, a reevaluation of the diagnosis and perhaps additions to the diagnosis are in order. A somewhat altered approach to instruction may be necessary to bring success.

A variety of remedial techniques should be used
There is an unfortunate tendency, once a form of remedial instruction has been prescribed, to stick to the use of that specific type of exercise to overcome a known deficiency. Basing a remedial programme upon a diagnosis does not imply that a given exercise can be used until the child's reading disability is corrected. There are many ways to develop each of the skills and abilities in reading. An effective remedial programme will use a variety of teaching techniques and instructional procedures.

Many sources of help describing teaching techniques are available to the remedial teacher. Professional books on remedial instruction in reading give suggestions for correcting specific types of reading retardation. Russell and Karp (1951) have compiled a helpful group of remedial techniques. Manuals and workbooks accompanying basal reading programmes are the most fruitful source of teaching techniques. The exercises suggested for teaching the skills and abilities when first introduced in such manuals and workbooks are the sort of things that prove beneficial for remedial programmes. If, for example, a fifth grade child has difficulty with finding root words in affixed words, the teacher can find many and varied exercises in second and third grade manuals to teach this skill. The remedial teacher could have the child start with exercises which have simple variant endings on words, such as *walked* or *looking*. As the child improves, the exercises can be increased in difficulty up to those found in fourth and fifth grade manuals or workbooks which involve words with prefixes and suffixes, such as *unlikely* or *reworkable*. Teachers' manuals and workbooks accompanying basal readers give exercises and suggested activities that may be used to teach all skills and abilities in reading. The newer basic series of books have lists of these exercises with page references. As she examines the teaching techniques suggested in such materials, the remedial teacher can accumulate a variety of exercises for each of the important types of disabilities. She can keep the programme dynamic and interesting to the child by using a variety of teaching techniques and at the same time be sure that the instruction emphasizes the skill development that is needed.

In attempting to use a variety of teaching methods and techniques, care must be taken that the teaching approaches do not confuse the child. The directions given him should be simple and the teaching techniques should not be changed too often. The exercises should be as nearly like the reading act as possible. Artificial or isolated drills should be avoided. The child should not have to spend time learning complicated procedures or directions. Enough variety should be introduced, however, to keep the programme stimulating.

An effective and interesting teaching technique should not be used too long nor so often that it loses its value. A fifth grade child, for example, may be weak in visualizing what is read. For him, the remedial work is planned to emphasize the ability to form sensory impressions and to stimulate the imagination. The teaching techniques used have him read a story and then draw some illustrations for it. This is an effective means of getting this particular child to visualize as he reads. But remember, if he should have to draw pictures of what he reads every day, he may decide that he would rather not read at all. Variety could be introduced by visualizing for different purposes. At one time, pictures for a play television show might be made; at another time, the child might describe how furniture could be arranged for a creative dramatic presentation; at another time, he might read and tell how he thought the scene of a story looked. All of these purposes would require visualization of what is read.

Basing treatment upon an understanding of the child's instructional needs means that the remedial programme is planned after a thorough diagnosis has been made. It does not mean that the programme becomes fixed or that further study of the child is unnecessary. It is true that if the basic principles of remedial instruction discussed in this chapter are followed, approximately 65 per cent of disabled readers will improve even without diagnosis. However, there will remain somewhere around 35 per cent of disabled readers who will not get along well. Aside from those children who are described as cases of simple retardation, there is no way of knowing which children will be among the successful and which will be among the 35 per cent for whom the remedial work will fail. Whichever children the failures happen to be, they will probably become even more stubborn cases than they were before the remedial instruction started. Those children who did improve without a diagnosis would have improved even more rapidly if the remedial programme had been designed to meet their specific needs. Mass training by common methods is unfortunate even if given the label of remedial instruction.

The reason most programmes that attempt to correct reading disability meet with some degree of success is because the children are treated individually and many desirable adjustments are made. Even artificial programmes, which are basically poor, will demonstrate a modicum of success if they are given by an enthusiastic teacher because they are given to individual children. Well-rounded remedial programmes based on careful and continuous diagnosis, using a variety of teaching techniques and taught by an equally enthusiastic teacher, will give far better results.

Remedial programmes must be highly individualized

A programme designed to treat reading disabilities is based on the assumption that children learn differently and need programmes that meet their individual requirements. Such programmes must be based on a recognition of a particular child's physical and mental characteristics and must be designed individually to be efficient in overcoming his difficulties.

The remedial programme should be in keeping with the child's characteristics
The expected outcomes of instruction and the methods used in achieving these outcomes will need to conform to the child's characteristics. If the child is lacking in general intelligence, he can neither be expected to reach the ultimate stature in reading of children of greater mental capability nor can he be expected to progress as rapidly. The remedial teacher will be wise to modify the outcomes of the programme. The prognosis for rate of gain is usually directly proportional to the general intelligence of the child. In addition to lowering the results she expects, the remedial teacher would be wise to modify the methods of instruction also to meet the slow-learning child's needs. Such children need more concrete experiences, more carefully given directions, and more emphasis on repetition and drill than do children of higher intelligence.

If a child has poor vision or poor hearing, modifications in methods will need to be made. Such limitations make learning to read more difficult but in no way preclude the child from achieving. Deaf children have been taught to read about as effectively as their contemporaries with normal hearing when methods of instruction were adjusted to their needs. Children with marked visual defects have learned to read well, but they are more likely to get into difficulty. The disabled reader with lesser degrees of sensory handicaps can be taught more efficiently if his limitations are known and modifications in methods of instruction are made.

Remedial instruction should be specific, not general
The remedial teacher should focus instruction upon the specific reading needs of the child. The diagnosis has usually indicated that there is something specifically wrong with the pattern of the child's reading performance. One child, for example, may have learned to read with speed but falls short of the accuracy required in certain situations. Such a child should be given material to read that has factual content and he should read it for purposes that demand the exact recall of those facts. Another

child may be so overconcerned with detail that he reads extremely slowly, looking for more facts than the author wrote. He becomes so concerned with the detail that he cannot understand the author's overall intent. The teacher, in this latter case, would be specifically endeavouring to make the child less compulsive so that the rate of reading and its outcomes can become compatible with the purposes of this particular reading.

The principle that remedial instruction should be specific and not general means that the remedial teacher should emphasize those phases of reading development that will correct the child's reading limitation. It does not mean that just one type of exercise should be employed nor does it mean that a specific skill or ability should be isolated and receive drill. In the case of a disabled reader who has an insufficient knowledge of the larger visual and structural elements used in word recognition, the teacher would be making an error if he used a method that gave isolated drill on word elements. A more effective procedure would be to have the child read a basic reader at the proper level of difficulty. He would read for the purposes suggested in the manual, but when he encountered a word recognition problem, the teacher would help him by emphasizing the larger elements in the word. When the exercises given in the manual for developing basic skills and abilities were studied, the remedial teacher would have this child do the ones that gave him experience in using the larger visual and structural parts of the words. The teacher could construct some additional exercises that would provide experiences with the larger elements in words the child already knew so that he could learn to use these in recognizing new words. Types of exercises suggested in manuals of other basic reading series using vocabulary known to the child could also be used in constructing these teacher-made materials.

Remedial instruction should be energetic
Growth in reading presupposes an energetic learner. Of course, the child must learn to read by reading. He must attack the printed page vigorously and often if he is to succeed. A fatigued child cannot be expected to make gains during the remedial period. Therefore, the length of the period for remedial instruction should be such that concentrated work is possible. The disabled reader frequently finds it difficult to attend to reading for any considerable length of time. His lack of attention may be due to a variety of causes. In one case it may be lack of physical stamina, while in another it may be that he is not getting enough sleep at night, or it may be that his emotional reactions to reading sap his vitality. His inattention or lack of vigour may be due to habits of escaping from an unsuccessful and uncomfortable situation. Whatever the cause, most children if properly motivated can apply themselves to the reading situation at least for a short period of time. Obviously, if the lack of attention and vigour result from a condition that can be corrected, the correction should be made. In any case, the length of the remedial reading period should be adjusted so that an energetic attack can be maintained.

Frequently it is necessary to divide the remedial sessions into short periods. The child may work with the remedial teacher for a period of forty-five minutes. At the start of the remedial training, it may be necessary to have him read from a basic reader for only ten minutes for specific purposes and then have him use the results of his reading in some creative activity, such as drawing, constructing, modelling, discussing or the like. Then the child might work on some skill development exercises which emphasize the training he needs. These exercises might entail rereading the material he read at the first part of the session or they may be word recognition drill on new words introduced in the basic reader. Finally, the child might be asked to tell about the book he has been reading independently. As he gains in reading growth, the length of concentrated reading time should be increased. Soon the child who has no physical limitation will be reading longer without interruption. When this is so, the use of creative activities can be less frequent. Then the child can read for several days during the remedial periods before he utilizes the results of reading. He will still need to discuss what he has read and do the exercises suited to him as suggested in the manual or as found in the workbook.

Remedial instruction must be organized instruction

Reading instruction in both the developmental and remedial aspects must be well organized. The skills and abilities grow gradually as the child meets more complex applications of each. There is a tendency for remedial teachers to neglect the sequences involved in teaching the child each of the basic areas. In word recognition, remedial work is often erroneously given in one phase before the child has developed the learning that should precede it. The child may, for example, lack ability to break words into syllables so the remedial teacher gives him exercises to develop that skill. A study of the sequence in word recognition techniques might show that the child had many other learnings to master before he could be expected to be successful in this relatively mature approach to word recognition.

In order that growth in word recognition may develop smoothly, with no undue burden upon the learner who is already in difficulty, a gradual, orderly sequence must be maintained. Such organization is necessary so that there will be no omissions in developing the essential skills, so that there will be little chance for overemphasis, and so that new skills are introduced to the child when he has the necessary prerequisites for learning them. In learning to recognize words, the child should first establish the habit of left to right orientation before he is allowed to employ any detailed analytical attacks. He should also learn to recognize word wholes when he knows them, rather than to employ analysis; to use the context and initial elements before he is encouraged to attend to variant endings; and to form the habit of viewing the word systematically from start to finish before he is required to visually separate the words into syllables.

The child who is in confusion in reading requires even more systematic instruction than does the child who is learning without difficulty. The remedial teacher must either be completely aware what sequence of learning is desirable in all the areas of reading growth or she must use the basic reading material in which the orderly development of skills has been carefully planned out. The remedial teacher cannot afford to use haphazard approaches. She must follow the sequence and explain carefully each new step in it. Therefore, the most successful remedial teachers find it expedient to use basic reading programmes, modified to fit the child's specific needs whatever they may be.

The reading processes must be made meaningful to the learner

One reason why the disabled reader is in difficulty is because he does not understand the processes involved in being a good reader. The remedial teacher has the responsibility not only for maintaining orderly sequences of skill development, but also for making the steps involved meaningful to the child. The teacher should not only teach the child to use context clues in word recognition, but also she should let the child see how helpful such an aid to word recognition can be. The teacher should show the child how to organize the material he reads for effective retention. She should, in addition, let the child understand why such an organization is effective. The child should be led to understand the importance of reading certain material carefully with attention to detail, while other material can be read rapidly to understand the general ideas it advances.

If the remedial teacher expects the child to retain a knowledge of word elements, it is important for her to show him how much they will aid him in recognizing new words. For too long, many remedial teachers have felt that if the child is stimulated to read material at the correct level of difficulty he will automatically develop the needed skills. This point of view can be seriously questioned. A more reasonable assumption is that the child should be shown how to go about his reading and how much use he can make of each added reading accomplishment. Suppose a child, for example, has learned by rote to pronounce prefixed words. How much better it would have been to point out to him the prefixes in those words and show him how they change the meaning of the root words.

The remedial teacher will find that making the processes of reading meaningful to the learner helps to solve his reading confusions. Drill on isolated parts of words is not as effective as is a meaningful approach to reading. Modern developmental reading programmes are planned to enable the child to develop the needed skills and abilities and to understand the usefulness of each. The remedial programme should be concerned even more with making reading processes meaningful to the child. The day has long since passed when it was assumed that if we but interested the child in reading, he would effectively go ahead on his own to develop skills of which he was unaware.

Consideration of the child's personal worth is necessary

The disabled reader frequently feels insecure and defeated in school. Any remedial programme designed to treat reading disabilities must make the child feel his successes from the start. It must also take into account the child's sense of personal worth. The child who is in serious trouble in reading is often antagonistic towards reading and thoroughly dislikes it. He would like to wake up some morning knowing how to read, but he believes there is something wrong with him that precludes his learning to read. Frequently he thinks that he is mentally incapable of learning or that he has some other defect. Often he has a poor estimate of himself as a person.

Remedial programmes should consider the fact that the disabled reader builds a barrier between himself and all reading instruction. One of the first tasks of a remedial teacher is to gain the child's confidence. Resistance to the remedial programme will be magnified if the child is classified in any unfortunate way. Whenever the remedial work is to be done by the classroom teacher, the child should be a working member of that class. He should be able to enter into the various activities even though his part in them is meagre.

If it is necessary to give a child remedial training in the school reading centre, great care must be taken when the work starts. Remedial programmes should be considered a privilege and should be entered voluntarily. When the remedial groups are made up, it is strategic to include in them the brightest children who are disabled readers. These children are known to be bright and capable in other areas of the school curriculum and so the other children will see that the programme is for able children who are having some specific difficulty. Another reason for selecting the more able children to start with, is that in their instances there is a greater chance for rapid improvement. This will enable the programme to get off to a good start and will make it possible to do the most service to the greatest number. Besides, such an approach will place the remedial work in its proper perspective of being special instruction in reading rather than a class designed for the mentally inept.

In many schools, cases are selected for remedial work by sending the four or five poorest readers from each room to the reading centre. This is an unfortunate practice. As has been previously explained, the poorest readers in the room are not necessarily the children who will profit from remedial instruction in reading. Many such children are essentially slow learners. They are not disabled readers. Only children who are properly classified as reading disability cases should be sent to the school reading centre for remedial instruction. Another tendency is to refer disciplinary and delinquent children to the reading centre for individual work or for work in the smaller group. While it is true that many delinquent and disciplinary cases are poor readers, it is unwise to give the remedial teacher too large a number of these children at any one time. The correction of reading disability is a difficult task and if too many kinds of problems are concentrated in any one group, the teacher cannot hope to be successful. Also, the reading centre will acquire a reputation as a place for misfits.

In general, it is desirable to inaugurate remedial work with children who have the following characteristics:

1 General intelligence of over an IQ of 90 as measured by suitable tests.
2 Children who have asked to be admitted after the work has been discussed with them.
3 Children whose parents have requested such service.
4 Children who are classified as having reading disability as their major problem.
5 Not too great a proportion of children with behaviour problems at any one time.

Frequently the disabled reader is emotionally tense or insecure. He has had no real opportunity to gain confidence in himself because most of the school day involves reading. For some time he has been much less effective in school work than his intellectual level would indicate that he should be. Such a child may become submissive or demanding, aggressive or withdrawing, or show his basic insecurity in a variety of ways. He may develop attitudes of indifference, dislike, or rejection. He may resist help, display few interests, and be antagonistic towards reading instruction. Remedial reading programmes must overcome these unfortunate attitudes and compensatory modes of behaviour. One of the first responsibilities of the remedial teacher is to develop in the child a need for learning to read. The second is to gain the child's confidence to such a degree that he will know a personal interest is being taken in him and that now his reading problem is going to be solved. A direct attack on the reading problem by a businesslike, considerate adult will do much to overcome tensions and faulty attitudes. When a child recognizes that an interest is taken in him and his problem, it will give him the much-needed sense of personal worth and the confidence in himself that he has hitherto lacked.

The reading programme must be encouraging to the child

Most disabled readers are discouraged about their failure to learn to read. They frequently think that they cannot learn. This lack of confidence in their ability to learn is detrimental to possible reading growth. The effective learner is a confident and purposeful learner, one who has a desire to learn and finds pleasure in working towards this goal. In order that a child may go ahead rapidly in learning to read, it is necessary for

G. L. Bond and M. A. Tinker

him to know that he can learn and to see that he is progressing satis-factorily.

There are several principles underlying remedial instruction that give the child this sense of confidence he needs. The following principles will help to give the child the necessary encouragement:

1 The teacher must be optimistic.
2 The child needs group as well as individual work.
3 The child's successes should be emphasized.
4 A positive approach should be used in pointing out errors.
5 His growth in reading should be pointed out to the child.
6 Remedial programmes should not be substituted for enjoyable activities.
7 Remedial programmes must be pleasant and free from undue pressures.

The teacher must be optimistic

A teacher who would help a child to overcome a reading disability should be a buoyant, energetic person. She must make the child sense her confidence in him. At times, the problems involved in correcting a complex reading disability may seem to her to entail almost insurmountable teaching problems. Nevertheless, the teacher must approach each disabled reader showing that she knows he will learn to read. Such an attitude is an outgrowth of a thorough understanding of the instructional needs of the child, that is, a sound diagnosis, and of having the remedial programme planned well enough in advance so that the general nature of remedial instruction is clearly in mind. In addition, the teacher gains immediate confidence through knowing exactly what is going to be undertaken during each remedial lesson. A well-prepared teacher who knows exactly where each session is going will instil confidence in the child. With this preparation, progress in reading ordinarily takes place.

There are periods during the corrective treatment of practically every remedial case when there is little evidence of new growth. But all the same, confidence in the child's ultimate success must be maintained even when things do not appear to be going well. Under some circumstances the remedial programme should be restudied and the diagnosis reviewed, but all this need not lessen confidence in the child's ultimate success.

The child needs group as well as individual work

The disabled reader needs to share experiences with other children just as much as, or even more than, the child whose growth in reading is normal. Not only should his classroom work be organized so that he can participate in some of the important activities with which the class is concerning itself, but also it is beneficial for the child who is in difficulty to see that there are other children who are having similar difficulties. It is therefore recommended that whenever possible disabled readers should work in groups. Much good can be gained by the disabled reader seeing other children around him who are in a like difficulty, and who are making progress in overcoming it. It is sometimes assumed that remedial reading instruction is a formal procedure in which the child is separated from other children and drilled until his disability is corrected. Such instruction is most unwise. It is a boost to the child to know that there are other children who are learning to read and who are able to use their newly gained proficiencies in group situations.

The child's successes should be emphasized
In order that the remedial programme may be encouraging to the child, his successes rather than his mistakes should be emphasized. Teachers have a tendency to point out errors to children rather than to make them feel that for the most part they are doing particularly well. A child whose errors are continually focused upon may become overwhelmed by a sense of defeat. A wise teacher will start the child in a remedial programme that is somewhat easy for him so that his successful performance will be immediately apparent. As he gains confidence, the difficulty of the reading situations may be increased. The teacher should always be quick to recognize when the child has put forth a real effort and has done something well. Many times, particularly at the start, recognition will have to be given for activities related to the reading rather than the reading itself. Gradually the teacher will find increased opportunities to give praise for the actual reading that is well done. At all times it should be remembered that the effectiveness of remedial instruction depends in no small measure upon the child's gain in confidence. This gain in confidence is brought about through successful experiences with reading which in the past had caused the child so much difficulty.

A positive approach should be used in pointing out errors
The emphasis upon success does not mean that errors are to be altogether overlooked. The faulty reading of a child must of course be brought to his attention. Errors in word recognition must be pointed out. Faulty habits in reading which limit his speed must be recognized by him before they can be corrected. Sometimes it is necessary to demand greater exactness in reading on the part of the child. While it is true that the teacher must point out the child's mistakes, she must at all times indicate that the child is improving and that for the most part he is really doing well. If, for example, a child should call the word *house, horse* in the sentence 'The dog ran up to the house,' the teacher should point out to him that he had the sentence nearly correct, but that in order to be exactly right he should have looked at the centre part of the last word a little more carefully. As a matter of fact, the child did recognize most of the words in the sentence. He made an error that indicated that he was using the context well and that his error was a very slight one indeed. The words *house* and *horse* do look much alike.

In a comprehension lesson, the child may give the wrong answer to a question. Instead of saying that the answer is wrong and calling on another child in the group, it would be far better for the teacher to say, 'Let's see what the book says about this' and then find out where the child made his error. It will frequently be found that he did not understand the meaning of a word or that he failed to notice a key word such as *not*, or that he had not grouped the words into proper thought units. Whatever the cause of his error, it should be located and the child should be shown the correct way to read the passage. The attitude of the teacher should be not one of pointing out errors but one of helping the child learn to read.

Growth in reading should be demonstrated to the child
The disabled reader needs to have his growth demonstrated to him. There are many ways in which reading growth can be shown. The diagnostician has isolated the child's needs in this regard and indicated the amount of emphasis that should be given. It will be recalled that the method for demonstrating the progress of the child to him depends upon the nature of the reading problem. If, for example, the child is trying to develop a sight vocabulary, he could make a picture dictionary of the words he was try-ing to learn. As the dictionary became larger, the child would recognize that he had increased his sight vocabulary. The child who is working on accuracy of comprehension could develop a bar chart (Figure 1) in which he would indicate his level of per cent of accuracy on successive periods. If such a child failed to gain over the period of a week, the teacher could simplify the material or ask more general questions so that accuracy

FIGURE 1   *An accuracy bar chart*

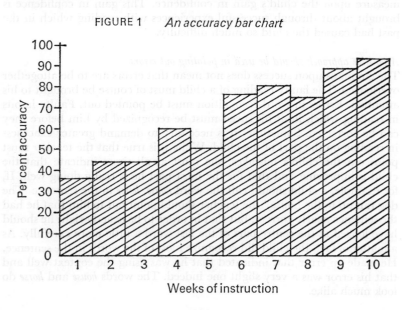

Weeks of instruction

222

would increase. Then as the child gained confidence, the difficulty of the material could be gradually increased again. It is a good plan for the child to go back, from time to time, and reread something that he has read previously. He will discover that material that was difficult for him a short while ago, is now relatively easy for him to read. This will be especially true if the teacher takes time to develop the necessary readiness prior to the reading.

Whatever the nature of the difficulty, it is important for the remedial programme to be organized to demonstrate to the child that he is progressing towards his goal of better reading. The child who has been in difficulty for a long time needs whatever encouragement can be given him. He needs not only to be in a comfortable learning situation, but also he needs to see that he is making effective advancement in reading.

Remedial programmes should not be substituted for enjoyable activities

The remedial teacher must so organize the periods of instruction that children are not required to come for training at a time that competes with other activities of great importance to them. For example, it is a frequent practice to have children come to a clinic for remedial instruction after school. This is a decidedly unfortunate time for a boy who enjoys outdoor sports with his friends, and who finds this the only time that such outdoor games are played in his neighbourhood. In scheduling summer reading programmes, it is wise to delay their start until a week or so after school is out and the children have found that they have time that they do not know what to do with. Even then the better scheduling time for classes is probably in the morning because the majority of things that the child likes to do, such as going swimming or playing baseball, are done in the afternoon.

The busy classroom teacher frequently finds it difficult to give an individual child attention he needs when the class is in session. She may therefore select recess time or the time in which other children have their hobby clubs, or are in the auditorium viewing a film, for helping a child with his reading. Such a practice is understandable but is unfortunate for the correction of a reading disability. A better time would be to work with the children needing reeducation while the rest of the children are busily engaged in studying or reading independently. Whatever time is used for giving remedial help, it is important that it does not conflict with activities which are important to the child.

Remedial programmes must be pleasant and free from undue pressures
An effective remedial programme must be one that is satisfying to the child, makes him feel that he is getting along well, and keeps at a minimum any anxiety which he feels about his reading progress. The teacher's responsibility in encouraging the child to read energetically is indeed great. She should neither unduly hurry the child nor allow him to dawdle;

she should be sure the child is working hard and yet avoid putting undue pressure on him. Most children, in fact practically all children can be expected to work intently in developing reading ability. This is especially true if the reading materials are at the right level, if the child is properly motivated, and if he is reading for purposes that are real to him. There should always be a friendly atmosphere, but an atmosphere that keeps uppermost the point of view that the child is there to learn to read.

Materials and exercises must be suitable to the child's reading ability and instructional needs

The selection of appropriate material for remedial work in reading is one of the most important problems the remedial teacher has to solve. Some teachers feel that the most important element in the problem is that the material should deal with a subject in which the child is interested. Others feel that the level of difficulty of the material is of even greater importance. Still others believe that having the type of material that is compatible with the nature of the remedial instruction is of paramount importance. There can be no doubt that all three of these elements enter into the selection of appropriate material for remedial instruction. Without trying to decide here between them, we may conclude that the more important considerations in selecting material are:

1 The materials must be suitable in level of difficulty.
2 The materials must be suitable in type.
3 The materials must be at the appropriate level of interest and format.
4 The materials must be abundant.

The materials must be suitable in level of difficulty
The child grows in reading by reading, therefore the material that is used for remedial instruction should be of a difficulty that enables the child to read comfortably and with enjoyment. The diagnostician will have suggested the level of difficulty of the material the child could be expected to read. The remedial teacher must pick out materials at that level to suit the child. The difficulty of material can be judged in many ways. Readability formulas, such as the Lorge formula (1944), the formula of Dale–Chall (1948) and that of Spache (1953) have proved useful in estimating the reading level of materials. Most of the basic readers are carefully graded and indicate the level of reading maturity necessary for their use. The difficulty of an ungraded library book may be judged by comparing it with the various grade levels of a basic reader. For example, a library book can be compared with a third grade reader. If it is judged to be harder, it may then be compared with a fourth grade reader, and so forth, until the approximate level of difficulty can be estimated. In making the judgment, the teacher should look at the number of unusual words it contains, the length of its sentences, the number of prepositional phrases,

the number of unusual word orders, the complexity of the ideas it includes. In judging level of difficulty, it is important that the remedial teacher remember that the results of standardized survey tests tend to give an overestimation of the skill development of a reading disability case. Therefore, it is usually wise to start remedial instruction with material that is somewhat lower than the child's general reading score as indicated by standardized tests.

The difficulty of the material that is suitable for remedial instruction will vary somewhat with the nature of the child's disability. The teacher should modify the general estimate of level of difficulty according to the outcomes of instruction to be achieved by the use of that material. For example, if the child's major problem is one of developing sight vocabulary, the material should be relatively easy with few new words being introduced. Those that are introduced should be used often in the material. For such a child, a relatively easy level in a basic reading programme would be desirable. On the other hand, for the child who is trying to analyse words effectively, a higher concentration of new vocabulary would be desirable. The child could well afford to meet one new word in approximately every 20 running words. This would give him an opportunity to employ the techniques of word analysis that he needs to develop and at the same time it will enable him to maintain the thought of the passage so that context clues can be used as a means of checking the accuracy of his word recognition.

A child who is trying to increase his speed of comprehension should use material that is for him definitely easy. Such material would have few if any word recognition problems for him. On the other hand, the child who is trying to increase his power of comprehension should use material with which he must tussle, but he must have a reasonable chance of successfully comprehending the material.

The materials must be suitable in type
It is often said that any kind of material that is suitable for teaching reading in the first place is suitable for remedial instruction. While this is true, it is important to recognize that the material must be nicely selected to meet the child's instructional needs. The type of material that is suitable for one kind of disability is not necessarily suitable for another. If the child's major problem is that of increasing his speed of reading, the most suitable material would be short stories whose plots unfold rapidly. The material should not only be easy in regard to reading difficulty, but the nature of the content should be such that the child can read it to gain a general impression or the general significance of the story. If, on the other hand, the child's problem is one in the word recognition area, a basic reader along with the exercises found in the manuals and the workbooks related to the word recognition problem would be the most desirable type of reading material to use. If the child's problem is in the comprehension area and it is desired to increase his accuracy in reading, material in

science or in social studies that has considerable factual information should be used. In every instance, the material should be at the appropriate level of difficulty, but also in every instance, the material should be of a type that is appropriate to the outcomes of reading expected.

The materials must be at the appropriate level of interest and format
A relatively mature and intelligent twelve year old will usually not find first and second grade material interesting, nor will he find the format very attractive. Such a child with second grade reading ability must nevertheless use material that he can read. The problem facing the remedial teacher in this respect is very great. The second grade book is designed for a child who is seven or eight years of age. The pictures in it are of small children and its print looks large and juvenile. The topics dealt with in the book are appropriate to the seven or eight year old and not to a twelve year old. Therefore, many books that are used for remedial reading instruction lose some of their value because they lack interest and have the wrong format. In such a case, however, there can be no compromise with the need for using material that is at the suitable level of difficulty. The problem resolves itself, then, into how to find material that is of a suitable level of difficulty and is as appealing as possible to a child of more mature age.

The materials must be abundant
In selecting material for remedial work, the first and most important consideration is that it must be of the proper level of difficulty. The second is that it should be appropriate in type. The third is that it should be interesting in format and meet the interest level of the child. Another consideration in securing materials to be used in remedial reading is that they should be abundant. There should be a wide variety of material meeting many interests and at various levels of difficulty. For any one child, there should be ample material suitable for him to read. There should be material for his remedial instruction and also material for his independent reading. The independent reading for a remedial reading case should be considerably easier than that used in giving him remedial instruction. The material for independent reading needs to be on a wide variety of topics because the children will have a wide variety of interests. The material that the child is to read independently should fulfil an existing interest which the child already has, while the material that is used for instructional purposes must be such that he can be motivated to take an interest in reading.

Sound teaching procedures must be employed

During the entire discussion of principles for treatment of reading difficulties, it has been implied that remedial instruction is the application of sound teaching procedures directed towards the specific needs of the child.

Instruction in remedial reading is not unusual in character nor is it necessary to use expensive and artificial equipment. The skills and abilities should be emphasized in actual reading situations free from isolated drill. Sound teaching procedures such as those used for introducing the reading skills and abilities in the first place should be used. The materials best suited to remedial instruction are those that are best for the developmental programme.

The difference between remedial instruction and the developmental programme is in the extent of individualization and in the study of the child rather than in the uniqueness of the methods or materials it employs. There are certain principles of reading instruction that are sometimes neglected in remedial work. Readiness should be carefully built for every topic and every selection to be read by the disabled reader. This includes the creation of interest in, the development of background for and the introduction of new words for each selection the child reads. The child who is in difficulty in reading, just as much as other children who are not, should have the purposes for reading well understood before the reading is done. He should also use the results of his reading in a creative enterprise of one sort or another. If, for example, he has read a selection about flood control to find what techniques are used, it would be important for him to make a diagram of a river bed illustrating what he had learned, just as it would be for children in the developmental reading programme. Seeing that children use the results of their reading is a good procedure for all children. It becomes an essential practice, though an often neglected one, for children who are in difficulty in reading. The form of use to which the results of reading are put may be a discussion, a picture drawn, a chart made, a map planned, or any one of many such enterprises. The relative amount of time devoted to these things should be small, however, and above all, the creative work should be the child's own.

Consideration must be given to the learning environment of the child both in and out of school. Whether the remedial work is done in the classroom, the school reading centre, or the clinic, only a small segment of the child's reading is done during the corrective lessons. If the remedial programme is to be successful, the rest of the child's reading day must be adjusted to his needs and reading capabilities. The effective work of the remedial periods can be destroyed if unfortunate demands or pressures are placed upon the child either in school or at home. As has been stated earlier, both the classroom teacher and the parents will be willing to co-operate if they are given an understanding of the child's reading problem. The parents are often endeavouring to help the child with his reading, and this is as it should be, but the remedial teacher should consult with them so that their work will be of the greatest benefit to the child. Bond and Wagner (1955) show many ways in which parents can help a child to grow in reading.

The remedial teacher will find it helpful to keep a cumulative account of the child's progress. The record should include the books read; the

G. L. Bond and M. A. Tinker

type of exercises used, and the success of each; any charts used to show the child his progress; and the results of periodic tests. In this connection, any indications of fields of interests and anecdotal accounts of the child's reactions to the remedial programme will be a help. By studying this record, the teacher can compare periods of rapid growth with the type of exercises used and books read at those times. A study of past records will recall to the teacher those approaches that were successful with other similar cases. The teacher can assemble a file of such folders, arranged according to the specific problem involved.

A carefully designed followup programme is necessary

When the child has made progress sufficiently to permit his release from the concentrated remedial programme, he should gradually be put into situations where he must rely to an increasing extent on his own resources. All such children should be carefully followed up by the classroom teacher. For many, continued reinforcements by means of further remedial help are most important. In a study of the long-term effects of remedial reading instruction, Balow (1965) found that continued remedial training, amounting to long-term treatment rather than a short-course programme, is desirable. He concludes that concentrated remedial work gives remarkable results, but that 'severe reading disability is probably best considered a relatively chronic illness needing long-term treatment rather than the short course typically organized in current programmes'.

Many of the children with less severe reading difficulties may be able to make the adjustment into regular classroom work. Even these children may become discouraged again if their work does not go well after they finish remedial instruction. Any indications of loss of interest or of confusions in learning should get immediate attention by the classroom teacher during the readjustment period.

References and selected readings

BALOW, B. (1965) The long-term effect of remedial reading instruction *The Reading Teacher* 18, 7, 581–6
BLAIR, G. M. (1956) *Diagnostic and Remedial Teaching* rev. ed. New York: Macmillan
BOND, G. L. and WAGNER, E. B. (1955) *Child Growth in Reading* Chicago: Lyons and Carnaham
BOND, G. L. and WAGNER, E. B. (1966) *Teaching the Child to Read* 4th ed. New York: Macmillan
BRUECKNER, L. J. and BOND, G. L. (1955) *Diagnosis and Treatment of Learning Difficulties* New York: Appleton-Century-Crofts
DALE, EDGAR and CHALL, JEANNE (1948) Formula for predicting readability *Educational Research Bulletin* 27 Ohio State University, Columbus 11–20 ff, 37–45

*DURRELL, DONALD D. (1956) *Improving Reading Instruction* New York: Harcourt, Brace and World

GATES, ARTHUR I. (1947) *The Improvement of Reading* 3rd ed. New York: Macmillan

HARRIS, ALBERT J. (1961) *How to Increase Reading Ability* 4th ed. New York: Longman

KOTTMEYER, WILLIAM (1959) *Teacher's Guide for Remedial Reading* St Louis: Webster

LORGE, IRVING (1944) Predicting readability *Teachers' College Record* 45, 404–19

RUSSELL, D. H. and KARP, E. E. (1951) *Reading Aids through the Grades* New York: Teachers' College, Columbia University

SPACHE, G. D. (1953) A new readability formula for primary grade reading *Elementary School Journal* 52, 410–13

*TINKER, MILES A. and McCULLOUGH, C. M. (1962) *Teaching Elementary Reading* 2nd ed. New York: Appleton-Century-Crofts

WATKINS, M. (1953) A comparison of the reading proficiencies of normal progress and reading disability cases of the same IQ and reading level Unpublished PH.D. thesis, University of Minnesota, Minneapolis

4.3 A method to meet the needs of backward readers

GEOFFREY R. ROBERTS

Department of Education, University of Manchester

Reprinted from Geoffrey R. Roberts (1969) *Reading in Primary Schools*
Routledge and Kegan Paul, pp. 72–85

Causes of backwardness

Many teachers of nine, ten and eleven year old backward readers have difficulty in finding a method which will help these children to forget their failure and restart the process of learning to read with ease and fluency. They will, of course, be aware of the fact that the backwardness may be caused by physical defects in sight or hearing, or by emotional disturbance (Vernon 1957), and the teacher should examine these possibilities by obtaining advice from the educational psychologist and using, with care, diagnostic tests and observations. However, it is not the purpose of this paper to examine testing or to prescribe methods for children with physical or emotional defects. There are many backward readers who, for one reason or another, have just not mastered the difficulties of reading. They have no physical defects which should impede their progress in reading and the degree of emotional disturbance does not appear to be sufficient to cause them any insuperable difficulties. To all outward appearances they are just slower children.

It may be that the methods employed when they were first introduced to reading were unsuitable or they may have failed to master crucial parts of their training in the basic reading skills. Dr Joyce Morris (1966) found some of the following deficiencies amongst poor readers: inability to tackle isolated words, insufficient knowledge of the names and sounds of the letters of the alphabet, limited ability in the analysis and synthesis of words in terms of their constituent sounds, lack of directional attack upon words, inattention to the details of words, and inadequate capacity to memorize words. Birch and Belmont (1964) have suggested that one of the difficulties retarded readers experience is that of integrating what is seen with the appropriate sounds. Blank and Bridger (1966) accept this finding, but they suggest that it may be more exactly explained by a failure to label the letters of a word. They do not exclude other explanations; for example, that retarded readers possess a knowledge of the labels but do not use them because they pay insufficient attention to detail, or that there may be a defect in the sensory systems. However, the important implication of these researches for classroom procedure is that a remedial method in general use should be one which emphasizes and helps both the application of the relevant verbal labels to the visually presented words and letters, and also the integration of auditory–visual information. In doing this it may enable the children to learn to accomplish those parts of the skill that they have missed.

Of course there may be other factors which have played their part. These children may not have been sufficiently interested in the content of the reading materials and lessons to want to learn to read; they may not have been compatible with their teacher; or there may have been any one or more of a number of influences working upon them in such a way as to distract them from reading—for example, home circumstances, where there was a lack of respect for reading. Any one of these factors could have prevented the child from concentrating upon learning to read at a vital stage and, thereby, he could have missed crucial parts of the instructional programme.

Requirements of the teacher

The teacher, in these circumstances, requires a method which rekindles the child's desire to read and enables that child to retrieve the situation by learning what he may have missed. It is not a clinical situation where one teacher is able to deal with one child. On the contrary, there are thirty to forty children in the class and, therefore, the method chosen must be comprehensive, even though, as in the case of unstreamed classes, the number of children requiring remedial teaching may be half a dozen at the most. In more homogeneous classes this number will be substantially higher. In these situations the main method or approach must provide a comprehensive coverage of a large number of possible deficiencies in reading and, at the same time, it must be simple to operate and control.

Fernald's method

One method which is sometimes suggested is that described and used by Grace Fernald (1943). Unfortunately, most of those who advocate this method stipulate that it is good 'as a last resort'. Why, it is difficult to understand, unless it is because it involves the teacher in a little extra unusual work! But then surely some deviation from normal practice is absolutely essential if children have reached the age of nine or ten and are still finding reading difficult. And most teachers in charge of children in such dire circumstances are only too pleased to adopt any method which may succeed. Fernald's method, described in chapter five of her book and designated as a method for total or extreme disability, has all the ingredients of a general and valid method of remedial teaching.

The needs of the children

When studying a remedial method for teaching children to read, it is important that the first consideration should be the general needs of the children. It must be remembered that these children have failed and that they know that they have failed. This creates a situation so critical that any feasible method must create the conditions in which learning will again be possible. In order to accomplish this, five general needs must be covered. They are:

1 The children need to be convinced that they can learn.
2 They need to be shown a mechanical process which will help them to learn and remember words and phrases and which gives them an insight into how words are constructed.
3 They need a totally different method of learning to read.
4 They need something which shows clearly and instantly any progress they make.
5 They may need specific help in certain aspects of reading.

Having defined the needs of the children and their requirements in broad terms of methodology, it is now possible to examine Fernald's method in detail and to see how it fulfils these needs.

The first and second needs

The first and imperative need is what Fernald called reconditioning: the teacher must convince the children that they can learn, that their failure up to now has not been their fault but rather the fault of the methods by which they have been taught previously. And to lighten the whole aspect of their expectation of the new burden about to be thrust upon them, they can be told that all that has been lacking is that they have not been shown the 'tricks of the trade' and that now they are about to be introduced to the secrets; everyone knows the strength of the human desire to belong to an 'in group'!

This leads to the second need. It is useless to tell these children to learn words or phrases without showing them how to set about learning. They need some framework of active participation in the learning process, which is mechanical and remains constant. It should also be capable of easy adaptation at later stages as the child progresses.

When one examines the details of the ways in which Fernald's method deals with these two needs, one sees that she spared no effort during the reconditioning period to convince the children that they could learn words. A reputedly retarded reader is asked to choose a word he thinks is difficult. This word is then written in large writing on a piece of paper and the child traces over the word with his forefinger. Simultaneously, he pronounces the syllables of the word, e.g. pen-cil.

The tracing and vocalization of the word are repeated, ten or twenty times, until the child thinks that he can write the word without copying. When he has tested himself on another piece of paper, and is satisfied that he knows the details of the word, he is asked to display his ability to the class by writing the word unaided on the blackboard. The effect of success on the child, and on the rest of the class is electrifying. All are keen to try this 'new trick'.

Failure by any child to write the word correctly can be redeemed by the teacher striking an optimistic attitude and asking the child to continue the tracing and vocalization a little longer. At this stage it is imperative that success is achieved, even if the child has to trace the word fifty times in all.

This method of learning new words is simple, direct, and whilst conforming to a single pattern which a teacher can impose upon a large number of children, it incorporates a wide variety of ways of learning words by visual, auditory, tactile and kinaesthetic means. As such, it is extremely useful for the teacher who knows little of the sophisticated ways of dealing with backwardness in reading, but who nevertheless has to face every day a class of children who desperately need help. The child's 'attention is not called to the words he does not know but to the fact that he is capable of learning any words he wants to learn' (Fernald). Furthermore, it seems reasonable to suppose that by constantly tracing and saying the parts of words, the child will gain an understanding of the construction of words. This knowledge will call the child's attention to the integration of visual stimuli and auditory responses and it will help him to make the predictions about clusters of letters, which Gibson (1963) found so important.

One note of caution should be introduced. It is absolutely essential to the whole of Fernald's method that the tracing should be done on the paper with the forefinger. Neither a pencil nor tracing paper should be used, for these impede learning through the tactile and kinaesthetic senses. Even adults find it difficult to copy letters, or anything else, through tracing paper. The concentrated effort that is necessary to hold the tracing paper in place and to follow the lines of the letters, divert the child's attention from the general kinaesthetic 'feel' of the word—i.e. the rhythmical movement involved in tracing the word with a finger. The experiment of Miles (1928) and Husband (1928) and Fernald's own comments show the advantages of direct unimpeded contact between paper and finger as a learning device.

The third and fourth needs

The third need is for something totally different from anything that they have had in the past. It should be a method or device which is within their ken, in that they can manipulate it with ease; it must hold their attention through manipulation; and it must, by its approach, hold their interest. It must, in effect, be something which gets away from the type of books on which they have failed and from the apparatus and all the paraphernalia of postinfant school doldrums, into which these children may have been cast.

Yet they need something which shows clearly and instantly any progress they make, and which constantly reminds them that they are making progress in *reading*—not in games, not in exercises, but in actually reading the written text.

Fernald's method gives them something totally different. It does not rely upon reading books (although it certainly does not exclude them) and it does not require any apparatus apart from pencil and paper. It is based upon the construction of their own reading material by the children. Once they have been reconditioned and introduced to the tracing–vocalization method of learning words, they are asked to write stories which will be placed, eventually, in their own 'reading book'. These stories can be written about any topic and can be of any length, from one sentence to as many pages as the pupil or teacher likes. Any words they cannot spell are written for them by the teacher and are learnt by the tracing–vocalization method before being used in the story. A record of these words is kept in a personal box file by each child. Other teachers may prefer to keep a record of these words by writing them on the back of the child's original story, storing them and periodically handing them back to the child for him to revise the words he has learnt. Both these ways of recording new words have their advantages. The former is neater, it forms an easy means of reference back to words already learnt, and it acquaints the child with alphabetical order. The latter is by no means an easy form for referring back, but for the purposes of revision it enables the child to reencounter all these words within the meaningful and perhaps vivid setting in which they were first encountered. Meaningful associations would be rekindled and the child's facility in their usage would be enhanced.

When the story is completed the teacher reprints it, with reasonable corrections to grammar and without any spelling mistakes, within twenty-four hours, if possible. It is then pasted into the child's 'reading book' and the child reads it aloud to the teacher.

As time goes on the tracing and vocalization may diminish and gradually disappear, so that the child is then left with a method of learning words which has evolved out of the tracing and vocalization and which is satisfactory to the child.

The advantages of this form of reading lesson are obvious. It is different, it is simple, and it is relevant to reading because it leads the child on, not only to reading, but to the construction of a book which he and others can read. The child is working to some purpose, he gains a sense of creative achievement, his interest is held by the objectives of the task and his concentration is ensured by the mechanical nature of the task. How often do we hear teachers complain 'If only he could concentrate for long enough.' Fernald's method is a constructive answer to this plea.

As the 'reading book' grows, so does the confidence of the child, for he is now able to give demonstrative proof of what he has always hoped was the case, namely that he can remember how to read what he has written. He can even secretly test his powers of transfer by trying to read some other reading book that is left lying around. And so his confidence grows visibly and quickly. Likewise, his understanding of the construction of written language grows. He learns to translate spoken into written language and to express his thoughts and ideas with increasing facility, and in doing so, he increases his understanding of language, especially written language, and thereby increases his ability to interpret other people's writing.

In chapter six entitled 'Partial disability' Fernald (1943) sets out her suggestions for the next stage, when the child passes on to read printed books. She suggests that the child should scan the current paragraph or page for unknown words before attempting to read it. These he lightly underlines and the teacher pronounces them for him. The child then learns the word, either by tracing and vocalization or by some other suitable method, and finally writes it without copying. Then he reads the text.

An adaptation of this procedure, which may be easier to operate in a large class, is one in which the child asks the teacher for help with any unknown words as they occur during the actual reading of text. The teacher merely pronounces the word for the child and writes it on a slip of paper. The child then continues reading but, at a convenient place to break the reading, for example, the end of a chapter or story, the child learns these words in the way suggested by Fernald. The slips of paper containing the words which the child has learnt are retained for reference and revision. A box file of all new words can be compiled.

The fifth need

Finally, the type of child with whom this chapter has been concerned may need specific help in certain aspects of reading or at certain stages in his progress. For example, he may find the irregularities of grapheme–phoneme correspondence disconcerting and the phonic conventions bewildering. Stott's *Programmed Reading Kit*, the appropriate SRA *Reading Laboratory*, some of the games and exercises from *Fun with Phonics* and *Sounds and Words*, or Monroe's emphasis on defining and dealing with specific deficiencies, all have something to offer, and the teacher should easily find enough here to supplement the Fernald method. But it is possible that children who are backward in reading, but who do not suffer from physical defects or severe emotional disturbances, may need specific help outside the normally accepted scope of reading schemes. They may need applied speech training to obliterate or compensate for irregularities in speech which distort the auditory interpretation of written symbols, or they may need to be brought to a clearer awareness of the meaning of language, through an understanding of the significance of stress, intonation and sentence patterns. Much can be done to imbue the text with life, individuality, significance and meaning, if children are shown how radically the meaning of passages can be altered merely by changing the manner in which they are read.

The importance of Fernald's method

Before leaving the contribution of Fernald to the alleviation of reading difficulty, it would emphasize the importance of her ideas if the reason for the success of her method were evaluated. Perhaps the most important factor is the motivational one. Her method is basically a language experience approach, but in its purest form—in that all the words read come directly from the child. This being the case, everything the child is asked to read is based upon his own experience or interest, and the whole edifice of learning is built upon familiarity.

As far as word recognition is concerned there are three advantages. It seems probable that this method helps the child to blend letter sounds by specifically training him in this procedure. This is particularly important because, as Jeanne Chall (1963) found, ability to blend letter sounds is closely related to reading ability. In the second place, young children and retarded readers have some difficulty in associating visually and auditorily perceived patterns (Birch and Belmont 1964 and 1965). In this case it seems probable that Fernald's method aids children to make this association.

Order and orientation of letters and sounds frequently are another source of difficulty in the early stages of reading (Vernon 1957). Fernald's method imposes a systematic left to right orientation and causes the child to note the order of grapheme–phoneme correspondences.

Finally, an advantage of this method is that it combines reading and writing and it incorporates spelling. Therefore it can form, for those children who need it, a major part of the work in English. The writing of stories replaces the more usual types of written English lesson, instruction in spelling is catered for; and the teacher, although he has to rewrite the stories for the children, is released from marking essays and other written work. Some teachers have in the past been deterred by the prospect of stories to be rewritten piling up, but surely it is up to the individual teacher to control the number of stories written under this scheme. Perhaps one of its most useful characteristics is that this method can be used to whatever degree thought necessary by the teacher. It can be used with small or large groups and it can be used periodically as an alternative to other types of reading lesson, without conflicting with them.

Other considerations

This paper has dealt with one method of teaching children to read at an age which is later than normal. It does not pretend to answer all the problems of backwardness in reading. All it suggests is that with some children, who are finding reading difficult, some degree of success will be achieved by engaging them in tasks, the performance of which will give them some insight into the nature of written language and its interpretation.

There have been some recent researches by Collins (1961) Lovell and others (1963) which may lead us to question some aspects of the long-term effectiveness of remedial teaching. It is imperative that all teachers who are in contact with children who have received some form of remedial teaching should not make the mistake of believing that once the child has begun to read with some fluency his troubles are over. This is obviously not so. There is no reason that we know of so far to suppose that having mastered the simpler subskills of reading he will find the later subskills within easy attainment. Indeed, the fact that he was slow to master the former should indicate that he may be slow to master the latter. Furthermore, just as it has been stressed that normal readers need a continuing programme of help throughout the stages when they are perfecting their already achieved reading skill, so backward readers will need such help and guidance in greater measure. It follows then, that if a child requires remedial teaching in the upper junior school, he also requires a programme of remedial instruction in the lower secondary school at least. This will be necessary no matter how great the improvement he made in the upper junior school, for even where this improvement is substantial, a programme designed to increase his ability in reading, as distinct from a programme designed to teach him to read, will be necessary. Once it has been found that a child has difficulty in learning to read, that child should be kept under close but discreet surveillance for several years after the initial remedial work has been undertaken, and the work that he does in school should be planned accordingly.

References

Birch, H. G. and Belmont, L. (1964) Auditory–visual integration in normal and retarded readers in *American Journal of Orthopsychiatry* 34, 853–61

Birch, H. G. and Belmont, L. (1965) Auditory–visual integration, intelligence and reading ability in school children in *Perceptual and Motor Skills* 20, 295–305

Blank, M. and Bridger, W. H. (1966) Deficiencies in verbal labelling in retarded readers in *American Journal of Orthopsychiatry* 36, 840–7

Chall, J., Roswell, F. G. and Blumenthal, S. H. (1963) Auditory blending ability: a factor in success in beginning reading in *The Reading Teacher*, November

Geoffrey R. Roberts

COLLINS, J. W. (1961) The effects of remedial education in *Educational Monographs IV* University of Birmingham, Institute of Education

*FERNALD, G. M. (1943) *Remedial Techniques in Basic School Subjects* New York: McGraw-Hill

FERNALD, G. M. and KELLER, H. B. (1921) The effects of kinaesthetic factors in development of word recognition in *Journal of Educational Research* 4, 355–77

GIBSON, E. J., OSSER, H. and PICK, A. D. (1963) A study of the development of grapheme–phoneme correspondences in *Journal of Verbal Learning and Verbal Behaviour* 2, 142–6

HUSBAND, R. W. (1928) Human learning on a four-section elevated finger maze in *Journal of General Psychology* 1, 15–28

LOVELL, K., BYRNE, C. and RICHARDSON, B. (1963) A further study of the long-term effects of remedial teaching in *British Journal of Educational Psychology* 33, 3

MILES, W. (1928) The high relief finger maze for human learning in *Journal of General Psychology* 1, 3–14

*MORRIS, J. M. (1966) *Standards and Progress in Reading* Slough: National Foundation for Educational Research

STOTT, D. H. (1962) *Programmed Reading Kit* Glasgow: Holmes MacDougall

VERNON, M. D. (1957) *Backwardness in Reading* Cambridge: Cambridge University Press

4.4 Teaching procedures

GILL C. COTTERELL

School Psychological Service, West Suffolk
Education Authority

Reprinted from A. W. Franklin and S. Naidoo (1970) (eds) *Assessment and Teaching of Dyslexic Children* Invalid Children's Aid Association, pp. 49–70

For the last four years I have had a unique opportunity of studying a minority group of intelligent children who have difficulty with reading and writing in varying degrees of severity. Many of them had been referred to child guidance clinics or had years of failure in remedial groups, despite individual help. They are children to whom reading and writing do not 'suddenly come'. The mastery of symbolic language needs to be a systematic, step by step process.

I have learnt not to expect a dyslexic to know anything which has not been specifically taught, because little is picked up incidentally in connection with language structure, and I expect some degree of overlearning to be necessary for everything taught. I have learnt that it is best to let the child set the pace, rather than for me to feel frustrated by his inability to go at mine. Initially I tended to teach too much too quickly, so that little was grasped thoroughly.

This work has been challenging as I do not like to be beaten by a child. In the ideal teaching situation detailed observations have been possible, and ways of helping children round their particular stumbling blocks have been explored. Because the majority of children assimilate the sound/symbol system of language comparatively easily, the teacher hardly has time to be aware of the exact problem of a struggling dyslexic in a large class. It is easier to think him lazy or stupid.

My paper will cover the whole range of reading and spelling disability from five to eleven years. The first section concerns the initial approach necessary to help the 'complete nonstarter' who has suffered several years of failure, whether he is a visual or an auditory dyslexic. This is dealt with in some detail and in the light of my own experience, because getting started is the most important thing of all.

In the second section I shall talk about my 'middle programme', the acquisition of the vowel digraphs and ways of lightening the learning load. The third section will deal mainly with the teaching of spelling in a more formal manner to the child who can read to some extent, but who is held back by his spelling disability.

The complete nonstarter

Many children with five year level scores on standardized reading and spelling tests have now passed through my hands, and all have had either a severe visual or auditory perceptual weakness, or both. These children are rare and you may never have come across one. They come to the Centre from far afield—Lincolnshire, Herefordshire, Bedfordshire, the south coast, as well as from the Home Counties, but there are certain learning profiles evident among them. They either have a temporary or permanent deficit in visual recall, or the auditory memory of a four or five year old on the Auditory Vocal Sequencing test of the Illinois Test of Psycholinguistic Abilities (ITPA) (Kirk *et al* 1968). One or two children have deficits in both areas and very poor auditory discrimination may be an added difficulty.

With all the children my approach, and that of other teachers at the Centre, is a creative one, as reading and writing need to be part of the total environment connected with a child's interest and with topical events. He learns kinaesthetically through writing. Sylvia Ashton Warner (1963), in her fascinating book *Teacher*, says that 'First books must be made of the stuff of the child himself, whatever and wherever the child.' In this way individual key vocabularies of 'organic words', loaded with interest, are built up.

Making a book gives an incentive to write, and this increases as the destroyed desire to write is reawakened. No driving is necessary from the teacher with this method. The child has complete interest and is fully motivated in the learning situation. Because what he is writing is related to experience, as his experience widens he gains an ever widening vocabulary. Spelling, reading and writing go alongside. The child opens up and gains confidence in his new found ability and writes more. Reversals tend to lessen as word form is understood. He asks for books to read to seek for information and generally 'comes to life'. When he says he has been to a library, a real desire to read has been created.

There is little danger of these severe dyslexics racing away with too many words too quickly. At first it may take them twenty minutes to think of one short sentence of four or five words, and write it correctly from memory. They can be painstakingly slow. I find that they usually know what they want to write, and may indeed be mines of information, but the problem is *how* to put it down. Small words, which may take so much teaching in isolation, are more easily learnt when used in interesting context, as learning becomes meaningful.

At first interests may be fleeting, so titles such as 'News', 'Things', 'My book of all sorts' appear. The launching of the book and the planning of the cover are important motivating moments, and discussion as to the contents can ensue. The 'organic word' on the cover may serve as a link with a difficult sound group later. It should stand out boldly. The boy who made 'An anything book' provided his own visual mnemonic for that difficult word *any*. It was also a prop for others, as his book was clearly displayed.

It is the approach to learning new words that varies according to the type of dyslexia. The visual dyslexic, who may be quite good auditorily and able to discriminate the basic vowel sounds, will benefit from a phonetic approach whereby he learns to recognize pronunciation units within words. He is able to work from the part to the whole. On the other hand this process may prove excessively difficult for the very severe auditory dyslexic, who profits from a whole word approach as he tends to notice the overall pattern of a word. His best beginning is to work from the whole to the part. I find a child is taught most profitably through his learning strength, if he has one, as one wants him to meet with success.

Mastering the English language, which can be thought of as one enormous jigsaw of words, presents a marathon task for a child who can barely remember one word. Progress will be more rapid if words containing like visual/sound units can be taken in groups. But for some dyslexics, usually of the auditory type, each word may have to be treated as a unique entity, no generalization taking place. It is no wonder that progress can be slow.

The visual dyslexic

For the visual dyslexic, who is weak in word recognition and visual recall, it is no good waiting for his sight vocabulary to develop before introducing phonics. Johnson and Myklebust (1967) in *Learning Disabilities*, say that instant recognition of whole words may not occur after months or even years of training. The purpose of reading instruction is to give the child a means of identifying words he sees. He needs to be taught the letter sounds systematically, then the digraphs, and how to blend them into meaningful words. This type of child is bound to fail by the 'look and say' approach in school and should be identifiable early on. The Stott *Programmed Reading Kit* (Stott 1962) is a useful collection of games for teaching this group of children letter sounds, blending, and then reading.

Visual dyslexics tend to reverse more letters and for longer than other children. Besides the b/d, p/b, d/g reversals they may have an up and down directional confusion too, u/n, m/w. I associate these latter confusions with the weakest dyslexics. On the window in my room I have a big w for Willy Window, a visual nonverbal clue to aid recall. I have never succeeded in fixing b/d for good. Many ways have been tried but the old error creeps back from time to time, always in a testing situation. It is no use spending overmuch time on this.

With the basic tools of phonics, visual dyslexics will be able to work out unknown words for themselves in reading and writing. The 'ar' is an

241

important unit to teach early on as it occurs in so many words, and the nonvisualizer will write 'brk' for bark. When these children learn the sound of 'ar' they are able to write almost any word containing the sound instantly, unlike the severe auditory dyslexic, for whom two or three rhyming words are an effort. For children who can perceive rhyme auditorily progress can be quite rapid. But there are fifty vowel digraphs or more to master, so it is bound to take at least fifty lessons before all the phonic tools are available for use. Time for revision and consolidation is necessary too, and ways to make these interesting are discussed in the second section.

It is the nonphonetic words that are going to trouble the nonvisualizer, 'come', 'was', 'done', 'mother' etc. I retain alphabetic spelling for these short words, the child spelling each word aloud as he writes it. Mnemonics may also be invented, e.g. '*Mother* catches moths.'

For the visual dyslexic in the beginning stages of topic work, I use the Edith Norrie Letter Case (Arkell 1970), a Danish method employed in the Word Blind Institute in Copenhagen. The child builds his sentence using the letters, working out words for himself in sound and syllable units, and he then writes the sentence, committing each word to memory. I usually 'flash' a nonphonetic word on a piece of paper to train visual memory. As difficulties in spelling occur, the next phonic point for teaching crops up naturally.

If a child is auditorily affected as well, it is wise to teach the long vowel sounds first, which are easier to differentiate than the short vowels. Kinaesthetic learning may be the strength here.

The auditory dyslexic
There are dyslexics with language/auditory difficulties. Among my present pupils at the Centre, aged between eight and sixteen years, twelve are in this category with varying degrees of severity. Some have been with me for over three years and others for three months. They are an extremely difficult group to teach, and the hardest task is getting them from a complete inability to read up to the nine year reading level.

On entry the most severe—those with an auditory memory below six years—are seldom able to write more than the first letter, if that, of a three letter word. Although the individual letter sounds may be known, the child has no idea at all how to build up or work out words that he has never seen. Early identification in the classroom is extremely important, and I want to give you as clear a picture of this problem as I can. Most of them have a higher Performance than Verbal Quotient on the Wechsler Intelligence Scale for Children (Wechsler 1949) (wisc), some being of superior nonverbal ability.

Many children with language disorders have no problem in understanding the spoken word, but are deficient in using it to express themselves. Words do not flow out of them and few in this group are lively chatterboxes. The severe auditory dyslexic tends to be slow, indistinct and hesitant in his speech, as if he is 'finding words'. Many have a deficit in reauditorization, that is words cannot be remembered for spontaneous usage. Questions tend to be answered monosyllabically, keeping words to the minimum. Many have a history of slow speech development and have received speech therapy in the early years.

Another interesting feature is the tendency to twist words in spontaneous speech, e.g. 'communication' may come out as 'mocunication', 'telescope' as 'stelecope'. The child is unaware of his error, but occasionally says 'No, that's not right is it? But you know what I mean.' Over the last four years I have listed these 'twisted words' and notice that they are all produced by those with a disturbance in auditory sequencing and poor auditory discrimination. A four or five syllable word cannot always be repeated accurately either until it is written down and divided into syllables. The visual symbol aids auditory recall.

Jeremy used to talk about a 'lash-eye' for an eye-lash, a 'barrow-wheel' for a wheelbarrow when he was six, and he was generally weak at picking up the grammatical structure of language, as are some dyslexics of either type, even those from a literary home background. They say things like 'I were there', 'You beated me', 'Have you tooken it?' A weak auditory memory is evident when the child cannot read back what he has just written, though the sentence was made up by himself. He is liable to forget what he is going to say at times and lose the thread of a story he is telling. An inability to sequence auditorily is evident in other ways. There may be difficulty in recalling the day of the week, the months of the year, the alphabet, and multiplication tables. If five-figure telephone numbers cannot be repeated, the problem is very severe. Factual verbal material may be recalled more easily. If the order of commands is confused at school, the teacher will think a child lazy or stupid.

Poor auditory discrimination is evident in speech. Roger told me one day that he was learning 'royal studies' at school when he meant 'rural studies'. It was hard to persuade him that he had heard the word incorrectly.

Discrimination of short vowels is one of the greatest problems of the auditory dyslexic. Although he understands words such as 'big', 'beg', 'bag', in context, he is unable to perceive differences when they are heard in isolation. Don't wait for the basic vowels to be mastered before teaching the long vowels, e.g. *oo, ar, ee, or, ow* etc. In spelling 'gr' and 'cr', 'gl' and 'cl' may be confused, and there is a tendency to omit 'n' as a letter, and 'r' and 'l' after another consonant. Constantly dyslexics must be made aware of their speech, and should learn to vocalize, articulating clearly as they write, from the beginning.

I warn them about the 'grunting' n behind the nose that may catch them out, and teach 'tent' after the word 'ten' and 'broom' after 'room'. You cannot assume that because they know all the letter sounds, they can recognize double or treble consonant digraphs in words for spelling. Another interesting error in some severe cases is the confusion between the sound 't', 'n' and 'l'. This has usually been made evident in the early Stott Morris Cards, when an 'n' has been placed on 'lighthouse' and an 'l' on 'nurse'. In the mouth these sounds seem to be produced similarly and the child with indistinct speech is unaware of which sound he is making. Speech rhymes to improve diction are necessary; 'th' and 'f', and 'f' and 'v' also cause difficulty, as the sounds are hard to discriminate auditorily.

An auditory dyslexic seems to lack the ability to recognize rhyme between two words, or think of words that rhyme, even at the secondary school level. He cannot listen for part of a word and think of another whole word with the same ending. Because of these auditory disturbances, rarely is he able to make generalizations about new words that he encounters. Each word is a unique entity.

Because of their difficulties in auditory perception, memory and integration these dyslexics are unable to deal with the skills required for phonetic analysis, and may only be able to develop auditory skills after having learned a sight vocabulary. They respond best initially to a whole word approach and syllables are easier to recognize than individual sounds. The greater visual strength should be utilized as far as possible, and in fact, they may be able to profit from a 'look and say' approach to reading, though at six years of age they may not have been ready for it. I can sympathize with the teacher who says 'I've tried to teach him his sounds, but he seems to get nowhere.'

Experience has taught me that the initial approach with very severe auditory dyslexics must be kinaesthetic 'whole word'. The Fernald tracing method is most successful, as it is intended to be related to high interest, and a new word of any length can be learnt straightaway.

The child selects the word he wants to use and the teacher writes it in large joined-up writing on a card. He traces over it with his forefinger, saying each part of the word as he goes over it, without distorting the word. The tactile-kinaesthetic and visual stimulation is reinforced by the auditory-kinaesthetic speech link. The word may have to be traced many times initially, before the whole word is committed to memory, but gradually tracing becomes less until a child can just look at a word and retain it. The words are filed in a child's own alphabetically indexed word file, and these provide useful flash cards as well. It is amazing how rapidly long words are mastered by children who are unable to deal with sounds in any way. It brings instant success and is a means of word mastery not dependent on phonics. I recommend this technique for use with children who fail by other methods although it means a slow word mastery. Each child needs to build up his own basic working vocabulary as quickly as possible, even if it is only two words in a lesson.

When Keith came to the Centre at 12 years 9 months, unable to read and write, the itpa revealed a five year level of auditory memory, and he was comparatively strong visually. In his first lesson he drew a motor-bike in great detail and I taught him 'motor' and 'bike' using the Fernald method. He traced each word five or six times, then wrote them from memory in rough before writing the heading above the picture. When Keith came for his second lesson, two days later, he had remembered both words and wrote them correctly on the blackboard. After 'motor' I asked if he could write 'motors', 'motoring', 'motorist', 'motor-car', overworking 'motor' as much as possible, and showing him how words can grow from a root. This was real achievement for Keith after six years of failure.

Keith did not understand rhyming, so when he had written 'bike', I suggested that he should write 'like' below, by changing just the front letter of 'bike'. Unless I mentioned this latter point he would be likely to write 'lbike', this is using a *visual* approach to rhyming. He needs to *see* similarities in words first, and later this is related to hearing the similarity. I should advise mastering two or three words that rhyme at a time, no long reading or writing of word lists, as this causes confusion and does not aid recall for spelling for this group.

When writing a word I encourage vocalization, with clear articulation, so that kinaesthetic, visual and auditory pathways to the brain are all engaged to strengthen the memory pattern for recall.

Overlearning is important and at every lesson I give Keith short tests on words he had learnt, from five to fifteen words at a time; when three consecutive 'ticks' are down, the word is taken off the testing list, as it is considered 'fixed'. In practice I find this has occurred 95 per cent of the time. Keith knows all the words he has been taught, which are several hundred now, but nothing beyond that. He is speeding up generally, but cannot be hurried. He must be allowed time to think. I used to feel that his brain had been inactive for too long, but that now it is slowly waking up and he is beginning to think for himself. In his first year he made two years' progress with reading and spelling and reached the seven year level. This may be considered quite successful, since he had grasped little from six years in a classroom.

When James came to the Centre at the age of eleven, with IQ of 98, he was a complete failure after two years in a remedial group. Like Keith, he had a five year auditory memory and was stronger visually. I taught him to read by 'look and say' using first the Ladybird *Key Words* scheme and flash cards (Murray 1964). After success with the first three books he went on to the *Beginner Books* which are humorous and have a controlled vocabulary. In the first lesson I usually ask a complete nonstarter to write all the words he knows. James wrote 'and', 'it' 'cat', 'the'. I taught him 'mum' and 'dad' writing each with a felt-tip pen, and then studying them. We called them 'sandwich words'.

When he came for his second lesson I asked him if he could remember his two new words, and asked him to write 'mum' on the blackboard. He wrote 'dad', and vice versa. He knew those two words, but had no idea how to remember which was which. It illustrates so well the complete lack of understanding about the sound/symbol system of language. I asked James what his mouth did in the middle of his name, and then I asked him to guess which of the words said 'mum'. The link between speech and symbol was begun.

When a child cannot read he has nothing to visualize, and with a four year old auditory memory sounds are meaningless units, so that his speech is the one thing that he always has to guide him. At least consonants may appear in the right place if he follows 'what his mouth tells him to do'. He is able to write words he previously thought were impossible, and light dawns. This link between speech and symbol is vitally important and it seems to be one of the basic ideas that is not automatically grasped by this severe dyslexic group. Although I talk about 'visual strength', it is not totally reliable and often only the general impression of a word is recalled, but speech can be used for checking, then 'was' is not written 'saw' and vice versa. (The visual dyslexic writes 'sor'.)

Blending is a skill which may need training for both visual and auditory dyslexics. Phonic Rummy, an excellent American card game containing 12 packs in all, is especially devised to do this. The packs cover the basic vowel sounds and all main vowel digraphs. It is an excellent remedial tool, as it acts as a means of reinforcing new sound units introduced, and has many remedial possibilities. The simplest pack, Junior Phonic Rummy, has a picture card for each basic vowel, which adds to the novelty of the game. It is through this that I introduce the basic vowels to the auditory dyslexics.

In the game, cards are collected in 'sound' families, and the aim is to read each word as quickly as possible. It will be played slowly at first, but as words and sounds become familiar, speed increases. Ten minutes of a lesson spent on this is time well spent and is usually enjoyed. It can also be played with a group of children. The idea of how to attack a word not recognized at sight is gradually developed. Severe auditory dyslexics are very much slower than the others when playing this and may have considerable difficulty with 'closing' on the third sound. A good lead into the idea of blending is by using Stott's 'portholes' and 'half moons' first.

Don't be afraid of introducing simple spelling rules to beginners as these are often helpful to those with logical minds. If rules can be mastered they cut down the learning load. By simple rules I mean:

1   no word in English ends in 'v' or 'j'
2   'qu' always go together
3   short words tend to end in double 'l', 's' and 'f'
4   the short 'i' sound at the end of a word is always 'y' as no English words end in 'i'.

Not all dyslexics fall into the clear cut categories that I have been describing, but I have been considering the rare complete nonstarter, who tends to be very severely underfunctioning in some area. It is important to use whatever strength he possesses to help him cope with his particular problem. If you can teach the most severe case then the less severe are comparatively simple.

As yet little has been said about reading because this activity is such a small part of a lesson. Apart from reading back everything he writes, only the last few minutes may be set aside for reading in the beginning. The child who can't read finds it a tiring mental process, and he is likely to be yawning within a few minutes of concentrated effort, because of the automatic response it requires. Gradually the length of time is increased, but seldom beyond a quarter of an hour.

The aim is always to read at 'talking speed' if possible. Books chosen must hold interest for the child, have clear print, not too much writing on a page and a controlled vocabulary. Hearing a child read is insufficient help on its own for dyslexics. Reinforcement by writing, using ways already mentioned, is necessary too. Discourage finger pointing as far as possible, though certain children seem unable to focus on a word without it. A card held below the line and moved down helps to maintain the place.

I think I understand why these severe cases fail when taught in groups, when I see how desperately slow they are and how long it takes them to think, recall, write and decide which sound comes next and which way up each letter goes in every word even in an ideal teaching situation when there is no external pressure on them. No teacher of a group could possibly wait for all the slow mental effort involved. The children *do* appear stupid, but can be taught at their own speed. Individual help is essential and for the child with a very weak auditory memory this needs to be daily. The 'terrible slowness' has to be lived through before any speed can be expected. Having broken the language up into so many minute step by step portions, I am left amazed how the process of reading and writing is so easily mastered by so many. They are indeed fortunate.

The structure of written language

When reading and spelling reaches the seven and a half year level, this usually indicates that a simple sight vocabulary has been acquired and that the basic idea of building short three or four letter phonetic words has been mastered. To know all the vowel digraphs and the possible symbol associations for the various sounds is the main difficulty that has to be tackled, as few of these are automatically deduced by the child.

Although practice in blending, rhyming and word building is still necessary, I tend to encourage much more written work in the topic book at this point. A more definite title may appear, such as 'Aeroplanes', 'Animals', 'Volcanoes and earthquakes' and 'Cars'. As new words and sound patterns naturally arise, these may become key words for future teaching, unknown being linked to known words. Spelling rules arise which are naturally introduced as learning props. To some children they cause confusion, so they need to be kept to the minimum and as simple as

247

possible. The general principle is that teaching must proceed in a slow systematic way, each point being securely grasped and overlearnt before rushing on to the next.

A book to be recommended is Spalding's *The Writing Road to Reading*. Here are clearly set out the basic tools of phonic knowledge which should be at the fingertips not only of every remedial teacher, but also of all teachers of English. The method, known as 'unified phonics', is a scientific method of teaching the basic techniques of language, requiring accurate speech, spelling, writing and reading. It is reported as highly successful in the United States with all children, and ideal for teaching beginners to read. It helps to prevent typical errors of reversals and sequencing because the pupil thinks of a word first as a series of sounds and later as syllables, as he speaks and writes.

Phonic tools must be mastered in order to decipher, pronounce and understand new words in print. No gadgets or expensive devices are needed for this system. The book contains many useful ideas for teaching and would be of value to students in colleges of education. Spalding's book lists Orton's 70 phonograms and recommends that individual cards be made of them, which provide an extremely valuable diagnostic tool.

Initially I drew up a list of the 70 phonograms for every pupil and marked those known and those not known. A check list with all the individual letters and consonant digraphs was constructed for each pupil. A quick record was needed of the child's weakness in phonic knowledge, and also of what had been specifically taught. Each child's check list is beside me throughout every lesson and spontaneous errors can be immediately noted. After working on a particular sound unit I place a tick at the side of it.

Often it is the *type* of error that needs to be noted rather than the actual word misspelt. If, for instance, 'broom' is written 'boom' I mark a cross by 'br'. Then when teaching, for example, the vowel digraph 'ow' at a later date, I see that 'brow' is inserted in the group. If I specifically wanted to work on 'br' words I would suggest that the child drew a 'brown broom by a brick bridge over a brook', labelling the objects and writing a sentence about the picture afterwards. When the check list is studied you find that the children who have no difficulty with the consonant digraphs, are usually those who are stronger auditorily, while others can deal with none of them automatically. Inevitably the need for much more teaching will make progress slower for the latter group.

On the list the sound units are printed in groups in alphabetical order. Each of the larger units represents a block of words. The teaching order will depend on the need to know a certain pattern of sound, those such as 'au', 'aught', 'are', 'ough' will probably not be among the earliest taught. If you do not have examples of words containing these sound units to hand, *Sounds and Words* (Southgate and Havenhand 1960) is an excellent set of six books for reference. Besides lists of words containing like sound units there are a few puzzles and word games for a child to do. I do not advocate reading long lists of words regularly as this word-calling is a somewhat dull occupation.

The work which emphasizes a writing or kinaesthetic approach with the child articulating clearly as he writes is of course multisensory. For six months at the Centre I taught two boys together. Both were eleven years old, reading and writing just below the nine year level, but one was an extremely severe auditory case, who relied on his visual strength to a certain extent, while the other seemed to be totally deficient in visual retention but was quick at dealing with any length of phonetic word.

What was so interesting from one lesson to the next was the way in which words were recalled in tests each week. The words we worked on were always written in several places and used in context by both boys, using a multisensory approach. Take for example the word 'aunt', initially spelt wrong by both children. Because it is a difficult word they overworked it by listing all their various aunts. In a test in the following session the visual dyslexic wrote 'arnt' (phonetic rendering) and the auditory child wrote 'anut'. The latter retains the general visual image and, as the last things he thinks about are the sound elements, does not realize that he has written 'a-nut'. The word was spelt correctly by him thereafter.

No amount of writing 'aunt' fixed the word for the visual dyslexic. He did not get it right until he studied the word further and said 'a-unt'. For the nonvisualizer, alphabetic spelling of nonphonetic words may be a help, and this method should be used. This particular boy never knew what to do with a list of 20 words he was given for homework each week in school. He was not likely to retain any by just 'looking' at them and nothing further was required of him. He would be expected to learn all these in one evening and would sure enough be in trouble the following day as the majority were incorrectly spelt. This is not surprising in view of the overdose of words. As the boy became extremely anxious we recommended that he should be allowed a week in which to master ten words at first, just being given two each evening. The important thing is that the teacher understands why he fails and tells him how to master these words. He must *do* something with them, carefully studying them and using them in context.

What a lesson consists of
A forty-five minute lesson will contain a variety of activities in which the child is encouraged actively to participate. The lesson must not be allowed to become dull routine, and changing the activity maintains interest and makes allowance for a limited span of concentration. Some external motivation may be necessary early on to combat past negative feelings of failure, but by degrees the child becomes totally involved in the learning situation, writing about things in which he is interested, reading books he likes and acquiring tools of learning which help him. As he

meets with success and encouragement internal motivation develops, but this can be as easily lost as it is gained.

Goals must be immediate and surmountable, achievement and success visible. A topic book gets thicker. It doesn't matter if there are only a few words and a picture on each page. The list of words known becomes longer; more lines are read to a given time limit, these are all small incentives, but the child is spurred on.

A lesson will include a quick test on words previously learnt. This may be anything from three to thirty, examples of different sounds and rules taught being included. Any errors are used in a new way and are likely to reappear in the test next time. After three successive ticks by a word it is generally 'fixed' and remains part of the basic vocabulary. Anything from 12 to 85 words may be mastered in a term, according to the child's ability and the speed at which he works. The amount of overlearning necessary varies from child to child.

I always teach something new each lesson, a sound unit, a spelling rule, a prefix, a suffix or maybe only a word or two. Sometimes several points may be taught, but they will be quite different in nature to avoid confusion in recall. They will be connected to the child's work in some way and must stand out in his mind afterwards. A statement of fact, e.g. 'or' makes such and such a sound, is usually insufficient for many dyslexics, though this method should be tried first before devising elaborate schemes to aid recall.

Part of the lesson may be spent playing Phonic Rummy to train blending and reinforce the teaching of a sound unit, or practice in syllabification may be necessary.

Time for topic work will be included somewhere. Often I keep it for the last ten minutes or quarter of an hour so that motivation is maintained. If a child arrives with pictures, drawings and ideas flowing out of him, then I should begin with it. He will learn the new words according to the technique best suited to his particular difficulty, and the word under consideration. The use of a variety of methods adds to the interest. Whatever is written should be read back afterwards by the child. Reading probably comprises about a quarter of an hour of the lesson at the most, although this is not a rule. Games of word recognition may also be included, and some language training.

Sometimes it is necessary to spend time teaching handwriting. Many letters may be formed in an extremely primitive fashion, preventing flow in the handwriting. The child who grips his pencil tightly needs loosening up with Marion Richardson writing patterns. He may fail to know that the weight should be on his left hand, if he holds his pen or pencil in his right hand and vice versa.

Each child has his own alphabetically indexed notebook in which to enter his new words. He can carry this round in his pocket and use it at school for reference.

Opportunity for oral work and exchange of ideas is an important part of the lesson. The child may need to be encouraged to articulate more clearly. The teacher should articulate clearly too. Speech rhymes can be used to improve his diction. With the use of a mirror he can watch himself practising certain sounds. Word meanings as they arise need discussion to aid comprehension.

The majority of children who have reading and spelling difficulties are able to deal with short phonetic words but lack knowledge of the vowel digraphs. These must be taught systematically, but not all in the same manner or recall is confused. Phonic teaching need not be dull and dry. I always aim at each digraph having its own association in the child's mind. The dyslexic tends to remember what he does—a drawing, a rhyme, a game or a story, more quickly than an individual word. Verbal tags aid his recall and many can be taught how to devise mnemonics for themselves. Active learning in a meaningful setting is superior to drills on word lists.

To 'fix' the vowel digraphs I usually wait for a key word to arise, such as 'car', 'boat', 'sports' or 'train'. For three weeks I once tried to teach a severe eleven year old auditory dyslexic the sound of 'or', asking him to recall the sound on arrival for each lesson. To my dismay it was always as if it had never been mentioned before, but I learnt that that was my bad teaching. Had I waited for 'sports day', when the sound unit was in an 'organic' word, the problem would have been dealt with more simply. I should keep revising 'sports' as a whole word, and then later point out the small unit 'or' inside it. This principle is one that I follow for the minority who cannot retain isolated sound units, working from the whole to the part.

It is worth considering whether a child's name, home address or school address, contains a clue to a sound pattern—Wendy, Timothy, are examples of the 'i' sound at the end of a word. In this way the memory load is reduced.

One digraph always difficult to recall is 'ew' but if Andrew, Matthew or Stewart can make up a rhyme about themselves, including other 'ew' words which must be given them, this sound can be mastered early. Illustrations add to the fun of rhymes such as:

> Andrew found a screw in the stew,
> He could not chew it,
> So he threw it
> Into someone else's stew!

A 'News' book with the title in large clear letters is another starting point for working on 'ew'. The object of all this is to fix the sound of 'ew' for reading, and at the same time to draw attention to the fact that the sound 'oo' is spelt 'ew' on the end of a word, whereas it is 'oo' in the middle. The latter is often easily mastered early alongside drawings of 'Soon to the moon with my balloon', 'The man in the moon in boots with a broom' etc.

The less common 'ue' words should be kept apart and taught *en bloc*.

In this way words support each other in the child's mind, if they contain the same visual and sound unit. On the wall we have a picture of 'Blue glue! Is it true? I haven't a clue'. The ability to associate ideas is important here. In the month of May, deal with 'ay' words, when it snows deal with 'ow'. 'Ea' has no sound of its own, it copies 'e' or 'ee'. The visual dyslexic has no means of knowing which of the 'ee' or 'e' sound units is used in a word, so they must be linked together to help him. A rhyme may be invented to cut down his learning load and act as reinforcement.

The 'ow' sound always tends to cause trouble. Inside a word it is usually 'ou' and at the end it is 'ow'. Rather than deal with 'ou' for the auditory dyslexic I teach the larger units of 'out' and 'ound', as these frequently occur.

Spelling rules such as 'dge, tch, ch, always follow short vowels' are very dull. Try to fix 'tch' with '*ca*tch the *ca*t', '*ma*tch the *ma*t', '*it it*ches'. Do not introduce irregularities at the same time. Certain generalizations can be given so that a logical attempt at spelling an unknown word can be made.

I have always found 'dge' very difficult to fix. Visual dyslexics write 'edge' as 'ege' (a phonetic rendering). Auditory dyslexics write 'egde' (having a vague idea of the general pattern). This is after the sound pattern has been previously taught supposedly! In fact everyone went on misspelling the word week after week. Finally a picture of 'Ed on the edge' helped to sort it out for everybody.

There are five common different ways of writing the sound 'er'. 'Her first nurse works early', a sentence cribbed from Spalding's book, gives examples of these. If 'er' is the most generally expected spelling of this sound then it is the others that have to be fixed in some way. Just giving examples of 'ir' words or 'ur' words is often not sufficient for dyslexics. From my observations I note that visual dyslexics just cannot remember whether a word contains 'er', 'ir' or 'ur'. The auditory dyslexic tends to include the correct vowel and may say 'I know there's a "u" in it' but writes 'Thruday', or 'Satruday', not checking on the sounds.

So it is with the visual dyslexic's problem in mind that 'ir', 'ur' must be taught. For 'ir' we have made up a story about 'a thirsty bird in a fir tree chirping', weaving in other 'ir' words. This may vary according to the child. What develops spontaneously is most beneficial, the teacher perhaps throwing in a few suggestions. Again illustrations can add to the enjoyment.

'Ur' words are linked in a story about 'a curly headed nurse in purple who lost her purse in church'. These stories must clearly be kept apart in the child's mind and not taught in consecutive lessons. One set of words should be firmly established before the other is introduced.

'Wor' provides a rule that can be followed. Most words beginning with 'wer' are spelt 'wor'. Here '*Wor*d Blind Centre' offers an immediate fixing point.

There is not time to deal with every digraph fully, but I have tried to show the way I have worked after studying the problem.

On the walls in each classroom at the Centre are visual aids to help master phonic units. These are made by children to teach children. The visual representation and its association stand out in the child's mind. In a test, how often they say, 'Oh, I remember, I did a picture of it', or 'It was up there on the wall', and the word is recalled. Because what is permanently displayed may make no impact, changes are made regularly to keep the children alert. New words and pictures are added, the work of one child helping another.

Syllabification, in the beginning adding endings 'er', 'ing', 'y' to simple words, goes alongside other teaching as, in the general course of writing, words of more than one syllable continually crop up. The auditory dyslexics may find syllable and whole word units simpler to deal with than thinking of individual sound units. Words such as 'ice', 'ape', 'all', 'age', 'art' are all useful if recognized as wholes. I always encourage auditory dyslexics to notice patterns of words rather than to think of the 'sound' units.

It is often simpler to teach short words from within longer words, e.g. 'some in sometimes', 'meet in meeting', so don't be afraid of introducing long words.

Good visualizers notice double letters once they are familiar with a word, whereas the visual dyslexic never remembers them and must try to master the rule to help him. Failing that he must split the syllables and say 'stop-ping', 'let-ter', 'ap-pear'.

Auditory dyslexics may show no progress on standardized word reading tests which demand phonetic analysis. Reading a piece of prose is often considerably easier because of the contextual clues. A boy may have mastered the spelling of forty or fifty new words in a term but his progress may not be apparent unless they appear in a standard test, especially when each word for him is a unique entity.

The visual dyslexic tends to miss double letters and misspells words containing 'ea, ai, oa, ew, au, aw, ou, ough, igh'. Once he is able to write any length of regularly phonetic word he needs much overlearning for the irregularities. If he cannot apply and remember spelling rules, alphabetic spelling alongside kinaesthetic learning is probably the answer, linking words containing like visual units together, e.g. 'I *eat beans* with my m*eat*', 'I *eat* gr*eat* m*eals*.'

Spelling rules, if they can be mastered, govern hundreds of words and cut down the learning load. Some of the most severe cases have very logical minds and can apply these systematically. Some of the most helpful rules are:

1 'all' only has one 'l' when followed by another syllable (also, although etc)
2 'full' only has one 'l' when it comes at the end of a word
3 a final 'e' is dropped before adding 'ing'
4 regular plurals add 's'

5   words ending in 'ch', 'sh', 'x', 'z' (hissing sound) add 'es' in the plural
6   the 'one and one' rule can be well demonstrated with the Edith
    Norrie Case, the red vowel standing out clearly, a useful and com-
    monly occurring rule to master.

The typewriter
The typewriter is a useful piece of apparatus as it is motivating in itself.
It is also an excellent means of kinaesthetic reinforcement. Sometimes a
child will type when he refuses to write. The words matter more than the
medium in which they are produced. The typewriter is not 'whole word'
learning and therefore should not be used with the Fernald technique.
    If a child is typing in his topic book, I suggest a rough copy first to
avoid errors. In the following lesson he reads back what he has written and
I dictate it as he types, so that his memory is being trained all the time. If
he is unsure of a word, he first tries it out on a piece of paper.
    The child who writes in a slapdash fashion, with little thought and
omitting many syllables, is slowed down by the typewriter. He says each
syllable distinctly before he types it, thus avoiding omissions and, as he
does not want errors in his work, he stops to think. This is worth the great
effort required because he develops better habits.

Language training
Those with a language problem who lack automatic use of language
should be given plenty of opportunity for oral work in the remedial training programme. Practice in finishing partial sentences or phrases, e.g.
'I write with a . . ., salt and . . ., bread and . . .' thus associating pairs of
words in common usage, opposites being especially effective. It is amazing
how limited these children are in their use of language. The other day a
fourteen year old could not tell me the opposite of 'black' and I am frequently told that the plural of 'mouse' is 'mouses'.
    Considerably more language training is now included. I have made sets
of 'general knowledge' cards on postcards to test knowledge of opposites,
similars, similes, plurals, collective nouns, meanings of expressions, sayings
and abbreviations. Only a few minutes of a lesson may be spent dealing
orally with one or two cards. The child unable to read tells me the answer
and then tries to find it on a card. I jumble the order of the answers. Time
is not spent memorizing nonsense syllables or series of digits, but verbal
responses are in a meaningful setting.
    Children with reauditorization difficulties cannot remember how to say
what they have in mind. In school they may raise a hand to answer a
question, but by the time the teacher calls on them, they have forgotten
what they intended to say. A disturbance in word recall is revealed by
hesitant speech, not quite a stutter, and it can also affect oral reading
which is done less well than silent reading. Meaning is associated with the
visual symbol, but fails to recall the correct auditory symbol. As a result
oral reading is filled with substitutions. The sight of even a known letter

does not recall the sound. It is often exasperating to hear such children read, for the simplest book is read slowly even when reading ability is at the nine year level.

A child's book must always hold his interest. Large print, short lines and a controlled vocabulary are recommended in the early stages. Humour makes the *Beginner Books* popular with all ages. James Webster's *Rescue Reading* (1968) is much enjoyed at the seven year old reading level and above. The *Ladybird Easy Reading* series offers a variety of nonfiction material. Knowledge of a subject and of a book's content helps any child to read more fluently. Stories become difficult for dyslexics when content is not controlled and virtually any word may appear at any time.

As mentioned previously, finger pointing is to be discouraged. It may keep the place, but it also holds back the eyes when they should aim at 'being ahead of the voice' in order to progress from the 'word by word' stage of reading. From the start I encourage the children to try to read at talking speed. When a new word is encountered I either tell the child so that he can continue with the story, or I stop and let him build it with letters and work it out for himself. It depends on the word. He enters the word in his notebook afterwards.

Some children have extreme difficulty in looking ahead and reading words in phrases. I cover the words as they are read with a white card to prevent regression and to give the feeling of 'moving on'. In this way words are being fed into the right visual field all the time.

I have noticed that the visual dyslexic has difficulty in reading in phrase units. His visual span is short and he reads word by word, just not sufficiently quickly to be fluent. Each word read has to be blended rapidly for few words may be sight words, and this may be the explanation.

Fluent readers, when encountering a long unknown word, read it as if it were a sight word but in reality they have blended it rapidly. It is difficult to get the visual dyslexic to 'look ahead' when reading and to read fluently at talking speed. The eye tends to be fixed on the word that he is actually saying. Hence he is also slow in moving his eyes back to the beginning of the next line. Because his difficulty is part of a neurological dysfunction he is liable to miss lines and words.

Very few children have come to the Centre under the age of nine, but those seven and eight year olds who have come, have been comparatively easy to teach. They had experienced no sense of failure and learning was still fun. I used the multisensory approach outlined earlier in this lecture, systematically covering each stumbling block as it showed itself. I found that little overlearning was necessary, but that the activities associated with the various sounds were sufficient to aid recall. One little boy remarked one day 'This is a funny reading Centre. I learn to read by drawing!'

There is no doubt that these young children are capable of learning the structure of language quite rapidly, but must be specifically taught as, unlike their more successful peers, they do not automatically grasp the sound/symbol associations. If I returned to class teaching of seven or eight year olds now, I should watch for any opportunity for fixing a 'pattern of sound' in the minds of the whole class, keeping a record of what I covered. Only one unit might be overlearnt in a week, but it would be an attempt at systematic, step by step teaching for the sake of the poor readers and spellers, and by the end of the primary school all the basic tools of phonics could be covered.

The seven year olds who came to the Centre were unable to read or write a word, were highly intelligent, but thought to lack reading readiness. At the end of two years, the $9\frac{1}{2}$ year level of reading and spelling had been reached. The children could hold their own in the classroom but were slightly slower than their intellectual equals and liable to twist words in writing. Jeremy, a year after discharge, had continued to make progress which was very pleasing as we feared he might regress. The importance of early discovery cannot be overstressed as the 'gap of retardation' is quicker to close, and behavioural problems accompanying years of failure are avoided. Time is an important factor in teaching.

The most difficult child of all to teach has been Dick, who has a four year old level of auditory memory and very weak visual retention. The problem here is not how to teach him the structure of language, but how to recall a word. What is known one day, then overlearnt, is completely forgotten a month later, as retention is so weak. The prognosis here is poor, even for a child of high average intelligence. Dick has made two years of progress with his reading in three years and he has tried terribly hard, but fifty minutes with me twice a week is insufficient, and for these children daily short spells of individual help are clearly essential.

Mild degrees of difficulty

This section deals with the 'mild dyslexic', that is one with mainly a spelling disability. Mild dyslexics may have acquired fluency in reading or they may still read haltingly at the nine year level or above. Many of my pupils have been boys of grammar school ability and university potential, strong usually in maths and science.

Their spelling level of at least three or four years behind their chronological age level fails to serve their needs, leading often to an anxiety state and culminating in referral to us for help. Some pass as boys of 'average ability' and receive no remedial help at school where their spelling handicaps all their written work, causing frustration and hiding their potential. Many of them are found in secondary modern schools, sometimes in the lowest streams. Two such pupils of the Centre have successfully mounted the hump of o level English and have taken A levels in science and maths.

When I first came to the Centre, among my pupils was an eleven year old boy, who had failed his eleven plus and was 33rd out of 40 in his primary school class. His headmaster said that he would get through life all right as he could 'talk the hind leg off a donkey', and that he could easily take a job on his father's farm. It would not matter if he was not academic. This boy, when tested at the Centre, had the highest scores on the WISC that the psychologist had ever seen. He was verbally in the top one per cent of the population. The boy is now doing well in a boarding grammar school.

Teaching these dyslexics is much more formal than teaching the beginners. They are given an opportunity for free writing without necessarily working at a topic, and cover in a forty-five minute session a tremendous amount and a variety of activities. The emphasis is always on *writing*, with constant reinforcement and overlearning when necessary. Whether the weakness is in visual or auditory perception, I teach in the first place through their ability to reason, so that recall is not dependent on 'rote memory'. Word structure, spelling rules and word derivation are studied. These poor spellers can frequently follow a logical structured approach to language. The work has the following aims:

1 To speed blending ability if this is required to speed up reading, using Phonic Rummy.
2 To teach each vowel digraph differently and in a different lesson so that it has its own association in the child's mind. Avoid saying for example, 'These are all the possibilities of the "ee" sound' as this can be confusing.
3 To introduce spelling rules and watch for their application. Some rules only need mentioning, whereas the more difficult ones can be entered in a special rule book, which is taken away at discharge for reference. Rules govern hundreds of words and cut down the learning load.
4 The systematic mastery of all short commonly used words.
5 To remove the fear of long words. These are shown to be simple, many being regularly phonetic and able to be broken up into small manageable syllables.
6 To give general language training, widen vocabulary and comprehension.
7 To help a boy to notice the tricky parts of a word for himself, to invent his own mnemonics and to learn new words in the way best suited to him. An alphabetically indexed notebook is handy for reference for spellings that have caused trouble.

Spalding (1957) recommends that individual cards should be made of all the phonograms. These form a useful diagnostic tool and in the first lesson help to show the standard of a dyslexic's phonic knowledge. The cards, placed in order of difficulty, are dealt and the child asked to make 'the noise'. It is frequently the vowel digraphs that are not known, and I wonder whether they are taught as tools necessary for writing. Good spellers seem able to recall visually or deduce phonetic analysis easily, but I venture to suggest that a short while spent on each basic sound unit during the years in a primary school might help bad spellers to be less severe. Dyslexics would need opportunity for overlearning, which would not hurt the other bad spellers, given an interesting approach.

A more formal approach for the mastery of vowel digraphs is advised with this less severe group, who need the main phonic tools as fast as possible. Most of them already possess a basic spelling vocabulary and examples of words are available to use for a working base.

Short words
It is the short words that cause so much difficulty for the dyslexic. Which of the 'o' or 'ee' sounds is it? After some teaching on the most frequently occurring digraphs I systematically screen *Fowler's Scientific Spelling Books* (Fowler 1962). They provide a foundation vocabulary of words which every child should be able to spell automatically by the age of fourteen and they include spelling rules.

Book One contains 533 one-syllable words for all age groups, followed by Book Two containing 300 words commonly used by 9–10 year olds. Books Three and Four provide words for the 11–12 and 12–14 groups respectively. The final section of Book Four contains vocabularies of scientific, geographical, historical and mathematical words. It also has revision lists of the most tricky words in the early books.

Screening words
When a mild dyslexic is spelling at about the nine year level, ten minutes of each lesson may be spent testing a block of twenty words out of Fowler Book One. These are given not in the alphabetical order of the book, which might give a clue to the spelling, but first those most likely to be correctly spelt, plurals and verb tenses being thrown in at the same time. Out of the basic list of twenty, two to six errors may occur and these are worked on afterwards, and studied. The 'tricky' part is underlined, possibly in colour, and entered in the notebook at the appropriate alphabetic page. A story or sentences are then woven round these words so that they are used in context. This is important. Sometimes a serial story is written, humorous or serious and continuing from lesson to lesson. The ingenuity required to link the words appeals to the imaginative child.

A list is kept of all the child's errors. These will come up in 'quickie tests' in the following weeks, and stay on the testing list until correctly written on three consecutive occasions. Sometimes an error leads to the teaching of a sound unit not yet mastered. In one of the early lists for example the word 'bruise' occurs and this can be linked 'bruised' to the more familiar 'fruit', pronounced clearly 'froo-it' to help recall of the pattern. This is revised later when 'cruise' enters the list. A rhyme or story can be woven round this difficult but small group of 'ui' words.

In working systematically through Book One and Two many irregular small words tested have not previously been learnt, so time is not wasted mastering words already known or phonetically regular. The boys are encouraged to notice words on their school spelling lists that follow regular patterns and so do not need to be learned, thus reducing the amount of learning needed.

Roger, a fourteen year old intensely keen on science, was found by his science master to be held back by the spelling of scientific terms. He was given a rather overwhelming list of sixty such words to take home to study. The boy brought it along to ask for help. Seeing that two-thirds of the words listed were regularly phonetic, I tested Roger to show him how easily he could deal with the majority which presented no real obstacle, when each syllable was spoken clearly and dealt with systematically. This was a great relief. His errors could be divided into three groups for learning: the soft 'c' group, 'ph' words and then only two or three words remaining that needed individual studying.

Long words
Besides short word mastery, right from the start I encourage the building up of long words. A root word, such as 'port' or 'tract' is taken to see how many words can be built round it by adding prefixes and suffixes. Sometimes there are forty words or more, none of which, it should be emphasized, needs to be committed to memory. 'Important' often causes difficulty, but I always talk about an 'important ant' to aid recall. In the notebook an ant is drawn beside 'important'.

Syllabification
Many dyslexics by habit omit or insert syllables. They often write the first syllable, think the next and write the third, which produces a very strange word for others to read. It is wise to tap out the syllables first, saying each clearly, and reading it back afterwards. Gradually, as his skill improves the child is able to progress to writing as he naturally speaks the word.

Many dyslexics can write a long word without hesitation whereas reading one requires a much quicker automatic response. This problem can remain even after a considerable level of reading skill has been achieved. Most dyslexics are slowed down by the long unfamiliar word. The first step is familiarity with the most common prefixes and suffixes, so that certain groupings are at once evident within a word. I have cards of these which I deal out rapidly from time to time. These range from simple units like 'con', 'ter', 'im', to more difficult 'cious', 'cial'.

If a child can apply the knowledge that each syllable contains a vowel and can split double consonants, he may with this skill in phonetic analysis break down and synthesize a long word quickly. The visual dyslexic, to whom the general pattern of the word matters little, is encouraged to cover each syllable with his left thumb as he says it, leaving the final syllables visible. The sounding out of individual letters must be discouraged, if this habit exists.

The severe auditory dyslexic tends to make a guess from the overall

Gill C. Cotterell

pattern of a word first, and to look at sound elements is his last idea! His auditory sequencing weakness is clearly evident in his inability to synthesize, even when all the syllables are known. He may read 'con-tin-ent' or 'in-ter-est' and not reach the meaning of the word until he has said it quickly several times.

I have not yet found how to overcome the inability to read an unknown long word quickly. Sometimes I write long unfamiliar words on small strips of paper, so that the letters are practically as small as print, and ask the child to chop off the syllables, reading each as he does so, hoping that this training may transfer into his reading later. Another way of helping is allowing him to mark between the syllables as he reads from a newspaper whenever he meets a difficult word.

Simple prefixes
After games in which compound words are paired, I introduce simple prefixes: 're', 'de', 'be', 'over', 'under'. I send the child home to think of ten words beginning with 'over' without consulting the dictionary. I stipulate *only* ten words because I don't want to deal with more than ten mistakes next time. On his return we usually add to the list. It is a way of reinforcing many simple tricky words at the same time. Giving a verbal clue instead of the word makes it into a game.

Scrambled meanings
This is a form of dictation made interesting. The derivation and meaning of any prefix or suffix, such as 'mis', 'bi', 'auto', 'aqua', are discussed. Ten examples beginning with 'mis' (meaning wrong) are taken, written in a list and read back. The meanings of the words are then dictated in the wrong order and each meaning has to be placed by the correct word. This is excellent for widening vocabulary and for the general understanding of words. Alternatively, meaning can be dictated first and the boy asked for the required word with only the prefix given as a clue. Those with high verbal ability can do this rapidly, unlike those with a language problem who produce the word so slowly.

Words beginning with 'att', 'app', 'ann' are usually regular apart from the double letters. How 'attend' was derived from 'adtend' is explained. The visual dyslexic is the one most liable to errors with these, so he needs to say 'at-tend'. These words can also be learnt using the 'scrambled meanings' technique.

Suffixes
The suffixes that are phonetic cause no problems. Others require specific teaching such as that 'ous' on the end of a word means 'full of', later 'ious' and 'tious' can be introduced. Without explanation 'us' is written which is what would be expected, especially from a nonvisualizer.

The suffix '-al' on the end of a word means 'to do with', e.g. topical, musical, historical. This suffix should not be introduced until the fact that

75 per cent of the words which end with this sound end in 'le' has been established and reinforced by playing Phonic Rummy D.

Once '-ick' is firmly mastered as an ending for short words, 'ic' needs pointing out on words of two or more syllables, such as 'comic', 'arithmetic', 'topic'.

The '-ate' suffix is obvious in dedicate, create, but not in 'delicate', 'desperate', 'immediate'. Train the children to say them literally, in order to recall the correct spelling.

'-ine' sounding 'een' is another pitfall. Words containing examples of this can be woven into a story. '-ice' as a final syllable, as in 'notice' and 'justice', causes trouble and needs special attention.

'Two-way words', which can be pronounced in two different ways, such as 'minute', 'record', 'subject' have recently been collected. This has a certain degree of transfer when reading, as attempts to try various syllable groupings when reading new words are more likely.

In this paper I have described my method of work with the mild dyslexic. My aims are to reduce to a minimum the amount to be memorized, to encourage the maximum of writing and of the overlearning of error. A wide usable vocabulary built up in this way leads to rapid progress.

To use ten minutes of an English lesson each week in this way would benefit not only the mild dyslexic but other poor spellers as well. The patterns within words are not automatically assimilated and need pointing out. A record of errors could be kept inside the back page of an English exercise book. The check list too could be adapted for classroom use as a record of points taught or to be taught. The class could discuss how the various members remember the spelling of words. Notice particularly what the bad spellers say!

There is little value in giving lists of twenty words to be learnt. When 'famous' is spelt 'famus', do not just write the correct spelling for the child to copy, but spend a few minutes collecting similar words. The good spellers will readily contribute words.

These mild dyslexics usually improved by three or four years' spelling age in a year, so that they left the Centre spelling at between the eleven and twelve year level. Beyond that they must help themselves. They will never spell every word correctly, but should have developed sufficient confidence to attempt words and to convey their thoughts to paper. That small words require as much thought as the longer ones handicaps the dyslexics most in examinations. Whereas spelling barely needs attention from the normal child, for the dyslexic every word needs thought.

Reading

Fluent reading of simple, interesting material is better than word by word reading of a difficult book.

Simon at 12 years 9 months was reading even simple material word by word. When I pointed out that there was no need to be looking *at* each word as he said it, but that he should be 'thinking' ahead, letting his eyes go ahead of his voice, he read fluently that first day.

In my experience English teachers are always held responsible for a child's spelling in all subjects. Couldn't the history, geography and science staff teach their own special vocabularies gradually over a year?

Important new words in a lesson should be written up clearly on the blackboard for the sake of the visualizing child, who may be unable to imagine how it is spelt from just hearing it. Seeing the word as a whole aids recall and when tests come along he may be more competent to attempt written answers. How, for example, could the word 'Parliament' be taught in a class?

1 The teacher should write it clearly on the blackboard.
2 It could then be written underneath, in syllables, Par-*li*-a-ment, with the tricky part underlined.
3 It could be pointed out that 'I am' is in the middle. Perhaps an MP might say 'I am in Parliament'. This mnemonic may help some.
4 Ask the class to write it without looking at the blackboard, on the desk with the finger, in the air with their eyes shut, on paper.
5 Recall it in the following lessons, asking a child to write it on the blackboard, or fill in missing letters.
6 Who can find out the origin of the word? Ask the French master.

A few minutes spent on a word is not wasted and this approach should be more beneficial than writing a word out three times which involves no mental effort on the part of the child. He needs a prop for recall and the ideas given above deal with the auditory, visual and kinaesthetic aspects of learning.

Mnemonics
Irregular words are likely to present difficulty to all children but especially to the weak visualizer. Dyslexic children often have good memories for facts. Mnemonics are frequently recalled more rapidly than the word itself, and are remembered best if devised by the children themselves with the help of the teachers. Children should not be given a list of them to cram, but they should be devised spontaneously when the 'problem' word arises. They can be used at all stages of learning and children can soon learn to invent their own ways of mastering their tricky words.

References

ARKELL, H. (1970) The Edith Norrie Letter case in A. W. Franklin and S. Naidoo (eds) *The Assessment and Teaching of Dyslexic Children* London: Invalid Children's Aid Association
*ASHTON-WARNER, S. (1963) *Teacher* London: Secker and Warburg
Beginner Books (various authors and dates) London: Collins

FOWLER, W. S. (1962) *Fowler's Scientific Spelling* Edinburgh: Holmes MacDougall

*JOHNSON, D. J. and MYKLEBUST, H. R. (1967) *Learning Disabilities* New York: Grune and Stratton

KIRK, J. *et al* (1968) *Illinois Test of Psycholinguistic Abilities* University of Illinois Press

Ladybird Books (various authors and dates) Loughborough: Wills and Hepworth

MURRAY, W. (1964) *Ladybird Key Words Reading Scheme* Loughborough: Wills and Hepworth

Phonic Rummy Buffalo: Kenworthy Education Service

SOUTHGATE, V. and HAVENHAND, J. (1960) *Sounds and Words* London: University of London Press

SPALDING, R. B. (1957) *The Writing Road to Reading* New York: Morrow

STOTT, D. H. (1962) *Programmed Reading Kit* Edinburgh: Holmes MacDougall

WEBSTER, J. (1968) *Rescue Reading* London: Ginn

WECHSLER, D. (1949) *Wechsler Intelligence Scale for Children* New York: Psychological Corporation

4.5 Some psychological and sociological characteristics of 'good' and 'poor' achievers in remedial reading groups: clinical case studies

HUGH LYTTON

Department of Educational Psychology,
University of Calgary

Reprinted from *Human Development* (1968) 11, 4, pp. 260–76

Introduction

As part of an investigation into factors relevant to the effectiveness of remedial education, the author carried out a large-scale study examining the achievements of remedial pupils in a Scottish county classified in various ways e.g. by method of selection, IQ, initial reading age etc (Lytton 1961, 1967). While it was found that some factors—IQ being one of them—were associated with significant differences in achievement, their predictive usefulness was limited, as many discrepant results occurred. It is evident that factors other than cognitive variables are related to success in remedial education. In order to understand them it was thought more fruitful to abandon group techniques and carry out clinical case studies, as suggested by Vernon (1960) and Zangwill (in Money 1962).

It was decided therefore, as part of the larger investigation, to obtain two groups of 'good' and 'poor' achievers in the remedial situation, matched for age, sex and initial nonverbal IQ, and to assemble by case study methods as detailed a picture as possible of each child's intellectual functioning, personality make up and home background. It was hoped that such an investigation in depth would throw some light on the factors in each child's situation that might be associated with good or poor achievement in the remedial group. By comparing contrasted groups it was also intended to arrive at some generalization, limited it is true, yet going beyond the individual case.

The literature on the personality patterns of retarded readers has been reviewed by Vernon (1957) and Money (1962). It does not seem to contain a study that attempts to distinguish between those who make good progress under remedial education and those whose disability is resistant to treatment.

Subjects

In the first place two contrasted groups of 12 good achievers and 12 poor achievers (8 boys and 4 girls in each group), matched for sex, mean age and mean nonverbal IQ were selected—(the G and the P group). The criterion for good achievement was a reading level, after remedial teaching, close to the age norm, assessed by the Burt–Vernon Word Recognition Test (Vernon 1938), and at least an 'average' assessment of reading by the child's teacher and the writer. The criterion for poor achievement was a 'poor' assessment by the teacher and an exceptionally long period in the remedial group in the attempt to remedy the disability.

The British reading tests used have norms derived from a school population from Scotland where the investigation was carried out. The norms are expressed as 'reading ages' (RA) based on the average reading achievement of the appropriate age group. Vernon (1938) gives details of the standardization procedures.

When the results were initially analysed by sex it became clear that the boys, particularly in the P group, showed characteristics quite distinct from the girls and that separate analyses for boys and girls were essential. The two boys' groups by themselves were well matched on mean age and mean WISC full-scale IQ (though no longer on nonverbal IQ); Table 1 shows the data. The number of girls was too small, however, to provide any significant results and the analysis of their data is therefore not reported here. The attainment data, for which the two groups were contrasted, are shown in Table 2.

Methods of assessment

WISC
This was administered in the normal way.

Rorschach (Klopfer et al 1954)
This was given in the normal way; the scoring was checked by an experienced Rorschach worker.

Drawing a person
This procedure was based on Machover's (1949) suggestions. Each child was asked to draw a person and, when he had done so, was asked to draw a person of the opposite sex. The drawings were evaluated in a qualitative way on shading, rigidity, maturity, size of drawing, position of drawing etc.

Story about the drawings
The story was analysed, again qualitatively, for length, the kind of hero represented and identification with him, the kind of action depicted and the general tone of the story.

TABLE 1   *Initial data on subjects*

	Matching variables	G Group (N:8)	P Group (N:8)
Initial CA	M:	8 yrs. 7 mths.	8 yrs. 4 mths.
	Range:	7:5–10:7	7:4–9:8
	S.D.:	1.3	0.8
WISC IQ, full scale	M:	97.3	97.0
	Range:	88–107	90–107
	S.D.:	7.3	4.9
	Other variables		
WISC IQ, verbal scale	M:	97.9[1]	95.5[1]
	Range:	86–110	87–106
	S.D.:	7.4	5.5
WISC IQ, performance scale	M:	96.6[1]	99.1[1]
	Range:	85–104	86–117
	S.D.:	7.6	9.2
Initial reading age (RA–Burt–Vernon Test)	M:	6 yrs. 9 mths.	5 yrs. 4 mths.
	Range:	5:7–8:8	5:0–6:6
	S.D.:	1.3	0.6
Initial achievement ratio (AR = RA/CA)	M:	78.7	64.2
	Range:	72–87	52–80
	S.D.:	6.0	8.2

[1] Differences between verbal and performance scales not significant.

TABLE 2   *Attainment data*

		G Group	P Group
Months in remedial group	M:	7.1	37.3
	Range:	3–15	19–57
	S.D.:	4.2	13.1
Gain per month of remedial period (in months of reading age— Burt–Vernon)	M:	5.11	1.04
	Range:	2.3–14.0	0.5–1.7
	S.D.:	4.0	0.5

Drive assessment
This was a persistence task in which the child was presented with a reading test that he had not met before (the Vernon Graded Word Reading Test, Vernon 1938). After ten consecutive failures when, in the normal administration, the test is stopped, the child was told: 'These are getting quite hard now. But you *may* carry on if you like. Just stop when you don't want to try any further.' In this way, the child showed the amount of voluntary effort he was willing to put into a comparatively uninteresting reading test in a school situation, providing a measure of his 'drive to master reading'. The score was the number of words attempted (right or wrong) in this voluntary period.

Junior Maudsley Personality Inventory (Furneaux and Gibson 1966)
This was given in an experimental form in accordance with the instructions provided by the compilers. When a child's reading level was too low to allow him to read the questionnaire, the experimenter read the statements out to him. Scoring was for extroversion and neuroticism.

Adjustment indicators
These derive from teachers' ratings of pupil behaviour which were obtained on a questionnaire evolved by Bowlby and his collaborators (Bowlby *et al* 1956), here called the teacher's report form.

Anxiety rating
This was a composite score based on four component parts: (a) an anxiety rating by the experimenter on a three-point scale, based on the child's behaviour during the two interviews he had with each child; (b) teachers' anxiety rating on a three-point scale based on some questions in the teachers' report form (see previous paragraph); (c) Rorschach—an anxiety rating based on the Rorschach record, taking into account the number of refusals, the percentage of 'sinister' responses and the (k + K + c) per cent; (d) parents' impression of their child's anxiety on a three-point scale. The combined scale ranged from 4 to 12.

Home environment, history
The investigator visited each child's home in the evening so that there would be a greater likelihood of the child's father being present which, in fact, was the case for the majority of boys. The interview was a 'guided' one, i.e. there were set questions, but opportunity was also given for a free discussion of the child's characteristics and difficulties. An account of the child's early history was always obtained. When ratings based on the interview record could be made after the visit, this was done by a psychologist unfamiliar with the children. Ratings were made in the following areas:

1 'Family—cultural aspects' combines scores for father's and mother's education, father's and mother's reading habits and the presence or absence of books in the home.

2 'Family—material aspects' combines scores for father's occupation (classified according to the Registrar-General's list of occupations), family size, living space index ('rooms per person') and condition of the home.

3 'Parental attitudes to education' is based on parents' attitude to full-time education, job aspirations and help with the child's homework (universal in Scotland).

4 'Adverse family relationships' is the sum of ratings on 'harmony of the home', 'acceptance of the child', 'permissiveness', 'punishment', 'protectiveness', the scales being derived from the Fels parent behaviour rating scales (Baldwin et al 1949).

5 'Instability in father or mother' is derived from the interviewer's impression of the parents' personalities. As this is based on a comparatively short interview the rating is probably the least satisfactory of all assessments.

6 'Child—cultural aspects' is a score derived from the parents' estimate of the number of hours per week the child watches TV (negatively scored), whether he watches 'children's hour' regularly (positively scored), whether he reads magazines, comics and books, and whether his leisure pursuits are constructive or purely of the passive variety.

7 'Child's behaviour' is a score derived from the parents' ratings of the child's characteristic manner, his conformity and obedience and his attitude to correction.

8 'Child's relations with peer groups' combines ratings of relations with siblings as well as with friends and school mates, as reported by the parents.

9 'Child's maladjustment symptoms' and 'reading difficulties in other members of family' as reported by the parents in answer to questions.

Characteristics of good and poor achievers

Reading
When these boys were given a followup test, between one and two years after their discharge from the remedial group, the good achievers usually read their class book with fair fluency and had roughly reached their age norms on the Burt–Vernon Word Recognition Test (Vernon 1938). Even where they were rather slower in oral reading, they had no specific pronunciation difficulties and had a good understanding of what they read. On a comprehension reading test (Schonell 1963) they did not measure up to their age levels quite so well.

The reading of the poor achievers was typically slow, halting and stumbling. A few more general trends emerged from a very varied range of individual errors. A number of the boys had specific articulation difficulties. One suffered from a particularly severe speech defect (dyslalia and stammer), but there were others who did not pronounce consonants or had difficulties with initial blends of consonants. One of the most persistent and recurrent features that characterized these boys was that in their reading they were agitated and jerky.

Linked with this trait, a certain impulsiveness was often noticeable, which resulted in erratic misreadings of known words, in the substitution of completely different words, similar in meaning, in losing the place etc.

Intelligence measures—verbal and nonverbal
The full-scale IQ shows the poor achievers to have very much the same level of general ability as the good achievers (Table 1). In the verbal test, however, the P group did consistently worse than the G group, except, surprisingly, in 'Similarities'. But the hypothesis that the P group would suffer from greater spatial–perceptual difficulties was not borne out, except for one individual (see below). Their average performance IQ exceeded their average verbal IQ (though the difference was not significant) and as a group they were superior to the G group in all performance subtests except 'coding', and very much superior in 'block design'.

Cerebral deficit
Two of the poor achievers showed a discrepancy of 20 points between the V and the P scale IQ. It seems that these two boys fit the definition of 'cerebral deficit' proposed by Kinsbourne and Warrington (1963). Boy J (verbal IQ: 96; performance IQ: 117) would come into the category of 'language or aphasic disorders' for which his severe dyslalia and stammer are additional evidence, as well as the fact that his speech development was reported to have been very late. Boy I (verbal IQ: 106; performance IQ: 86) fits into the 'Gerstmann syndrome group'. He was also left-handed, as were several other members of his family, he showed directional confusion in reading and his exceptionally low scores on 'object assembly' where he was unaware of an obvious reversal (standard score: 6) and 'coding' (standard score: 5), further demonstrated perceptual deficit. It should be noted that there were other boys, without such striking signs of organic defect, whose reading retardation was equally severe.

Handedness
This was observed during testing and parents were asked about it, but differences between the two groups proved not to be significant. This finding is in line with the results of Douglas, Ross and Cooper (1967) who discovered no difference in reading scores between right- and left-handers.

Home environment (Table 3)
Since the study was carried out in an area where mining and agriculture are the chief industries, the social background of the whole group of backward readers was exclusively manual working class. It is noteworthy that

the poor achievers as a group did not suffer from poorer home conditions from the material point of view than the good achievers. Amongst both groups more fathers were semi- or unskilled workers. The average family size was high for both groups—5.0 children for the G group and 4.25 children for the P group. The average number of rooms per person was 0.71 for the G group and 0.74 for the P group. In all the material aspects of the home taken together—father's occupation, family size, living space, condition of home—the two groups did not differ significantly.

TABLE 3   *Family assessments*

	G Group Means	P Group Means	Significance Test
Family-cultural aspects	1.5	1.0	
Family-material aspects	6.3	6.6	
Parental attitudes to education	4.1	4.1	
Child-cultural aspects	4.5	3.4	
Hours watching TV per week	10.1	16.25*	U-Test (2-tailed)[1]
Child's behaviour (parents' report)	2.1	1.25	
Child's relations with peer group (parents' report)	4.75	3.50	
Adverse family relationships	0.43	1.00§	U-Test (1-tailed)[1]
Instability in father or mother	0.71	0.88	

Note: A 1-tailed test was used where a hypothesis predicted a difference in a certain direction
Significance levels of differences:

$$\S - 10\% \text{ level}$$
$$* - 5\% \text{ level}$$
$$** - 1\% \text{ level}$$

[1] Tied scores present. They were counted once for and once against the hypothesis and the average value of U was taken. If they had all been counted for, significance would have been greater, if counted against, it would have been less.

The cultural characteristics of the homes of the two groups were very much alike. Whilst all homes took a daily paper or a weekly magazine, it was only a minority of parents who read a book and the possession of books in the home was very rare indeed. The cultural atmosphere of the homes even of the good achievers therefore offered little encouragement. Parents would rarely encourage their child to stay at school beyond the minimum leaving age of fifteen, but in this they probably adopted a realistic attitude, since they associated a longer school life with passing academic examinations, which their children were not likely to be capable of doing. Again, the help with homework which the children received was about the same for the two groups. In none of these facets of home background was the group of good achievers distinguishable from the poor achievers. But whilst none of the parents of the poor achievers reported any education beyond the age of fourteen, even in night-school, five of the parents of the good achievers received at least some education a little beyond the age of fourteen.

Unstable traits in father or mother were no more noticeable with one group than with the other. On the other hand, adverse family relationships seemed to exist in only one family of the good achievers. The fact that they enjoyed on the whole a comparatively normal and supportive emotional climate was a distinguishing mark of the group, since adverse relationships of varying degree existed in five families among the P group.

The good achievers read comics, and a number of them also books, and spent about ten hours a week (a rough estimate only) watching television. In their own 'cultural' activities they were not outstanding.

As would be expected, the poor achievers read no books at home (other than as homework) but, as if to compensate, watched television on the average for sixteen hours per week. The hypothesis that amount of watching was related to personality factors such as anxiety rather than to sheer lack of outlet in reading, is strengthened by Himmelweit's conclusion, based on her large-scale study of children's viewing habits (Himmelweit *et al* 1958):

> Children who view a great deal do so (particularly the intelligent ones) because they have difficulties in making friends or problems in their family relationships.

Personality assessments (Table 4)

On the teachers' report form the good achievers received a rather high maladjustment rating—well above Bowlby's average score for 'normal' children (3.64). The negative traits noted by teachers were chiefly such things as: 'He is inclined to pay too little attention to criticism' and 'His attention wanders rather frequently', the antisocial, nonconformist traits attracting the greatest amount of attention in school.

The parents, on the other hand, when asked about behaviour traits that tend more in the neurotic direction, such as nightmares, fear of the dark, weepiness, attention-seeking behaviour, attributed comparatively few of these to the good achievers. They also found the boys' general manner and conduct on the whole fairly acceptable ('cheerful, active' was a typical comment), and thought that they got on reasonably well with their siblings and friends.

The composite anxiety rating shows the good achievers to have been moderately anxious. In the light of this, as well as of the maladjustment rating given by the teachers, it can be said that the G group boys displayed

Hugh Lytton

TABLE 4 *Personality assessments*

	G Group Means	P Group Means	Significance Test
Drive assessment	33.38	9.00**	U-Test (1-tailed)
Junior Maudsley Personality Invent. extroversion score	14.1	10.90	
JMPI neuroticism score	7.75	8.40	
Adjustment indicators-plus (teachers' report form)	12.0	8.38*	U-Test (1-tailed)[1]
Adjustment indicators-minus (teachers' report form)	6.13	10.50§	U-Test (1-tailed)[1]
Child's maladjustment symptoms (parents' rating)	2.63	4.90*	U-Test (1-tailed)[1]
Composite anxiety rating	6.90	9.10**	U-Test (1-tailed)[1]
Reality aggression rating	0.9	0.9	
Fantasy aggression rating	0.25	1.10*	U-Test (1-tailed)[1]

Significance levels of differences:

§ — 10% level
* — 5% level
** — 1% level

[1] Tied scores present. They were counted once for and once against the hypothesis and the average value of U was taken. If they had all been counted for, significance would have been greater, if counted against, it would have been less.

a medium degree of maladjustment, occupying an intermediate position between the average child and the poor achievers.

The very high maladjustment rating which teachers gave the poor achievers is perhaps somewhat suspect, as an inverted 'halo effect' may have been partly responsible for it. However, it is in line with the large number of symptoms of maladjustment which parents reported for their children. A similar unfavourable trend was seen in the poor achievers' general manner and conduct and in their relations with siblings and friends. Their general anxiety level was also typically high, as well as their fantasy aggression. These findings parallel those of Ellis (1949) who found a correlation of 0.33 between the severity of psychiatric diagnosis of 100 clinic cases and their improvement under remedial teaching.

A number of the poor achievers in this study attended a Hospital Child Psychiatric Department where for a variety of reasons, no long-term therapy was available for them. It may be of course that it was their considerable emotional disturbance which prevented them, in the absence of psychotherapy, from benefiting from the remedial teaching offered (Blanchard 1935).

The motivation of the good achievers to do well in a reading task (drive assessment) was extremely high, and this characteristic, one is tempted to judge, was a large part of the explanation why they overcame their reading retardation so successfully.

The very low motivation of the poor achievers, on the other hand, is very striking. While one is tempted to regard low drive as a very important contributory cause of their lack of success in the remedial group, it may be that it is in fact its consequence, as it has been shown (Sears 1940) that children who have experienced failure tend to have a very low (or sometimes unrealistically high) level of aspiration.

Spache (1957) suggested that retarded readers show resistance to adult suggestions and negativistic attitudes towards a remedial programme. The very low motivation shown in drive assessment would seem to support this, as well as the poor achievers' high S per cent in the Rorschach. On the other hand, teachers did not report that the poor achievers had any worse direct relations with them than did good achievers.

Rorschach and stories

The striking fact about the good achievers' Rorschach record was that they produced fewer responses than the poor achievers and rejected far more cards (Table 5). However, the responses they did produce were disciplined, more integrated and form-bound. The good achievers, it would appear, were more conscious of the dictates of reality, less ready to give way to their own impulses. Their tendency to reject cards suggests that their characteristic way of dealing with their tensions and conflicts was to suppress them and keep them under tight control rather than run the risk of their expressing themselves in disorganized, unsocialized actions. It may well be that translated into the world of school and reading achievement, this means that the good achievers' reaction to the remedial situation was to put their conflicts out of sight and to conform—by fulfilling expectations in the reading field.

Quantitative scoring was not attempted for the stories about the drawings and the following are qualitative impressions. On being asked to tell stories about their drawings, good achievers showed comparatively little evasiveness or resistance. It may be that they found this more familiar, and to them more realistic, world of drawing less threatening than the Rorschach inkblots. The tone of the stories was positive and wholesome, and the heroes they created showed that their self-image, the self-ideal they could aspire to, was that of active, successful people. This attitude would naturally be reflected in their efforts to overcome their initial disabilities.

The Rorschach test released a flood of responses from the poor achievers (Table 5). The fact that $(CF+C)$ considerably exceeds FC, as well as the large number of 0—responses, indicate that the poor achievers react to the diffuse quality of shading and colour rather than to the disciplining aspect of form. They appear to have great difficulty in combining the stimuli of

TABLE 5 *Rorschach*

	G Group Means	P Group Means	Significance Test
Number of responses	15.4	26.1*	t-Test (2-tailed)
% of good Ws	34.8	35.5	
F %	64.3	59.5	
Weighted form level rating	1.3	1.4	
Number of Ms	1.3	2.2	
Number of FMs	4.3	7.3	
M: Sum C	1.3:0.4	2.0:2.1	
FC: (CF+C)	0.5:0.5	0.4:2.4§	U-Test (1-tailed)[1]
(k+K+c) %	1.5	4.0	
A%	50.3	47.1	
Anatomy	6.8	2.8	
S%	1.4	2.9	
Number of additional Ss	2	32	
Sinister %	8.9	14.3§	U-Test (1-tailed)[1]
'Colour Shock' indicators (Alcock 1963)	1.5	2.1	
'Shading Shock' indicators	3.0	2.3	
Number of rejected cards	1.4	0.6	
Number of P responses	4.1	4.9	
Number of O responses	0.6	2.0	
Number of O responses	0.4	2.0§	U-Test (2-tailed)[1]

Significance levels of differences:

§ — 10% level
* — 5% level

[1] Tied scores present. They were counted once for and once against the hypothesis, and the average value of U was taken. If they had all been counted for, significance would have been greater, if counted against, it would have been less.

form and colour into a reality-based concept, thus corroborating Gann's (1945) conclusions.

On the whole it was the investigation of content rather than the usual Rorschach scores which brought out differences between the groups most clearly. It seems that the greater and more violent conflicts and tensions of these boys break surface in the imaginative open situation created by the blots. Their turbulent inner world takes control of their perceptions. Their conflicts are translated into threatening fantasies ('sinister' content), externalized expressions of their impulses, which challenge the world of authority and proclaim how little the boys are ready to conform to school expectations and demands.

One could glean an idea of how the poor achievers saw themselves from the 'draw a person' test and the stories based on it. The number of minute pathetic figures drawn at the edge of the paper was greater than among the good achievers (3 as against 1), the self-confident successful hero in the stories was much less frequent. Accidents did not feature very largely in the stories, but many had a certain tone of flat discouragement. It seems as if the poor achievers had resigned themselves to a colourless and unsuccessful existence.

TABLE 6 *Child's history*

	G Group	P Group	Significance Test
	N:7[1]	N:8	
Birth abnormal or premature (number of children)	1	2	
Delayed speech development (number of children)	0	5*	Fisher exact (1-tailed) probab. test
Number of serious illnesses	4	10*	Fisher exact (1-tailed) probab. test
Temporary separation from home (number of children)	4	7	
Reading difficulties in other members of family (number of children)	0	6**	Fisher exact (1-tailed) probab. test
	N:8	N:8	
Number of left-handers	0	2	
Speech defects (number of children)	2	4	

[1] One boy in care of local authority.
Significance levels of differences:

* — 5% level
** — 1% level

One of the most interesting findings concerned the involvement of physical and constitutional factors—apart from handedness—in this group (Table 6). A definite syndrome appeared to be associated with *severe* reading failure, as opposed to the milder, more easily remediable kind. The syndrome consists of:

1 delayed speech development in infancy
2 large number of physical illnesses, e.g. pneumonia, scarlet fever,

osteomyelitis (the greater number of serious accidents reported for the P group is also noteworthy: e.g. one boy broke his arm four times)

3   reading difficulties in other members of the family.

The nonphysical correlates of the severe reading retardation were a high degree of maladjustment and of disruptive anxiety.

Discussion and conclusion

Stott in several papers (1957, 1959a, 1959b) has demonstrated how close an association exists between several interrelated conditions: adverse factors in pregnancy, early illness, 'unforthcomingness', mental retardation and low achievements. He considers the postnatal handicaps to be evidence of 'multiple congenital impairment' in the child, an impairment of which the adverse factors in pregnancy are the cause.

Kawi and Pasamanick (1959) and Pasamanick et al (1956) similarly find a relationship between adverse factors in pregnancy and behaviour disorders and reading disorder in childhood. Chazan (1956) compared maladjusted ESN children with nonmaladjusted children and found that adverse physical factors—though not pregnancy or birth factors—were associated with maladjustment.

A recent survey of children on the Isle of Wight also showed that severe reading retardation was associated with delayed speech development, pronunciation difficulties, poor right–left differentiation and motor clumsiness—disorders in the physical field. In addition there frequently was a family history of reading difficulties (Rutter, private communication).

As early as 1935, Castner reported reading difficulties in other members of the family, emotional instability and delayed speech development as ascertained in preschool children, to be prognostic of later reading difficulties.

It is in the context of these investigations that the present study must be seen. Small as the sample is, the results are in line with those of the other researches and there exists therefore considerable converging evidence that physical factors, symptoms of emotional maladjustment and severe reading difficulties are all implicated together. Furthermore, the investigation suggests that this combination of factors, plus low drive level, as well as a history of reading failure in other members of the family, differentiate those whose difficulties are resistant to remedial treatment from those whose retardation is more easily remediable.

We see that the male poor achievers are distinguished by a generality of handicap stretching across the psychophysical domain from vulnerability to physical illness at one end to severe reading retardation at the other. Whether this is due to prenatal stresses in the mother or to constitutional factors is not clear: Stott's data leave room for doubt on this point, since pregnancy stress may itself be related to the mothers' constitution, and the present study did not investigate the question.

It may be thought that remedial teaching in the case of the poor achievers was hardly worthwhile. However, perhaps we have to revise our attitudes to remedial education and realize that in most cases it may have to provide more long-term support for the failing child than we had hoped. On further inquiry, it might indeed be shown that the good achievers could have been helped to fairly normal accomplishments in the ordinary class and that it is precisely the poor achievers who needed the extra help of the remedial group even to achieve their poor gains.

The emotional support and the glimmer of hope that each poor achiever received in the remedial group should not be underestimated.

Summary

The intellectual functioning, personality and home background of two contrasted groups of 8 good and 8 poor achievers (boys) in remedial groups, matched for age and IQ, were subjected to clinical study. The poor achievers were distinguished by a considerably lower drive level in a reading task; a higher degree of disruptive anxiety; a personal history that is characterized by delayed speech development in infancy, a large number of physical illnesses, and reading difficulties in other members of the family; to a lesser extent, by a more adverse parent–child relationship. The relations between the reading difficulties and the psychological and physical factors are discussed.

References

BALDWIN, A. L., KALHORN, J. and BREESE, F. H. (1949) The appraisal of parent behaviour *Psychological Monograph* 63, 299

BLANCHARD, P. (1935) Psychogenic factors in some cases of reading disability *American Journal of Orthopsychiatry* 5, 361–74

BOWLBY, J. et al (1956) Effects of mother–child separation: a followup study *British Journal of Medical Psychology* 29, 221–47

CASTNER, B. M. (1935) Prediction of reading disability prior to first grade entrance *American Journal of Orthopsychiatry* 5, 375–87

CHAZAN, M. (1965) Factors associated with maladjustment in educationally subnormal children *British Journal of Educational Psychology* 35, 277–85

DOUGLAS, J. W. B., ROSS, J. M. and COOPER, J. E. (1967) The relationship between handedness, attainment and adjustment in a national sample of school children *Educational Research* 9, 223–32

ELLIS, A. (1949) Results of a mental hygiene approach to reading disability problems *Journal of Consulting and Clinical Psychology* 13, 56061

FURNEAUX, W. D. and GIBSON, H. (1966) *The New Junior Maudsley Inventory* London: University of London Press

GANN, E. (1945) *Reading Difficulty and Personality Organization* New York: King's Crown Press

Hugh Lytton

HIMMELWEIT, H. T., OPPENHEIM, A. N. and VINCE, P. (1959) *Television and the Child* London: Oxford University Press

KAWI, A. A. and PASAMANICK, B. (1959) Prenatal and paranatal factors in the development of childhood reading disorders *Monograph of the Society for Research into Child Development* 24, 4

KINSBOURNE, M. and WARRINGTON, E. K. (1963) Developmental factors in reading and writing backwardness *British Journal of Psychology* 54, 145–56

KLOPFER, R., AINSWORTH, M., KLOPFER, W. G. and HOLT, R. (1954) *Developments in the Rorschach Technique* 1 New York: Harcourt

LYTTON, M. (1961) An experiment in selection for remedial education *British Journal of Educational Psychology* 31, 79–94

LYTTON, H. (1967) Followup of an experiment in selection for remedial education *British Journal of Psychology* 37, 1–9

MACHOVER, K. (1949) *Personality projection in the drawing of the human figure: a method of personality investigation* Springfield: Charles C. Thomas

*MONEY, J. (ed) (1962) *Reading Disability* Baltimore: Johns Hopkins Press

PASAMANICK, B., ROGERS, M. E. and LILIENFELD, A. M. (1956) Pregnancy experience and the development of behaviour disorder in children *American Journal of Psychiatry* 122, 613–18

SCHONELL, F. J. (1963) *Diagnostic and attainment testing* Edinburgh: Oliver and Boyd

SEARS, P. S. (1940) Levels of aspiration of academically successful and unsuccessful children *Journal of Abnormal Social Psychology* 35, 498–536

SPACHE, G. (1957) Personality patterns of retarded readers *Journal of Educational Research* 50, 461–70

STOTT, D. H. (1957) Physical and mental handicaps following a disturbed pregnancy *Lancet* 272, 1006–12

STOTT, D. H. (1959a) Infantile illness and subsequent mental and emotional development *Journal of Genetic Psychology* 233–51

STOTT, D. H. (1959b) Evidence of prenatal impairment of temperament in mentally retarded children *Vita Humana* 2, 125–48

VERNON, M. D. (1957) *Backwardness in Reading* Cambridge: Cambridge University Press

4.6 Reading and speech: an incidence and treatment study

CHARLOTTE SONENBERG and GERALD GLASS
Adelphi University, New York

Reprinted from *The Reading Teacher* (1965) December, pp. 197–201

There are many studies in the literature concerning the relationship of speech and reading (Jones 1951, Monroe 1932, Sommers *et al* 1961, Weaver *et al* 1960). These studies, however, in the selection of their samples and in the testing of reading through oral presentation alone may not have gone far enough in investigating the relationship of speech and reading ability. Since many studies based their findings on tests of oral reading (Monroe 1932, Sommers *et al* 1961, Weaver *et al* 1960), certain reading defects diagnosed as 'reading' omissions and additions may in fact have been speech errors. Many of the subjects of previous studies were not old enough to have matured sufficiently for such a complex skill as reading: Sommers *et al* (1961) studied first grade children, and Weaver *et al* (1960) used subjects under six years and three months of age.

The purpose of the first part of the present study was to discover the incidence of functional articulatory speech defects among a group of remedial readers. (By remedial reader is meant a child who is reading below grade and expectancy level and who is in need of specific instructional aid. By functional speech defect is meant a defect which has not been caused by organic disturbance, demonstrated or inferred.) The second part of the study was designed to compare the progress in reading of children with functional speech problems who were given both speech and reading therapy with the progress made by a matched group who received only reading therapy.

Procedure

The population for the incidence study consisted of forty children ranging in age between seven and sixteen. They were referred to the Adelphi University Reading and Study Centre by teachers or reading specialists for admission to the centre's summer session.

Information received from the various schools on these referrals included intelligence quotients obtained from either individually administered tests or paper and pencil group tests. With the exception of one child, who was dull normal, all of the children were within the normal and bright normal range.

The director of the centre administered to each student the Durrell Analysis of Reading Difficulty Test (1955), which allowed for a diagnosis of the reading strengths and weaknesses of each child. Weaknesses in word analysis and in aided and unaided recall were specifically noted, as well as a generalized instructional level of each child.

The senior author, a speech therapist, was present at the interviews and the administering of the reading tests. This provided her with an opportunity to analyse speech patterns employed during conversational speech as well as in oral reading. Notations were made of articulation difficulties. Following each reading diagnosis, a clinical evaluation of articulatory competency in both directed and spontaneous speech was made. The instrument used for testing directed speech was the Hejna Picture Card Test. Only disorders of articulation that could be classified as substitutions, omissions, distortions or additions, as defined by Van Riper (1913), were recorded. The number of errors possible, considering an error of position (initial, medial or final) as one misarticulation, was 64. Fourteen blends were also tested, bringing the total possible misarticulation errors up to 78.

The director of the centre retested several of these subjects as a check on the initial articulation testing, and the results of the retesting corroborated the initial findings.

Of the 40 children tested (poor readers), only 2 (5 per cent), were free from articulation errors; individual articulation errors in the remaining 38 children ranged from 5 to 55.

A test of auditory discrimination was administered, for which the section of the Durrell test titled 'Sounds (Hearing Sounds in Words)' was used. The examiner said the test word aloud, in full view of the child. The words from which the child was asked to select the word which began or ended with the same phoneme as did the test word were read aloud by the examiner. The examiner's mouth was obscured from the child's vision, so the experimenters could feel sure that only auditory cues were given.

After the completion of the reading and speech tests, the data were examined to select matched pairs, who were to be equated on chronological and mental age, grade and reading levels and number and type of functional articulation defects. Case records suggested that organic and/or psychological concomitants were present in 6 of the 38 poor readers with articulation defects. From the remaining 32 subjects with both reading problems and functional speech defects, five pairs met the rigid requirements necessary for the second part of this study.

A pure tone hearing evaluation was made of each subject, using a Beltone 15A audiometer in a soundproof room. The hearing of all was within normal limits. The ages of the subjects ranged from ten to fifteen.

The grade levels ranged from completion of the fourth up to and including the ninth grade. Their IQs placed them within the normal range. The number of misarticulations ranged from 18 to 55. The number of individual consonant sounds affected ranged from 10 to 18. There was nothing in the records, and nothing was observed during the interviews to lead one to suspect the presence of any organic or psychological problems that might influence the results of this part of the study.

The control group consisted of children who received only reading therapy. The experimental group was made up of children who received both reading and speech therapy.

Each pair of matched subjects received reading therapy for one hour daily, five days weekly, for a six week period, a total of 30 hours. The reading therapy was designed to increase skill in word analysis and silent reading comprehension. The reading teacher gave reading therapy to both the control subject and his matched counterpart in the experimental group. Each matched pair was part of a reading group not larger than five in number. One teacher taught two groups in which two of the matched pairs were enrolled. Three other teachers each taught one group in which one pair of matched subjects was enrolled.

The experimental group, in addition to the reading therapy, received an additional twenty minutes daily of individual speech therapy. Each of a child's defective speech sounds was dealt with in the course of the six-week instructional period. The technique used during the speech therapy could best be described as the phonetic-placement approach as described by Van Riper (1913). This therapy included: auditory training; production of individual sounds in isolation and in nonsense syllables; sounds in initial, medial and final positions in words, sentences and jingles. Emphasis was placed on the correct use of a sound in conversational speech. Speech notebooks were used for home assignments. Daily detailed records were kept of the therapy sessions and of observations noted for further reference in regard to this study.

At the completion of the six-week session, both the control and the experimental groups were retested in reading by the original reading examiner under conditions similar to the original test conditions. The reading examiner tabulated reading improvement based on performance on the Durrell Reading Test administered at the completion of this experiment compared with test performance before therapy. The tabulation was shown on a continuum of Q-10, with 10 being the greatest amount of improvement shown. This was a blind evaluation since the reading examiner was unaware of which children made up either the experimental or the control group. Six weeks following the posttesting still another evaluation was made by the reading examiner, which yielded the same evaluations as those he had made during the first retesting (indicating a high reliability between ratings).

Results

The data obtained during the first part of this study were examined to determine the incidence of speech defects among the remedial readers who served as the population for this study. The data showed that 80 per cent had functional speech defects (although 95 per cent had speech defects including ones other than functional). These percentages contrast with the relatively low percentages of speech defectives among the normal school population, as cited in such reports as the Midcentury White House Conference on Children and Youth (1952). These percentages are particularly interesting since incidences of reported speech defects in the school population have never exceeded the level of 10 per cent.

In this study of the 32 remedial readers with functional articulatory defects, articulation errors ranged from 5 to 55 out of a possible 78. The mean number of articulation errors was 26.4. The number of individual consonant sounds affected by these articulation errors, excluding blends, ranged from 2 to 18, out of a possible 23. The mean number of consonant sounds affected was 9.2.

The tests of auditory discrimination showed that 47 per cent of the remedial readers with functional speech problems had some trouble in the area of discrimination. Of the 15 children who gave evidence of problems of auditory discrimination, 11 had difficulties in articulating the sounds which were producing auditory discrimination problems. It is interesting to note that many of the letters associated with those sounds were cited by Munroe (1932) and Hermann (1959) as letters which often appeared as reading reversals, such as p/b, and f/t. The following sound substitutions were made by subjects of this study during the auditory discrimination test: k/g,* b/d, p/d, t/k, w/wh, m/s, f/t, d/t, t/l, t/unvoiced th, f/unvoiced th, p/m, p/g, f/v. The authors noted that many of the sound substitutions manifested in this study frequently show up as reading reversals.

The second (treatment) part of this study revealed the following data. Based on the comparisons made by the reading examiner of the student performance on the pre- and post-reading tests, four of the five experimental subjects made greater improvement in their reading skills than did the matched subjects in the control group. This improvement was noted in the areas of word analysis abilities and/or silent reading comprehension, as measured by their ability in aided and unaided recall of grade level paragraphs. Although all of the children showed some improvement in their reading skills, the evaluation described earlier indicated that the experimental group showed more discernible reading improvement than did the control group.

* Read k/g as 'k was substituted by the g sound'.

Discussion

First, there appeared to be a high incidence of functional speech problems among the children referred to the centre for remedial reading at the time of this study.

Second, many poor readers with defective articulation have problems of auditory discrimination. The sounds which the subjects found most difficult in auditory discrimination were for the most part included among those sounds which were giving these same subjects difficulty in articulation. Many of the letters representing these sound substitutions have been noted by reading teachers as 'reading reversals'. The similarity between the sounds which present problems of articulation as well as problems in auditory discrimination, and finally the letters symbolically representing these same sounds, which often appear as reading reversals, poses the possibility that all these problems are in fact one and the same problem. Many reading specialists recognize poor auditory discrimination as a deterrent to the development of beginning reading skills. Although some reading teachers present words containing the letters which appear as reading reversals to the child for further study, the letters are rarely isolated from the words and then studied in isolation. The reading teacher's approach to auditory discrimination differs from that of the speech therapist in that it does not usually include the technique of ear discrimination. Since the ear training described by Van Riper has been successfully employed in dealing with problems of auditory discrimination, it is suggested that this approach may be of help to the reading specialist.

Third, speech therapy given in addition to reading therapy to remedial readers with functional speech defects tended to improve reading skills beyond the improvement shown by remedial readers with functional speech problems who received only reading therapy.

The findings of this small-scale study suggest the need for further studies with more subjects. If new studies support the implications of the present study, we would need to work more actively on the correction of faulty articulation as an aid in the improvement of reading skills, and since most classroom teachers are not specifically trained to identify functional speech defects, we might conclude that speech improvement work should have a part in teacher training.

References

ASHA COMMITTEE ON THE MIDCENTURY WHITE HOUSE CONFERENCE (1952) Speech disorders and speech correction *Journal of Speech and Hearing Disorders* 17, 129–37

DURRELL, D. (1955) *Durrell Analysis of Reading Difficulty* Chicago: World Books

HERMANN, KNUD (1959) *Reading Disability* Springfield, Illinois: Charles C. Thomas

C. Sonenberg and G. Glass

Jones, M. V. (1951) The effect of speech training on silent reading achievement *Journal of Speech and Hearing Disorders* 16, 258–63

Monroe, M. (1932) *Children Who Cannot Read* Chicago: University of Chicago Press

Sommers, Cockerville, Paul, Bowser, Fichter, Fentum and Cupetas (1961) Effects of speech therapy and speech improvement upon articulation and reading *Journal of Speech and Hearing Disorders* 26, 27–38

Van Riper, C. (1913) *Speech Correction, Principles and Methods* Englewood Cliffs New Jersey: Prentice-Hall

Weaver, C. H., Furbee, C. and Everhart, R. (1960) Articulatory competency and reading readiness *Journal of Speech and Hearing Research* 3, 176

4.7 Breakthrough to Literacy in the remedial situation

DAVID MACKAY, BRIAN THOMPSON and PAMELA SHAUB

Adviser/warden ILEA Centre for Language in Primary Education; Deputy head Lionel Primary School, Hounslow; Head of remedial department Mayfield School, London SW15

Reprinted from 'The materials' in D. Mackay (1971) Breakthrough to Literacy in J. E. Merritt (ed) *Reading and the curriculum* Ward Lock Educational and a revised version of chapter 9 from D. Mackay, B. Thompson and P. Schaub (1970) *Breakthrough to Literacy Teacher's Manual* Longman

The *Breakthrough to Literacy* scheme was designed by a research team in the Department of General Linguistics at University College London as part of the Initial Literacy Programme set up under the Nuffield Foundation and later transferred to the Schools Council. The programme was intended to see what relevance there might be in the study of linguistics for the teaching of English in the classroom. The materials are intended for children in the infant class but have applications for remedial work at various levels.

The materials

The *Breakthrough to Literacy* materials do not claim to be entirely new; they make use of ideas and techniques which are a new departure in the teaching of literacy as well as using those that have been used before. They do, however, change the emphasis from *reading* to *composing* and as a result they dispense with the need for simplified texts on which to start children reading. They use our traditional orthography.

The prereading materials, the magnet board and accompanying figurines are intended as a means of encouraging talk, discussion and story telling in children who have had too little of such experience of language. Some written language may be incorporated with this material at an appropriate stage.

The crux of the Breakthrough to Literacy is the Sentence Maker. The teachers' version is an enlarged version of the children's and is used to establish basic understanding of the English writing system, to train the children in the use of the materials and to enable them to learn how to use about fifteen to twenty words *of their own choice* to make sentences *of their own choice*. These are recorded for each child so that he is composing his own book. The twenty-four illustrated books, the nursery rhymes and the two simple reference books reflect and extend children's ability to compose their own text.

The Teacher's Sentence Maker is a word store, a collection of 132 items arranged approximately in groups of nouns, adjectives, pronouns, verbs, prepositions. Word endings ('s', 'ed', 'ing') and punctuation (. ?) are included. Roughly half the items are grammatical items (words like 'and', 'when', 'of', 'am') and the remainder are lexical (words like 'school', 'dad', 'paint'). All the words included were found to be those most frequently asked for by children of five to six years old who used the materials during two years of trials.

The child's Sentence Maker is a triptych which stands in front of the child. The first two pages (as in the teachers' model) are printed with the entire word store, and children transfer to this personal model with the words they have learned to use with the teacher. The third page is blank in order to provide each child with items which are chosen personally. In this way each Sentence Maker has a common, shared store and a personal store which is likely to vary considerably from child to child. Introductory work in phonics is made possible with the Word Maker.

Breakthrough in the remedial situation

It is not for a moment suggested that *Breakthrough* replaces any of the specialist advice which a remedial child may need or that it makes up for lack of cultural enrichment. The *Breakthrough* materials can however help any individual child to overcome the difficulty of starting to read and write, and are flexible in use so that each child can work individually.

Although the materials have been designed for the use of infant children in the normal school situation, two of the key items—the Sentence Maker and the Word Maker—are of considerable help to slow learners. They can be used with children of any age, including those at secondary level, to enable these children to compose their own texts and read them back. The books accompanying the project materials and also the nursery rhyme cards and record have been used with benefit and pleasure with older children, but their relevance to the situation must be assessed by the teacher. Since *Breakthrough* was first published a Project Folder has been added to the materials as well as further books particularly suitable for older children. The Project Folder is identical in format to the pupil's Sentence Maker but without any word store so that children in the remedial situation work from their own particular language needs.

One aspect of literary learning is usually accentuated in the remedial situation: teachers very often refer only to remedial *reading* groups (and parents are anxious that their child should at least be able to *read* a little). The children themselves are presented for a very long period with other people's texts. Writing is often taught by asking the child to fill in blanks in other people's sentences, from a list of words supplied. Yet experience shows that these are the very children who find the greatest difficulty in learning in this way. They are the very ones who need a great deal of opportunity for production (composition of texts) in place of the struggle with the reception (reading) of special primer texts.

With *Breakthrough* materials the child produces his own reading material and quite soon he may also show interest in the work of other children. This is nearly always easier to read than the texts in books, because sentences are constructed in ways that are natural to children of the same age and embody common interests and experiences.

It has been found that the first result of using Sentence Makers with the older retarded children is a notable improvement in the amount and quality of their written work. Instead of filling in gaps in prearranged texts the children have now to grapple with the composition of complete sentences. Teachers have found that many opportunities are provided for discussing with a child any mistakes that have been made in a sentence— if it is incompletely made, if the tense is wrongly constructed, if there is an error in word recognition. All such occasions are opportunities for teaching and talking about aspects of the English language, and this discussion is a most important part of the learning situation.

When the wrong word has been used by mistake, this is time to begin the use of the Word Maker. Teachers in special schools will judge for themselves to what degree the Word Maker can profitably be used, but with children in remedial groups in the ordinary schools it is a great help. It is used in exactly the same way as with infant children. As is the case with the Sentence Maker, the Word Maker allows for the physical handling of the symbols and this makes a far deeper and more lasting impact on the child than the attempt to write the word (with subsequent crossing and rubbing out). Certainly it has far greater impact than copying down someone else's spelling and attempting to 'learn' it; a procedure which for most of these children has met with little success in the past.

Breakthrough in junior remedial groups

In junior schools the usual practice is for a remedial teacher to have groups of children (the smaller the better) for some time each day. If the children concerned can take their Sentence Makers back to the classroom and use them there after their group time, this is ideal, but this is a decision for both the class teacher and the remedial teacher to make. One practical difficulty in this situation is the acquisition of new words; the materials will probably be kept wherever the remedial teacher works and this may mean that children have to go to her to get new words. What happens may depend on how many children are involved and for how much of the day the remedial teacher is present.

In most cases the work with the Sentence Maker is likely to be limited to the remedial group period and it is recommended that this time be taken up initially with as much sentence making as possible and with writing these down and reading them back.

By the time they reach the junior school, almost all children (including those with no reading age) know a number of words to be found in the Sentence Maker. Each child can, therefore, start work with his own Sentence Maker, once the teacher has ascertained the words he knows and supplied him with the cards.

He may not be able to make a simple sentence with the words he has first recognized—for instance they may be *mum, school, baby, little, the, a, and*. In this case he should start by making phrases like 'mum and a baby' to enable him to see how the materials are used. Where a child recognizes rather more words, sentence work can flourish from the beginning. In schools where *Breakthrough* materials have been tried with junior remedial groups, although all the children were able to make some start with individual Sentence Makers, it has also been found that work with the Magnet Board is a great help in encouraging children to experiment with new words and new ideas.

Junior children who meet these materials for the first time are helped by the fact that these are quite different from the books which they already associate with failure. They will have some immediate success no matter how small it may be. Every sentence which is attempted—both the well-formed *and* those not so well-formed—will be the occasion for praise and encouragement, and the child will very soon become involved in the work. It has been found that even those children (well known to every remedial teacher) who seem to have no ability to concentrate, can be intrigued long enough to make one or two sentences and, that with patient encouragement, this span gradually increases—especially as sentence making of this kind involves them in playing an active and creative part.

The use of the Sentence Maker and the Word Maker, the sequence to be observed in teaching punctuation and the part played by books composed by the children follow the same principles as in the use of *Breakthrough* with infants.

The part played by the *Breakthrough* books, however, has sometimes to be modified. Some of the twenty-four *Breakthrough* books may be suitable for these older children: *People in stories, My story* and *In Bed*, for instance, would all be quite suitable for young, slow juniors. Some others may not seem to be suitable but in practice children have been found to enjoy them in spite of the fact that they were written for younger children. The subject matter does not worry them when they find the language used is similar to their own. They may also have another reason for liking a book: one remedial secondary girl said of *Things I can do*, which is aimed very definitely at the interest of infants' school children, 'I like this book.' When asked why she liked it she replied, surprised by the question, 'Because I can read it.' She may also have meant that the book measured up to her expectations of what books, and the language of books, should be like.

As in all learning processes, fast progress in working with the Sentence Maker may be followed by a period of consolidation and apparent stand-still. When such a point has been reached, the teacher should not try to hurry children away from the work. Sometimes children who have started to write quite freely, without first making the sentences in the stand, revert to simple sentence making for a time. Any slow child should be allowed to use the Sentence Maker for as long as he wishes. Even when he does not need to build up the sentences first, he may still find it helpful to have his word store to refer to, to make sure of spellings.

Breakthrough in the secondary remedial department

The number of illiterate children entering the secondary schools is com-paratively small, but for them the problem is severe. Consistent failure for six years of their lives leaves a mark on their personalities, quite apart from the educational loss it represents. Remedial teachers will be familiar with the symptoms these children show—ranging from the hardened 'If I can't do it it's not worth doing' outlook to the blushing, sweating nervousness of the child who is still trying desperately despite his conviction of failure. Sentence work is not just a form of therapy but it *can* provide what may be the child's last chance of entering the world of the written word.

Secondary children who are illiterate are usually given extra help in small groups. A small experimental group of such children used the *Break-through* materials with encouraging results. Work with the Sentence Makers was found to follow the same course with these children as with those in the Junior remedial groups.

The following is an example of the way the work of one child developed: September 1968. She made these sentences in her Stand:

> I like to run and play.
> I like to play with my friend.
> some teachers are horrible.
> some girls are horrible.
> some boys are horrible.
> I am not horrible.
> I am a good girl.

May 1969. Written without making the sentences in her Stand:

> One day was a witch who live in a old house and three was gold shoe in the princess garden and the witch wanted the gold shoe but the princess didn't give her the gold shoe. the princess wanted to give

the gold shoe to a little girl the witch didn't like the little girl but the princess didn't care. The little girl was frightened of the witch the next day the princess give the little girl the gold shoe. In the end the little girl was going home and the witch take the little girl away.

(aged 12)

This girl could only draw a picture and label it with one word from a given list of words when she first came to the secondary school. After she had graduated from the Sentence Maker she was able to write stories using it only as a reminder of her earlier work with it. Occasionally she had queries about spelling.

Working with the Sentence Maker with these children brought to light points at which they had become enmeshed in difficulties and completely blocked by them. It is often said that the writing of a remedial child is nonsense; but very often this 'nonsense' was found to be similar to the first sentences made by infants' children—grammatical parts of the sentence omitted and the importance of word order not yet fully understood in the written medium. The possibility of moving words around and of discussing their order was found to be of the greatest importance in furthering children's understanding of what they were doing. *The more everything was discussed the greater the progress they made.*

The sentences they composed were made to look more like adult reading matter and closer to the printed word, by being typed on loose-leaf paper. They then had a book in which they wrote the sentences they had just made in the stands, as well as a file with a typed version of the same sentences. (It may be argued that the secondary child could type his own sentences but, apart from the shortage of typewriters, this is a slow process which causes him to become impatient and leads him to make many mistakes. At this stage the aim is to enable the child to jump the hurdle of initial literacy—not to involve him in typing lessons.) The file of typed sentences was very useful in helping them to produce some written work in other contexts. After a short time it included a wide range of English sentence patterns and these were adapted for use in subject lessons as though they were items in a foreign language phrase book. Among their own sentences the children found the useful phrase, the correct spelling of a word they wished to use, and wrote with regained confidence.

The transition to printed books was difficult for children of this age because so few of the available books were simple enough and relevant to their interests. Some of them read the *Breakthrough* books quite happily after they were told plainly 'These books were written for much younger children than you. Have a look at them and see what you think about them.' Their opinions and comments were taken seriously. No one had spent longer looking at infants' reading books than they had; they were not likely to accept any they did not like. In this critical frame of mind most of the children in the group read the *Breakthrough* books quite happily and with undisguised relief at achieving success at last. Some of the children also used the books as a source for words needed in their writing (for example *People in stories* for fairy stories and *The Christmas tree* for seasonal writing).

Once sentence making was well established the Word Maker became very important. It was also used with groups of children who were already reading and writing to a fairly adequate standard but who still had difficulty with spelling. Some of them arrived at their secondary school not only with no idea about regular spelling patterns but with the additional burden of ingrained misspellings. Handling the symbol cards and re-arranging them until a word appeared in its correct spelling increased the confidence of these children. With a pencil on paper the old faults seemed inevitable; the pencil seemed to lead the hand into well learned mistakes whereas the arrangement of the symbols in a stand gave word making a 'new look'.

All the work with the Word Maker suggested for infants should be taken with the secondary child at this stage. Some of the more complex patterns should be practised as well. For instance, a group might make the word *fight* and then change the first symbol to make as many words as possible. They might agree about *light, might, night, right, sight, tight*; but *bight, dight* and *wight* might lead to further discussion and to the further possibility of making *chight* or *gight*. (The section on spelling rules in Appendix 1 of the manual helps the teacher to make full use of the Word Maker.)

Breakthrough in the ESN school

In the educationally subnormal teaching situation and in that which confronts teachers of the severely subnormal, it may be a mistake to describe literacy teaching as *remedial*. The development pattern of these children is normal—for them. That it is accompanied by the delayed onset of literacy learning and by a slower learning rate presents teachers with special problems. The children whose failure to read and write has been noted earlier, have problems of quite different origins. It may be helpful to consider the problems of slow learning and delayed learning separately from those of remedial learning.

The successful teaching of children with delayed development calls for concentrated attention on what has to be learned and on how such learning takes place. The difficulties most children must overcome are intensified in the case of subnormal children. Their solution can bring a special insight not only to the remedial and the subnormal teaching situations, but also to the way in which children normally acquire literacy.

No member of the team had any qualification or special training for dealing with subnormal children nor were such children in mind when the *Breakthrough* materials were designed. Nevertheless it was gratifying that one ESN school joined the project for the experimental year. The materials

D. Mackay, B. Thompson and P. Shaub

and their use were explained to the staff concerned who were then left to use the materials in the way they thought best.

They worked very much in the way an infants' teacher would, but with slightly older children. The Magnet Board was found to be very helpful for starting both discussion and sentence work. In this school too, attention concentrated on sentence work and it developed well. Near the end of the first term each child who had started composing sentences independently was given a book with one sentence typed on each page. The child took this book home to read to his parents and to illustrate during the holidays. This evidence of progress encouraged both the parents and the child.

No child had any difficulty in handling and arranging the Sentence Maker words, but some children made more progress than others. The teachers' impressions of the results of this work were that each child had progressed further with *Breakthrough* materials than with any others they had tried previously, that the children had become very much involved in the work and had greatly enjoyed it. (A fuller account of this work appears in H. L. Cleaver and P. Schaub (1972) A breakthrough to literacy in *Special Education* 61, 1.)

Breakthrough and children in a Training Centre

One Training Centre also tried the materials. Children in a Training Centre, because of the severity of handicaps from which they suffer, present a most difficult educational problem and one which we would not have ventured to consider had not the Centre concerned requested to experiment with *Breakthrough*. Originally the staff thought that only the Teacher's Sentence Maker would be of any use to their children. However, a group of the most able children used individual Sentence Makers with success. They also read several of the books. The enjoyment which these children get from their work was impressive and the success they achieved surprising. Most of them were not expected to be able to take any steps towards literacy and, indeed, if they had found it too difficult or in any way upsetting, it would have been inadvisable to have expected them to do so. However, they showed the greatest delight in the work and there was every evidence that they understood what they were doing. They read with meaning and they were able to link words and sentences in *Breakthrough* books to the appropriate pictures.

Experience so far therefore suggests that the *Breakthrough to Literacy* materials provide a fruitful source of help both for retarded readers and for educationally subnormal children.

4.8 The English Colour Code programmed reading course

DAVID V. MOSELEY
Consultant educational psychologist

Reprinted from Vera Southgate (1972) (ed) *Literacy at all levels* Ward Lock Educational, pp. 168–74

Research background

A survey of 1,254 children, carried out in 1967, revealed that the following symptoms were characteristic of retarded readers:

1 inability to blend three or more phonemes
2 limited awareness of single-phoneme differences between words
3 poor visual analysis of figures consisting of three or more elements.

At least 75 per cent of retarded nine year olds had one or more of these difficulties although very few (5 per cent) had all three.

These results influenced the design of a remedial reading and spelling programme, recently published by the National Society for Mentally Handicapped Children. If phoneme–grapheme relations were made explicit by auditory prompts and visual cues, it was thought that the majority of slow learners would be able to make the necessary links.

This rationale led the author to experiment with colour-coded grapheme tiles. As Lee (1960) has shown, consonants are much more regular in spelling than vowels. It was not necessary, therefore, to use separate colours for consonant sounds. The English Colour Code consists of fifteen colour-cues used for vowel symbols, with the exception of neutral vowels. The name of each colour includes the appropriate vowel sound, e.g. red *e* (short vowel), green *e* (long vowel). An essential point was that every possible combination of letters used for vowel sounds was included, and a single grapheme tile always stood for a single sound. The complete set of consonant and vowel graphemes was used for word-building, with the teacher providing the necessary items and giving phonic prompts as required. For example, if a pupil wanted to build the word 'launch', the teacher supplied him with the following symbols: au n l ch. The pupil would work out the correct order, and perhaps copy the word.

The grapheme tiles were used for six months by twenty-nine children

David V. Moseley

(aged 7–10 years) entering remedial groups. The children were selected from a considerably larger pool of entrants, on the grounds that they performed badly in blending and discriminating sounds or in copying designs. At the end of the six-month period, the average improvement in word recognition was twenty-one months on the Burt test, and this was accompanied by improved blending scores.

While these results were encouraging, the procedure necessarily involved one-to-one teaching. However, if the teacher's prompts and feedback were recorded on tape, and printed worksheets were supplied, the student would be able to work without close supervision. But would separate graphemes be recognized as such in printed words, in the same way as before, when separate tiles were used? Before proceeding to publication, it was important to determine by experimental means whether coloured vowel symbols and various other typographical cues simplified the decoding process.

Five versions of the same *ar* worksheet were randomly distributed among 290 normal eleven year olds. Sentences were read out on tape, and missing letters and words filled in to phonic dictation. No mention was made of the different graphic cues, which included colour, as well as fine, bold and italic type. Comparison of pre- and post-test spelling scores showed that the scarlet *ar* was not confusing, but that both fine and italic type gave poorer results than no cues at all. However, bold type helped to reduce errors in polysyllables by 61 per cent, although it was not effective when used as a cue for neutral vowels. In fact, all special cues used for neutral vowels and silent letters tended to confuse rather than clarify. For a more detailed account of this research, see Moseley (1969a). In the published version of the worksheets, colour and bold type are the only cues which have been retained.

A duplicated version of the complete course was used by ten backward secondary children for a period of seventeen weeks. The phonic prompts were supplied by a teacher, not by a tape recorder. In addition, a second group of eight children followed the same course, with recorded instruction played back by the (Edison's Responsive Environment) Talking Typewriter. Both groups showed substantial gains in reading, spelling, phoneme-blending and spatial analysis. As with junior children, it was very unlikely for a pupil to exceed a seven year level of attainment if he were unable to blend four phonemes reliably. Full details of programme content are given in a report by Moseley (1969b). The strong emphasis on phoneme-blending, first as a listening skill, and then linked with precise visual analysis of word structure, appears to be fully justified. So, too, does the claim that recorded phonic instruction can to a great extent take the place of the live teacher.

Application

The course has undergone two extensive revisions since the duplicated version was compiled. Each type of exercise has been tried out both at the

Centre for Learning Disabilities and in schools. While some parts of the course are specially intended for teenagers, the scheme is suitable for any pupil of eight years or more who can make sense of a phonic approach. This will exclude some educationally subnormal children who have inadequate powers of analysis or generalization.

As writing plays an important part in the course, a spelling test rather than a reading test should be used to decide where a student should begin. Spelling scores are sometimes significantly lower than reading scores, but the reverse is almost never true. A table of spelling ages and recommended starting points, covering attainment levels between five and nine years, is given in the manual.

If a tape recorder and headphones are available, the course may be used in a normal classroom as well as in a small group setting. Additional sets of worksheets may be purchased, so that more than one pupil can follow the same tape. If a tape recorder is not available, the teacher can present the material from duplicated notes.

The length of study periods will vary according to age and ability, but will probably be between fifteen and thirty minutes. It is not intended that a complete programme (or even a complete page) should always be worked through in a single session. The slowest rate of working is likely to be one programme per week. This allows three or four sessions per week for supplementary exercises and activities which will ensure enough repetition at each stage of learning. When the student shows his completed worksheet to the teacher, and reads out certain sections, the teacher decides how much followup work is needed. Some suggestions are given in the manual, and many other useful ideas have been put forward by Jackson (1971).

The worksheets are nonexpendable. They may be cleaned with a damp cloth, but before doing this the student should enter the words he has written in his own 'spelling dictionary'. He will then have lists for revision and for reference during free-writing. He should be encouraged to add new words on his own initiative. A colour-coded reference system is described in the manual.

Progress tests are given at three key points in the course. If a student does not reach the levels indicated, he should not be allowed to proceed.

Stages of learning

The practice of 'sounding out' never fails to attract criticism from holists. And yet the ability to blend phonemes is the most important single correlate of word-recognition (once a basic sight vocabulary has been acquired). Blending can fail to occur for a number of reasons, among which are the following:

1   poor auditory discrimination

David V. Moseley

2 indistinct articulation
3 limited memory for a sequence of sounds.

All three defects can be trained by audio-vocal practice.

Additional visual and association processes are involved in decoding the printed word. Immediate recognition of two- and three-letter graphemes becomes very important at a reading age of seven plus. Another essential development is flexibility in assigning sound-values to graphemes. In fluent readers these processes are automatic, although even fluent readers analyse new words subvocally, usually in syllable units.

It is obviously better for a child to rely on rapid subvocal analysis of a new monosyllable than to 'sound it out aloud' with grunts and groans. However, good subvocal habits are best acquired by listening to the voices of competent models. Quiet conditions are essential. A headset shuts out unwanted background noise.

The first five programmes are concerned with letter recognition, initial consonant sounds and short vowel sounds. No prior awareness of serial position is needed. No initial consonant blends are given in the examples for auditory discrimination, so the single consonant sounds may be as salient as possible. Many phonic programmes make the mistake of asking for responses to first, middle and final sounds at too early a stage. As Carver (1970) has shown, children do not normally master sequential aspects of decoding, including auditory discrimination of initial multiple consonants, before they reach an attainment age of $6\frac{1}{2}$–7 years.

More than 100 written responses are made in each programme, and the print size has been chosen to match the handwriting of a young child. The first side of each sheet deals with a group of five letters, which have dissimilar shapes and sounds. On the 'rhyme side' the range of letters to be recognized and written includes those which have been studied in earlier programmes. Here the student writes whole words and also copies simple sentences. A total of forty words is used. If both the letters and the words are to be thoroughly learned, supplementary exercises and games will be needed. Some of these should be designed to help make reliable discriminations between very similar sounds (e.g. m/n) or very similar shapes (e.g. i/j).

The next stage (programmes 6–10) gives a great deal of emphasis to the serial aspects of words and sentences. Both whole-word and phonic exercises are used. While more than seventy common words are learned without analysis, at least three times as many are shown to make sense phonically. Important sight words are taught in groups of four. The student has to put a mark beside the appropriate word whenever he hears it in a story. Frequent pauses are made so that the student can rehearse the phrase or sentence he has just heard. This trains him to try out various possible solutions, without forgetting the context in which a word occurred. It is most important that concentration on single words or sounds should not preclude listening for meaning.

The aim of the picture exercises in these programmes is to promote rapid blending of phonemes as a listening skill, and to link the dictation of sounds with visual scanning. The sounds are articulated at the rate of two per second. At this speed, the burden on immediate memory is greatly reduced and closure is easily achieved. The only motor response required is underlining one of two words, most of which differ by the omission or addition of a letter. If the sequence of sounds is rehearsed, the only visual aspect of the exercise is scanning the words and determining how many graphemes are present. This visual analysis is facilitated by the use of extra bold type to indicate graphemes of two or more letters.

Context clues are included in the phonic dictation exercises which follow. Here the student is asked to write in the letters as he hears the sounds. In each case he knows which word he is writing, and as the rate of dictation is slow he should be able to anticipate each sound subvocally. Attention is drawn to all letter positions in four-phoneme words. At first, the student has to write in only one or two letters per word but this is gradually extended to a maximum of four. At this level he may begin to analyse initial or final consonant combinations as single units. However, he is not yet expected to decode new words with any degree of fluency.

On the 'story side' of each programme, the student applies what he has learned in previous exercises. He listens to an episode featuring Ted and his friends and then writes in most of the words, which he can find in an alphabetical reference list at the top of the sheet. At each point the preceding words are read out on the tape, so the student can look back at what he has just written and keep the context in mind. The few words he does not have to write are those which are outside the sight vocabulary and grapheme patterns with which he is already familiar.

The structure of programmes 11–20 is constant, and at this stage the pupil learns how to decode words of three or four phonemes, including those with consonant digraphs and long vowels. Colour-coding facilitates the immediate recognition of vowel digraphs, and once a particular spelling pattern has been studied, it should be recognized without the aid of colour. Only one new combination of letters (qu) is introduced in these programmes; otherwise they serve to consolidate the spelling patterns which occur in programmes 7–10.

Throughout the course, the words to be written include only those spelling patterns which have been previously studied, together with one new pattern from programmes 20 onwards. There are also some sentences for the pupil to read, where the same restrictions apply. New demands are made on the student every three or four lines. Most of the sentences on the sheets include words with missing letters, which are filled in to phonic dictation. Sometimes the word is illustrated by cartoon-style pictures, and recorded sound effects are provided where appropriate. The student has to listen to the phonemes very carefully in order to get the full meaning of each sentence. After time has been given for him to complete the word, it is then spoken normally on the tape, and the student copies it at the side of

David V. Moseley

the sheet. Dashes indicate the number of letters, and the position of digraphs is indicated by the usual cues of bold print for consonants and colour for vowels. Phonic dictation is used for words which include the particular grapheme which is being studied. All the other words written by the student are excluded from analysis.

Each programme includes thirty or more examples of a particular spelling pattern. The words are taken from a 5000 word source list, compiled by the author from seven well known vocabulary and spelling lists. It is clearly not possible to provide enough repetition of individual words for learning to take place on a word-by-word basis. There has to be generalization on the basis of grapheme-patterns if the pupil is to progress beyond a reading repertoire of more than about 200 words. The worksheets are designed to familiarize the student with the full range of graphemes in a gradual progression. The order in which new graphemes are introduced is determined by frequency counts (number of different words rather than occurrence in continuous text), but some concessions have been made to the normal practice of teaching certain patterns in groups.

The teacher should provide ample opportunities for reinforcement of new words after the student has completed each programme. Games and exercises should be available requiring discrimination between short and long vowels, and including some of the more difficult consonant combinations such as *spr* and *str*. After programme 20, reading will come to play a major part in providing reinforcement, particularly if a phonically graded scheme is used. Most words will be read without hesitation, subvocal phonic analysis being used for those patterns which are as yet not fully automatic.

Increasingly, the whole syllable becomes the basic unit for word-building, and to prepare for this, extra bold print is introduced at programme 21 for cueing syllables which are stressed in speech. Separate phoneme cues are phased out, and dropped altogether after programme 35. The grapheme patterns studied towards the end of the course are of relatively low frequency, and include most combinations with silent letters. An attempt should be made in followup work to learn most of the examples.

A supplementary spelling course entitled *Syllable Study* concludes the programme. This is suitable for older and more intelligent students. It covers some rather complicated spelling rules, and teaches the meaning of common prefixes and suffixes.

References

CARVER, C. (1970) *A Group or Individual Word Recognition Test* (Manual of Instructions) London: University of London Press
JACKSON, S. (1971) *Get Reading Right* (Handbook) Glasgow: Gibson
LEE, W. R. (1960) *Spelling Irregularity and Reading Difficulty in English*

Occasional Publication no 2 Slough: National Foundation for Educational Research

MOSELEY, D. V. (1969a) Graphic cues for spelling in *Education*, 14th May

MOSELEY, D. V. (1969b) The Talking Typewriter and remedial teaching in a secondary school in *Remedial Education* 4, 196–202

4.9 ita and slow learners: a reappraisal

JOHN DOWNING

Professor of Education, University of Victoria, British Columbia

Reprinted from *Educational Research* (1969) 11, 3, pp. 229–31

Vernon (1967) in *The ita Symposium*, commenting on my (1967a) report of the original ita experiment, states:

> Contrary to Downing's conclusion, there *were* fewer children of poor reading ability in the ita than in the to group. (p. 158)

The conclusion referred to by Vernon was summarized by me (1967b) as follows:

> The slower-learning children do begin to show some benefit from ita at the end of the third year, but the poorest 10 per cent show negligible improvements in test results. (p. 293)

This conclusion was based on the average scores for each of ten 'achievement categories'. These were established by first ranking the scores separately in the experimental (ita) and control (to) groups and then dividing them into the ten equal achievement categories. Average scores were then computed for each of the ten categories to allow a comparison of ita and to results for each category (e.g. the bottom 10 per cent of the ita group was compared with the bottom 10 per cent of the to group).

This procedure helped to compress and summarize a great deal of data collected in the experiment but, because of the insensitivity of most reading tests at the lower scoring levels, this treatment of the data may have made the tests still less sensitive and thereby concealed real differences. Vernon's criticism draws attention to this problem and suggests the new analysis which follows.

Full information on the design and method of the experiment is provided in Downing's *Evaluating the Initial Teaching Alphabet*. The present article is confined to a reanalysis of the data along the lines suggested by Vernon's criticism.

Following her approach, instead of comparing the average scores of fixed proportions of slow-learners in the ita and to groups, the proportions of children in each of these groups who made low scores on each test will be compared.

Transfer results

Vernon's reference was to results of testing all children in both ita and to groups on to forms only of the tests. Thus for the ita pupils the measures are of transfer of learning from ita training to to reading. Table 1 shows how the ita group and the to group compared on the proportion of low scores on all tests administered *in to only to both groups* after the middle of the second year.

TABLE 1   *Proportion of low scores on to tests in ita and to groups*

Test	Time of test	Scores	Total number of children tested in each group	Percentage of children in low-scoring category	
				ita group	*to group*
Reading:					
Neale Accuracy	midsecond year	0–10	457	40.9	42.0
Neale Speed	midsecond year	0–10	457	22.8	19.5
Neale Comprehension	midsecond year	0–5	457	50.8	56.0
Schonell GWRT	beginning third year	0–10	291	21.3	23.4
Neale Accuracy	end third year	0–10	194	9.8	17.5
Neale Speed	end third year	0–10	194	4.6	4.1
Neale Comprehension	end third year	0–5	194	14.9	24.7
Standish NS 45	end third year	0–5	175	17.7	24.6
Spelling:					
Schonell GWST	midthird year	0–14	374	17.4	24.9
Schonell GWST	midfourth year	0–14	102	3.9	13.7

In six out of eight reading tests and in both spelling tests the trend is the same as that noted by Vernon. The two exceptions to this trend were in the Neale test of reading *rate* in midsecond year and at the end of the third year. The differences in the proportions of low scores are quite small in the first four reading tests administered in the middle of second year and at the beginning of third year, but at the end of third year they seem more important. Generally, by this time there were approximately only two-thirds as many low to scores in the ita group as there were in the to group. There were also substantially fewer very poor to spellers in the ita group in comparison with the to group.

But these comparisons are the least important in the original research both for theoretical and practical purposes. The pretransition scores of the ita group are the vital data for the essential aim of the ita experiment.

John Downing

Pretransition results

The original purpose of the research was to investigate the effects of t o on learning to read. To accomplish this, the experimental group not only learned i t a but were *tested in i t a*. Their results were compared with those obtained from testing t o pupils on parallel tests in t o. In this way the effects of t o as compared with regularized and simplified English as represented by i t a could be determined. The results of applying Vernon's approach to these more important data are shown in Table 2.

TABLE 2 *Proportion of low scores on i t a tests in i t a group and t o tests in t o group*

Reading test	Time of test	Scores	Total number of children tested in each group	Percentage of children in low-scoring category	
				i t a group	t o group
Basic Reader reached	end first year	Below Book III	651	61.6	81.1
Basic Reader reached	after 1½ yrs.	Below Book III	580	31.0	54.8
Basic Reader reached	after 2 yrs.	Below Book III	333	17.7	35.7
Basic Reader reached	after 2⅜ yrs.	Below Book III	278	10.1	25.9
Schonell GWRT	end first year	0–4	660	36.2	62.3
Schonell GWRT	after 1½ yrs.	0–4	585	14.4	27.7
Neale-Accuracy	after 1½ yrs.	0–10	459	27.7	54.5
Neale-Speed	after 1½ yrs.	0–10	459	17.4	19.4
Neale-Comprehension	after 1½ yrs.	0–5	459	46.8	69.3

Here, every one of the tests showed the same trend noted by Vernon, although once again the speed of reading seems least affected. On most tests the degree of difference is greater at the pretransition stage. For example, in four of the nine tests there were only half as many i t a pupils as t o pupils in the low scoring category.

Discussion

This reappraisal of the data related to the problem of the differential effects of i t a and to on the slower-learning pupils in the i t a experiment confirms Vernon's point. All the tests, except speed of reading, show that *i t a generally reduces the incidence of poor reading and poor spelling both before and after transition to to.*

Nevertheless, this does not seem to confound the original finding that the difference between i t a and t o is smaller among slow-learners than among average and above average pupils. Nor does it change the fact that in the weakest 10 per cent of the population any statistical difference between i t a and t o cannot be detected by conventional reading tests.

From the practical point of view, the original analysis and Vernon's approach question the effects of i t a on slow-learners in different ways. The ita and slow learners

original analysis attempted to answer the question: 'Does ita make a difference for the weakest 10 per cent?'

Vernon's criticism suggests the question: 'Does ita reduce the incidence of the poorer levels of attainment?'

The original analysis showed, in fact, that objective tests are unable to detect any difference between ita and to in the weakest 10 per cent of pupils tested.

This reappraisal suggested by Vernon's criticism answers the second question; ita does in fact reduce the incidence of poorer reading and poorer spelling attainments. In view of the lack of sensitivity of conventional tests to differences in the early stages of learning to read, this second answer may be more important to teachers of classes containing slower learners. A recent survey (Downing 1968) of the opinions of teachers in ESN schools using ita gives further support to the view that ita gives important help to slower learners who otherwise become confused by the irregularities of to, or are overwhelmed by the feats of memory involved in learning to.

References

*DOWNING, J. (1967a) Research report on the British experiment with ita in J. Downing, et al The ita Symposium. Slough: National Foundation for Educational Research

DOWNING, J. (1967b) Evaluating the Initial Teaching Alphabet London: Cassell

DOWNING, J. (1968) The initial teaching alphabet and educationally subnormal children Developmental Medicine and Child Neurology 10, 200–5

NEALE, M. D. (1963) Neale Analysis of Reading Ability London: Macmillan

SCHONELL, F. J. and SCHONELL, F. E. (1956) Graded word reading test in F. J. Schonell, Diagnostic and Attainment Testing London: Oliver and Boyd

SCHONELL, F. J. (1956) Graded word spelling test in F. J. Schonell, Diagnostic and Attainment Testing London: Oliver and Boyd

STANDISH, E. J. (1960) Reading Test (7+) Form NS 45 London: Newnes

VERNON, M. D. (1967) Evaluations—11 in J. Downing, et al The ita Symposium Slough: National Foundation for Educational Research

4.10 An experiment with ita in remedial reading

NICHOLAS J. GEORGIADES
Birkbeck College, University of London

Reprinted from *New Education* (1967) September, pp. 11–12

Most of the published work of the Reading Research Unit has been confined to the evaluation of ita with beginning readers. For two reasons this is not surprising. First, Pitman developed the writing system for just such children and secondly most of the grants to the Reading Research Unit were confined to evaluations of the medium with beginners.

However, in 1964 the Department of Education and Science allocated a sum of money to the Unit to assess the value of ita with children who had previously failed to master the skills of learning to read. This article represents the bare bones of a 30,000 word report presented to the DES after the completion of an experiment using ita in remedial reading classes (Georgiades 1969).

Much has been said and written of the value of ita with beginning readers. Many hoped for similar success with those who had previously failed to learn to read and that ita would become the final solution to much retardation.

The first paper suggesting that ita might be of value in the remedial situation was by Downing and Gardner (1962). They suggested that their first stage results seemed 'to provide positive support for the view that the complexity and unsystematic nature of the traditional spelling of English is an important cause of reading failure'. However, they urged caution, since a total of only 14 experimental and 30 control children were involved.

Gardner (1965) reported on experiments he had conducted in Walsall and suggested that certain observable facts could not be denied: that there had been a 'real improvement in classroom performance', that the problem of illiteracy 'had been virtually eliminated where the problem had been severe'.

Gardner further reported the progress of 75 pupils who had been matched with a control group and who were taught in groups by a peripatetic remedial teacher. The ita group gained 2.4 years (in reading age) in six months, the to group 1.8 years in the same period. However, no data was provided on the matching of the two groups, on the selection criteria or on such variables as intelligence and home background.

Others, during the period 1961–6 have indicated success with i t a in remedial situations (see Harrison 1964, Yeates 1963). However, most of the work thus far reported is predominantly anecdotal. Experiments that have been conducted represent no more than a first attempt at controlled evaluation. On controlled evaluation we are reminded by Campbell and Stanley (1964) that:

> Educational experimentation is the only means of settling disputes regarding educational practice, the only way of verifying educational improvement.

The experiment

Space precludes discussion of certain aspects of our decision-making processes with respect to the conduct and design of the experiment. It is hoped that the full report will be published and available in book form later this year (Georgiades 1969).

Two general considerations, however, should be borne in mind. First, that we attempted to evaluate i t a in a situation which would generate as much useful information as possible to as many interested parties as possible. Secondly, and arising out of our first consideration, we attempted a balance between our external validity (the extent to which our results could be generalized to a wider population) and our internal validity (the scientific value of our study). To facilitate such a balance our decisions about the design and conduct of the experiment were taken in the closest collaboration with the educational psychologists and teachers involved in the field. No decision of importance was taken independently of their views.

The design

It was decided to establish a design which could be analysed statistically by means of the analysis of variance technique, equating and balancing through the design such variables as the rural/urban environment of our subjects; the peripatetic or centre-organized system of remedial teaching and finally the oft encountered problem of differing teacher-abilities. Table 1 shows how this balancing was accomplished. It will be seen that the two former variables are balanced throughout the design as nearly as possible, and that each teacher taught i t a and t o groups.

The children

We adopted the following objective definition of children who were in need of remedial reading classes. A child retarded in reading for the purpose of

TABLE 1   *Total size of classes after dropouts and distribution of sex within classes*

		Experimental *ita* classes		Control *to* classes		
Area:	North	Boys	8	Boys	4	
System:	Peripatetic	Girls	1	Girls	5	Teacher Set: I
Locale:	Urban					
Teacher:	Mr A.	TOTAL	9	TOTAL	9	
Area:	East	Boys	6	Boys	8	
System:	Centre	Girls	3	Girls	2	Teacher Set: II
Locale:	Rural					
Teacher:	Mrs B.	TOTAL	9	TOTAL	10	
Area:	South	Boys	4	Boys	4	
System:	Centre	Girls	2	Girls	2	Teacher Set: III
Locale:	Urban					
Teacher:	Mr C.	TOTAL	6	TOTAL	6	
Area:	South	Boys	3	Boys	3	
System:	Centre	Girls	–	Girls	1	Teacher Set: IV
Locale:	Urban					
Teacher:	Mrs D.	TOTAL	3	TOTAL	4	
Area:	West	Boys	4	Boys	3	
System:	Peripatetic	Girls	4	Girls	5	Teacher Set: V
Locale:	Rural					
Teacher:	Mr E.	TOTAL	8	TOTAL	8	
Area:	West	Boys	1	Boys	2	
System:	Peripatetic	Girls	3	Girls	3	Teacher Set: VI
Locale:	Rural					
Teacher:	Mr F.	TOTAL	4	TOTAL	5	

TOTAL Boys: 51   Girls: 30   TOTAL: 81

this study would be a child of either sex, between chronological ages of eight and nine years at the start of the experiment (October 1965), who demonstrated on a full-scale Wechsler Intelligence Scale for Children a score of between 85 and 115 and who at the same time scored between 5.5 years and 6.5 years on the Burt (rearranged) Graded Word Reading Test. This definition represents a retardation of between two and three years in reading age below the chronological age of the subjects—a widely used criterion in assessing the need for remedial treatment.

The teachers

The teachers to be involved in the experiment had already been selected by their lea as competent remedial teachers, and had thus all attained high standards of professional competence. To a large extent the selection of the leas in the experiment predetermined the teachers who were to take part and virtually no control could be exercised by the experimenters. It should be remembered, however, that the teachers in fact taught both ita and to groups for the duration of the study.

Materials and methods

In autumn 1965 very few suitable parallel (ita and to) texts or library books were available. However, by the end of the second term of the experiment the groups were provided with 47 titles in both to and ita. In the third term 27 titles all in to were provided. All the children in the experiment received brand new reading materials in parallel identical versions. The teachers were actively discouraged from using any material other than that provided, although to what extent this discouragement was effective is difficult to estimate. Further, during the first term parallel versions of a workbook were also distributed.

In the past there has been severe criticism of the lack of control of teaching method in experiments evaluating ita. Teaching method is, of course, one of the most difficult of all experimental variables to control. However, all six teachers were exponents experienced in remedial reading instruction, and one would expect a great deal of common ground in their approach to the problem. In the earliest discussion it was decided that a pragmatic approach should be adopted, using whichever method of instruction seemed most appropriate at the time. The teachers were, however, continually reminded that the treatment of ita and to groups should be as similar as possible.

Apart from the tests used in defining our groups, other measures of reading and spelling ability were used throughout the experiment. The Neale Analysis of Reading Ability Forms A, B and C; the Schonell Graded Word Reading Test and the Schonell Spelling Tests Form A and B were given to the children at different times throughout the experiment as well as the Burt (rearranged) and the wisc.

Besides these attainment tests each teacher completed a Stott Social Adjustment Guide (used as a measure of adjustment) on each child. Further, data was collected on parents' occupations, type of home, size and position of children in family. This information enabled us to make satisfactory assessments of home backgrounds; the matching of the two groups seemed to be more than adequate.

Time limits

Before discussing the results of the study we should concern ourselves briefly with the time limits imposed upon the evaluation. Teachers involved with remedial reading instruction have in the past restricted the length of their regimes to approximately one school year. The reasons for this are quite understandable. The pressures on the service are always great, the waiting list seemingly unvarying in length. In the past those concerned have been anxious to keep the children for the shortest possible time commensurate with reasonable progress. On average then it seemed appropriate to examine the value of i t a in a course lasting one school year.

Teachers' records show that throughout the school year the t o groups had an average of 93 hours teaching; the i t a groups 96 hours teaching. During the remainder of the time the children were taught normally in their own parent schools.

In summary it can be said that the data presented in Table 2 and previous statements indicate that the two groups were matched with respect to the background variables of age, intelligence, socioeconomic class, adjustment and initial reading age.

TABLE 2 *Summary of data for to and i t a groups for chronological age, intelligence and two Graded Word Reading Tests*

	to			ita		
	NO	*Mean*	*SD*	*NO*	*Mean*	*SD*
Chronological age in years	42	8.50	0.34	39	8.40	0.29
Wechsler Intelligence Scale Score (Full Scale)	42	96.40	6.66	39	99.20	7.71
Burt Rearranged Reading Ages (1)	42	6.10	0.37	39	6.10	0.32
Burt Rearranged Reading Ages (2)	41	7.45	0.81	37	7.42	0.90
Schonell Reading Test no. of words correct (1)	42	14.10	4.90	39	13.00	3.90
Schonell Reading Test no. of words correct (2)	41	30.60	6.30	39	30.70	8.40

Results

It is not possible to give all the figures concerning attainment in the space available. However, Table 2 gives representative results on two of the tests concerned with word recognition. These results are representative in ita in remedial reading

the sense that the lack of significant difference between the means of the two groups was characteristic of all the attainment tests administered. On all but one test there proved to be no significant difference between the groups.

The single exception was a test of reading rate administered halfway through the experiment in which the t o group read significantly faster than the i t a group. This difference had disappeared by the end of the experiment.

As a measure of general progress, the Burt score indicates a mean gain of 1.35 years in reading age for the to group and 1.32 years for the i t a group. Such progress is not out of line with what many remedial teachers would expect.

Conclusions

What can we determine from the results of the value of i t a in remedial reading classes? We should remember that the experiment that was conducted was 'situation specific'. It dealt with a particular group of children in highly defined circumstances. Although the conditions were clearly specified they did represent to a large extent current practice amongst a great many remedial reading services. Further, we should remember that the children were spending only approximately one-tenth of their school time in one year being exposed to remediation. The i t a children returned to their parent schools where they were taught in to. However, as stated before, this situation is rather typical.

Given these conditions then, the results indicate that there is little to be gained by using i t a—similar results will be obtained by using the traditional orthography.

We should repeat that under different circumstances (say by using i t a intensively for a three month period of remediation) we might well have obtained different results. The fact remains that under the conditions described all too briefly above, i t a does not appear to offer any advantage over the traditional orthography in helping to remedy previous reading failure.

References

CAMPBELL, D. T. and STANLEY, J. C. (1964) Experimental and quasi-experimental designs for research in teaching in N. L. Gage (ed) *Handbook of Research on Teaching* Chicago: Rand McNally
DOWNING, J. A. and GARDNER, W. K. (1962) New experimental evidence on the role of the unsystematic spelling of English in reading failure *Educational Research* 1, 69–75
GARDNER, W. K. (1965) Remedial reading with i t a in England in A. J. Mazurkiewitz (ed) *i t a and the World of English* New York: Initial Teaching Alphabet Foundation

N. J. Georgiades

GEORGIADES, N. J. (1969) *ita in Remedial Reading Groups* London: Harrap
HARRISON, M. (1964) Hope for the hopeless in *The Teacher* 28th February
YEATES, R. G. (1963) Curing backwardness in reading *The Teacher* 16th August

4.11　The effects of counselling on retarded readers

D. LAWRENCE
School Psychological Service, Somerset County Council

Reprinted from *Educational Research* (1971) 13, 2, pp. 119–24

The aims of this study were to investigate the effects on reading attainment of individual personal counselling compared with the results obtained by a traditional remedial reading programme, and to consider the association between certain personality characteristics and reading retardation. Four groups, each containing twelve primary school children retarded in reading, were matched, and each group subjected to different treatments. At the end of a six month period the children in the counselled group showed a significant rise in reading attainment over all other groups, together with improved self-images as measured on the Children's Personality Questionnaire.

'Educational failure is personal failure' (NFER 1968). The retarded reader sees himself not only as an inferior reader but as an inferior person. Since reading is a skill which adults around him regard as important, failure in this area tends to invade the whole personality. The result is a child who has come to accept failure as inevitable and whose natural curiosity and enthusiasm for learning remain inhibited.

The retarded reader comes to the learning situation poorly motivated and lacking in confidence in his ability to learn. Apart from the adoption of a generally encouraging attitude, however, there is rarely a systematic attempt on the part of the teacher to improve the child's level of motivation. It is suggested in this article that in the treatment of retarded readers more attention should be paid to the child's emotional life. The usual system is to focus primarily on cognitive factors—on the diagnosis and treatment of perceptual disabilities, for instance, despite the fact that one of the retarded reader's most outstanding characteristics appears to be his poor emotional adjustment.

Dr Joyce Morris concluded in the Kent Survey (1966) that many poor readers became withdrawn, depressed, anxious for adult interest and affection, hostile, indifferent to adults, anxious to gain acceptance and

D. Lawrence

prestige among other children, hostile to other children and generally rest-less. The results of the experiment referred to in this article would seem to confirm Dr Morris's observations. On the o Factor of the Cattell Children's Personality Questionnaire, retarded readers scored significantly higher than good readers. Cattell describes a high score on this factor as indicating an 'apprehensive, worrying, depressed, guilt-prone' tendency.

A School's Council report (1970) emphasizes that much educational retardation occurs as a result of psychological deprivation. These children come to school already lacking in enthusiasm and curiosity for learning and probably with unsatisfied emotional needs. Whether the self-image and poor emotional adjustment of the retarded reader is a consequence or a cause of his reading problem, the end result is the same—poor motivation.

The recent work of Rosenthal (1969) illustrates the effect on the child's attainments of the particular attitude adopted by the teacher. The results of the experiment referred to in this article would seem to further confirm the importance of the quality of the personal relationships and the need to focus attention on the child's emotional life. The counselling method outlined in this experiment suggests a technique which could be used by any sympathetic person interested in the remedial treatment of retarded readers. Various writers have shown that personal counselling can be carried out by nonspecialists (Carkhuff 1968).

There is extensive evidence to indicate that lay persons can be trained to function at minimally facilitative levels of conditions related to constructive client change.

This experiment was carried out to investigate the hypothesis that it would be possible to improve the child's general level of motivation and ulti-mately his reading attainment by allowing him regular opportunity to express his personality in the company of a sympathetic adult.

Design of experiment

Four schools were selected as being typical village schools in a rural community. The children in these schools who were considered by their headteachers to be retarded in reading were then given the Schonell Word Recognition Test, the Sleight Nonverbal Intelligence Test and the Porter and Cattell Children's Personality Questionnaire. The cpq was also given to a random sample of good readers.

It was found possible to match twelve children in each school on chronological age, sex, mental age and reading attainment. Each group contained eight boys and four girls.

Group 1 received remedial reading from a specialist teacher for six months. Group 2 received remedial reading plus counselling for six months. Group 3 received counselling only for six months. Each child was seen individually for 20 minutes each week. Group 4 was a control group and received no special treatment.

All children were retested after six months in the Schonell Word Recognition Test. The Children's Personality Questionnaire was also given again at the end of the experiment to assess any significant change in personality profile.

Parents were not interviewed as it was felt that interviews could not easily be controlled and some parents would not possibly be able to cooperate. If this kind of counselling programme was to be of any practical value to teachers it also had to be as simple as possible.

Method used with counselling group

Basically this involved a responsible, sympathetic adult, with status in the eyes of the child, communicating to the child that he enjoyed his company.

1 The counsellor introduced himself as a person interested in children and who liked to ensure that they were happy in school.
2 The establishment of an uncritical, friendly atmosphere, involving total acceptance of the child's personality was attempted.
3 The counsellor tried to provide a sounding-board for the child's feelings—direct interpretation was avoided (Rogers 1965).
4 The interview was child-centred throughout.
5 As a rule direct questioning was avoided. Questions that were asked were posed in a general way except when presenting the Self-Concept Questionnaire (Table 7).
6 Discussion at first was sometimes only possible through the medium of drawings and pictures. The child was asked to draw a picture. In later sessions other pictures were used as a further stimulus to feelings, e.g. Children's Apperception Test pictures (Bellak 1954).
7 Early in the period he was asked for three main wishes and each discussed more fully.
8 Throughout the interview the counsellor tried to be alert for opportunities of praising the child's personality (not his skills), and in so doing, building up his self-image.
9 The following areas of the child's life were covered over the counselling period: relationship with parents; relationship with siblings; relationship with peers; relationship with other relatives; hobbies and interests; aspirations, immediate and long-term; worries, fears, anxieties; attitude towards school, and attitude towards self.

This procedure and framework were flexible and varied with the particular child and his needs as well as his moods.

D. Lawrence

Individual summary record of counselled group

Case 1 (RS)

R presented as a shy, timid, but friendly little boy. This shyness was confirmed on the CPQ test with a score markedly deviating from the average. On a self-concept questionnaire he revealed that he always felt stupid. R was the eighth of ten children and was insistent that he preferred school to home, where his parents were infirm—father with arthritis and mother with varicose veins. He seemed to accept that they could not spare him much time. It was probably significant that he said he often dreamed of his girl-friend. He loved to talk of this person, but only in later sessions did he confess that she was married.

It seemed that his need to feel affection was being projected onto this person. His three wishes were for a bicycle, a car and a football. Throughout the programme he revealed a strong compensation for inferiority feelings, e.g. 'I can climb trees better than any of my family.' In the CAT pictures his interpretations were notable in that the baby was always getting into trouble through doing stupid things, i.e. standing on mother's foot and causing her to drop her basket; mother smacking baby for playing in mud. There was also indication of his feeling of rejection i.e. parents unhappy because they wanted a different baby.

This boy made the most progress in reading (SWR 5.1–7.3 years).

Case 2 (SR)

This boy came out on the CPQ test markedly introverted with strong guilt feelings and a poor self-image. His stories on CAT pictures revolved around 'not being liked by other people'. This made him angry. He makes a mess in the home and his mother is cross. He worries about this, wishing he could be good. He is told off in front of visitors and this makes him angry. On a self-concept questionnaire he indicated that he felt it was always best to be a nice person—he did not feel this. S shone at drawing and his parents praised him for this. He insisted he disliked drawing and one day confessed that he only said this because he knew they were only trying to make him feel better since it was reading which he really cared about. This he worried about in bed at night. He also worried about the house father was rebuilding while they lived alongside, in a caravan. He wondered if it would fall. He worried about his parents' talk of going to Australia to live. He worried about his younger sister being cleverer—she could read. He worried about his mother being pregnant and perhaps another competitor. There were flashes of compensation for these feelings of inferiority e.g. 'I can now run 100 yards in 11 seconds.' He had no hobbies apart from drawing which he resented (SWR 7.7–8.7 years).

Case 3 (SB)

On the CPQ test all this boy's scores lay within the average range. He presented on interview as a pleasant, cheerful boy lacking in drive. Whatever type of conversation was introduced he had no strong feelings about it. On the CAT picture test, all his stories emphasized this attitude—no tensions, strains or stresses e.g. the fierce tiger was portrayed as benevolent at first, but later given the opposite role. He was not sure whether his parents knew that he was a poor reader: 'They have never asked me.' He talked easily about his life on the farm where he helped his father and intended to become a farmer himself one day. He said he did not mind being a poor reader. All the interviews were notable for the completely relaxed atmosphere he created. This boy made the least progress in reading of any in the group (SWR 7.9–8.1 years).

Case 4 (TS)
This girl on the CPQ test came out as markedly introverted with high guilt score. The first session was notable for her total inability to converse, confirming the high introversion score. In later sessions, however, she chattered incessantly about herself, her poor school work and her family. She indicated that she always felt stupid and that 'to be clever' was the most important thing. 'Daddy says I'm stupid' was an often repeated statement, said with no feeling, just acceptance of the inevitable. This child showed more worries and anxieties than any other member of the group. She was not an unattractive child to look at but wore glasses and hated it—'I'm so different from the others.' The CAT stories were notable for their recurrent themes of anxiety and family insecurity. I later found that her father had been blinded in an accident and her mother had left home. She was looked after by her grandmother. Throughout she insisted on saying 'I cannot read and I never will be able to read.' In fact, she did make some progress but again she denied this (SWR 5.3–6.1 years).

Discussion

The original hypothesis that it is possible to raise the level of reading attainment in a group of retarded readers through a process of individual personal counselling would appear to have been confirmed. The counselled group made the most progress in reading attainment compared with all other groups. The difference between this group and the other groups proved to be statistically significant in each case, except when compared with the group which received remedial reading combined with counsell- . ing.

The children in the counselled group were judged by their teachers to be more enthusiastic and confident in class the longer the experiment progressed.

The personality testing on the Cattell Personality Questionnaire at the start of the experiment indicated that all but two retarded readers in the counselled group had a higher than average o factor score. Cattell regards this as an indication of 'troubled, guilt-prone behaviour associated with a poor self-image'. It is interesting that a randomly tested group of good readers in the same school tested on the same test had without exception a below average score on the o factor. That poor performance in reading would appear to be associated with a poor self-image received further confirmation from the conversation of the individual children in the counselled group. At the conclusion of the experiment only two children in the counselled group had a higher than average o factor score. It would appear to be a further indication of the success of the programme.

From the individual summary record of the counselled group it looks as if retarded readers tend to have unsatisfied emotional needs but without specific symptoms of emotional maladjustment. None of the group was considered by his teacher to be emotionally disturbed or in need of treatment.

The two children in the counselled group who did not show a high guilt score at the outset were the two members of the group who had made the least progress at the end of the experiment. All the responses of sb (Case 3) seemed to be within the normal range. This boy appeared to be unusually content, even with his school failure, but not in an apathetic way. It might just be possible that some children are retarded in reading but with no associated emotional dissatisfactions. Increased motivation in this case would perhaps have been better achieved by making more demands on the child in the learning situation, rather than through a counselling programme.

The second child who made least progress in the counselled group showed a very high level of anxiety on the Cattell test and it was later discovered that she came from a particularly disturbed home background. She seemed a tense, restless child throughout the experiment and would probably have been better helped by referral to the Child Guidance Centre for a fuller psychiatric diagnosis. Counselling at this level of help could not be expected to help the severely emotionally disturbed child, and more specialist treatment would be indicated.

A third child who made less progress than all but the two just mentioned was later shown to have a neurological handicap and to be receiving medical treatment.

Most of the children's problems appeared to stem from the family relationships. This was not unexpected but the fact that the children appeared to derive benefit from talking of their problems to the counsellor without his involving the families raises interesting possibilities.

Given that educational retardation is often the result of poor home conditions we seem to be faced with the mammoth task of having to improve the home background before being able to effect any change in the child's attitudes. With the present general shortage of personnel in the educational and social fields this presents an almost insurmountable problem. The present experiment into the effects of individual counselling would seem to indicate that we can tackle the problem at this level of help without necessarily needing to interview parents.

Conclusion

In most cases of reading retardation it should be possible to increase the general level of motivation by planning a personal counselling programme. Where possible the selection of children for a counselling programme should be made in consultation with the school psychologist to eliminate those children who may, in fact, be in need of more specialized help.

The personal counselling described in this study probably could have been carried out by any sympathetic, intelligent layman, with a brief instruction in the techniques outlined. Expert psychological or psychiatric knowledge is not necessary.

TABLE 1 *Showing means and standard deviations for chronological age, intelligence and reading age as matched at the beginning of the experiment*

Group		Chrono-logical age	Mental age	Reading age
R	x̄ = 8.6		7.7	6.7
	SD = 1.18		1.04	1.36
R + Co.	x̄ = 8.6		7.7	6.9
	SD = 1.14		1.32	1.19
Co.	x̄ = 8.7		8.4	6.8
	SD = 1.04		1.18	1.09
C	x̄ = 8.9		7.9	6.5
	SD = 1.26		1.54	1.27

Results

R	= Remedial reading only
R + Co.	= Remedial reading + counselling
Co.	= Counselling only
C	= Control group. No treatment

Results from 11 children only were treated statistically owing to the fact that one child left the area from the R Group and also from the R + Co. Group.

TABLE 2 *Reading ages before and after treatment together with calculated gains*

| R + Co. | | | Co. | | | R | | | C | | |
Before	After	Gains	Before	After	Gains	Before	After	Gains	Before	After	Gains
5.1	5.9	0.3	5.3	6.1	0.3	7.2	8.1	0.4	6.6	6.9	−0.2
5.7	7.2	1.0	7.0	8.2	0.7	5.7	7.5	1.3	5.8	6.5	0.2
7.7	8.3	0.1	7.7	8.7	0.5	5.8	5.9	−0.4	6.7	7.2	0
7.7	8.6	0.4	6.6	8.1	1.0	5.5	6.0	0	8.7	8.6	−0.6
8.1	9.1	0.5	6.5	8.0	1.0	7.4	8.1	0.2	5.2	5.2	−0.5
7.9	9.0	0.6	5.1	7.3	1.7	7.6	8.2	0.1	5.4	5.4	−0.5
5.6	6.4	0.3	7.3	8.0	0.2	8.9	9.1	−0.3	5.5	6.3	0.3
8.1	8.5	−0.1	8.6	9.7	0.6	8.2	8.1	−0.6	6.7	7.4	0.2
8.3	9.2	0.4	6.6	7.9	0·8	5.4	7.3	1.4	5.6	5.5	−0.6
7.9	left	—	7.5	8.1	0.1	7.3	7.7	−0.1	8.2	9.0	0.3
6.0	7.3	0.8	7.7	8.4	0.2	6.4	left	—	5.4	5.6	−0.3
5.4	6.0	0.1	5.5	6.8	0.3	5.1	5.5	−0.1	8.7	9.0	−0.2
	$\bar{x} = 0.40$			$\bar{x} = 0.62$			$\bar{x} = 0.17$			$\bar{x} = 0.16$	

N.B. 0.5 was subtracted in each case to allow for the fact that the children were 6 months older at the end of the experiment.

TABLE 3 *Comparing 'O' factor score (on CPQ) of counselled group with randomly selected group of nine good readers in same school*

Counselled	Good readers
9 out of 11 had above average score	All had below average score

Reading attainment

		Poor	Good	
'O'	−	2	9	11
Factor				
	+	9	0	9
		11	9	20

chi-square = 10.3   p = approx. 0.001

TABLE 4 *Comparing change in 'O' factor score in counselled group (on CPQ) before and after treatment*

Before	After
9 with above average score	2 with above average score

Reading attainment

		Before	After	
'O'	—	2	9	11
Factor				
	+	9	2	11
		11	11	22

chi-square = 8.1   p = 0.01

TABLE 5 *Comparing average differences in gains in reading attainment*

Mann–Whitney 'U' Test

Group	'U'	Sig. level
R & Co. & R	34	NS
Co. & C	12	0.001
Co. & R	30	0.01
R & Co. & Co.	50	NS

D. Lawrence

TABLE 6 *Self-concept questionnaire*

I always feel STUPID	Sometimes I feel CLEVER and sometimes I feel STUPID	I always feel CLEVER
I feel I am NOT very GOOD-LOOKING	Sometimes I feel GOOD-LOOKING and sometimes NOT GOOD-LOOKING	I feel I am VERY GOOD-LOOKING
I am NEVER a NICE person	Sometimes I am NICE but sometimes I am NOT NICE	I am ALWAYS a VERY NICE person
I am ALWAYS AFRAID of things	Sometimes I am AFRAID and sometimes I am NOT AFRAID	I am NEVER AFRAID of things
I am a VERY NAUGHTY person	Sometimes I am NAUGHTY and sometimes I am GOOD	I am ALWAYS a VERY GOOD person

References

BELLAK, L. (1954) *The TAT and CAT in Clinical Use* London: Heinemann
*Cox, M. (ed) (1968) *The Challenge of Reading Failure* Slough: National Foundation for Educational Research
*MORRIS, J. M. (1966) *Standards and Progress in Reading* Slough: National Foundation for Educational Research
PORTER, R. B. and CATTELL, R. B. (1959) *Technical Handbook for the CPQ* Illinois: IPAT
ROGERS, C. R. (1965) *Client-Centered Therapy* Boston: Houghton Mifflin
ROSENTHAL, R. and JACOBSEN, L. (1968) *Pygmalion in the Classroom* New York: Holt, Rinehart and Winston
SCHOOLS COUNCIL (1970) *Cross'd with Adversity* Working Paper 27 London: Evans/Methuen

4.12 Some effects of the remedial teaching of reading

ASHER CASHDAN and P. D. PUMFREY

Faculty of Educational Studies, Open University;
Department of Education, University of Manchester

Reprinted from *Educational Research* (1969) 11, 2, pp. 138–42

Since 1944 many leas have set up remedial education services to assist children who, while remaining within the normal school, fail to learn to read. A considerable amount of research has been concerned with the short-term and long-term effects of treatment on attainment and on the child's social and emotional adjustment (see Chazan 1967 for a useful review). Substantial short-term gains in reading attainment of 2–3 months of reading age per month of remedial treatment are frequently found. However, these gains are usually recorded on Word Recognition tests; on Reading Comprehension tests, gains are rather smaller. Followup studies for varying periods up to three years after treatment have indicated little or no difference between children who had received remedial education and those who had not, in terms of their attainment. The relatively rapid progress made during remedial education is not continued when treatment ends. This failure of the remedial teaching of reading to improve children's attainments in the long-term is naturally somewhat disappointing to remedial teachers.

Some slight evidence exists that the longer the remedial teaching of reading continues, the greater the children's gain in terms of attainment (Cashdan, Pumfrey and Lunzer 1967). To return children to the situations which precipitated their initial failure and selection for remedial education is likely to result in some falling off in their progress. And remedial groups which have become too large and are taken by peripatetic teachers also cease to benefit the children.

Kellmer Pringle (1962) has stressed the importance for some children of remedial education as an 'emotional reeducation'; this is hard to measure and in Dunham's (1960) study his attitude scale brought out no improvement in the children studied, although their reading attainment had increased.

This article summarizes a small, but fairly well-controlled experiment in which both attitudes to reading and changes in reading attainment were examined in three groups of retarded junior school boys. Special features of the study are the comparison of once-weekly with twice-weekly teaching, comparisons between different reading tests, and the use of an improved version of Dunham's (1960) attitude scale. The aims of the experiment were to answer the following five questions:

1 Would second year junior school boys failing in reading make greater progress in attainment if given remedial help twice-weekly compared with a matched group given remedial help once a week?

2 At the end of the initial two-term treatment period, would the groups receiving treatment have significantly higher reading attainments on two criterion tests compared with a control group receiving no remedial help?

3 Would a differential practice effect favouring the boys' attainments on the Burt–Vernon Graded Word Reading Test (hereafter called the Burt test) compared with their attainments on the Standard Test of Reading Skill be found after two terms of remedial treatment?

4 Would any significant differences in attainment in reading be found between the three groups two years after the end of the initial treatment period?

5 Would any significant differences in attitude to reading be found between the treated and untreated groups two years after the initial treatment period?

The investigation

Twelve boys were selected from sixteen backward second year junior school children who were taught in groups of four as part of the practical work of a university diploma course. Two other groups of twelve boys were matched individually with the university group. The thirty-six boys chosen to take part in the investigation were of low average ability as measured by the Moray House Picture Intelligence Test. All had reading ages on the Burt test at least two years behind their chronological ages, and came from the Registrar-General's socioeconomic groups IV and V.

The three groups were named A, B and C. The twelve boys in Group A were given remedial teaching in reading in groups of four twice-weekly for 30–60 minute sessions at the university. All the teachers engaged in the work were qualified and experienced in remedial or special education. Members of Group B were taught in groups of from four to six children for sessions of similar length once-weekly by teachers of the local authority's remedial education service. Group C was a control group of children selected from the records of the remedial centres, and receiving no special help in reading. Some characteristics of the three groups are set out in Table 1.

There were no significant differences between the respective group means.

The initial experimental period lasted for two terms. At the end of the second term (spring 1964) all 36 boys were tested on the Burt test as well as on the Daniels and Diack Standard Test of Reading Skill. Twenty-two months later (spring 1966) as many of the subjects as could be found were tested again with the Burt test and with the Neale Analysis of Reading Ability, which allowed assessments for accuracy, comprehension and reading speed to be obtained. The boys were also tested on a Thurstone–Chave attitude to reading scale constructed by Williams (1965), a development of Dunham's (1960) scale. The Williams attitude scale

TABLE 1   *Characteristics of the groups at the start of the investigation*

Group	N	Mean CA	SD	Moray House Picture Intelligence Test Mean IQ	SD	Burt-Vernon Reading Test Mean RA	SD
Group A (University)	12	8.6	0.40	89.5	4.97	5.4	0.86
Group B (Remedial Service)	12	8.6	0.37	90.3	4.57	5.5	0.57
Group C (Control)	12	8.6	0.26	89.6	5.78	5.7	0.73

contains twenty-five statements with scale values ranging from 0.5 for the most positive attitude to reading to 10.5 for the statement indicating the most negative attitude.

As the investigation was based on the organization of a functioning educational service, the boys continued with remedial treatment for varying lengths of time after April 1964.

Results

The general school attendance of all thirty-six children during the two-term period was checked. There was great individual variation but no group differences. The mean number of remedial attendances for the two experimental groups was also examined. The university group, who attended twice weekly, should have made twice the number of attendances that were registered for the remedial service group. In fact, the discrepancy was even bigger—Group A (university) had a mean attendance of 37.1 and Group B (remedial service) of only 14.1, the discrepancy being due to absences and to organizational differences. These attendance differences were statistically clearly significant.

On the Burt test, the mean gains at the end of two terms were: Group A, 1.24 years, Group B 1.25 years, and Group C (control) 0.86 years. There was no significant difference between the groups, though the controls did appear to have made fractionally less progress than the other two groups.

Because gains in reading attainment attributed to remedial education might have been due to practice effects on the Burt test, the boys were also

A. Cashdan and P. D. Pumfrey

tested on the Daniels and Diack Standard Test of Reading Skill at the end of the initial experimental period. Scores obtained by the three groups are given in Table 2.

TABLE 2 *Group mean scores on the Burt Test and on the Standard Test of Reading Skill, obtained after two terms*

	N	Burt Test mean score	SD	Standard Test mean score	SD
Group A (University)	12	6.65	1.27	6.40	0.94
Group B (Remedial Service)	12	6.73	0.78	6.03	0.72
Group C (Control)	12	6.57	1.37	6.33	1.18

The small mean discrepancies between the tests for each group indicate little practice effect in the Burt test result. There is more indication in Group B than in the other groups, but even here it is slight. There was no significant difference between the groups in the numbers of children gaining higher scores on the Burt test than on the Standard Test of Reading Skill.

Although the initial experimental period ended in May 1964, all the boys in Group A continued to receive remedial treatment until July 1964, and six boys in this group received remedial help for a further twelve months. Most of Group B also received help until July 1964, and two members of this group continued to receive treatment after that date. The mean length of remedial treatment was 14.8 months for Group A and 9.5 months for Group B. The mean chronological age for all three groups at followup was 10 years 11 months. Because of extensive rehousing only 32 of the original 36 boys could be located.

Burt Test results
The mean gains of the three groups on the Burt test over the 22 months of the followup period were: Group A 2.52 years, Group B 1.46 years and Group C 2.50 years. There were no significant differences between the groups.

The mean rates of progress of the three groups on the Burt test were calculated in months of reading age per month of followup period. The results for the three groups were: Group A 1.36, Group B 0.80 and Group C 1.36.

Burt Test Results compared with the Neale Analysis of Reading Ability results
In order to see whether any tendency towards a differential practice effect favouring the boys' performance on the Burt test existed, the results obtained by the three groups were compared. None of the mean differences were significant. The scores of the three groups are given in Table 3.

TABLE 3   *Group mean reading ages at followup*

	N	Burt–Vernon test		Neale Analysis of Reading Ability					
				Rate		*Accuracy*		*Comprehension*	
		Mean	SD	Mean	SD	Mean	SD	Mean	SD
Group A	10	9.17	1.87	8.69	1.44	8.68	1.14	9.03	1.64
Group B	11	8.20	1.19	8.08	0.92	8.17	0.76	8.25	0.90
Group C	11	9.07	2.33	8.63	1.57	8.79	1.59	9.26	1.90

Attitude to reading

The boys' attitudes to reading were assessed, using the Williams (1965) attitude scale, in which a high score denotes a 'poor' attitude. The means for the three groups were 4.33 for Group A, 3.95 for Group B and 3.72 for Group C. The difference in scores between the groups was not significant. The correlations between attitude score and final reading ages were also not significant.

Discussion

In the light of our results we can now look at the five questions raised earlier.

The suggestion that boys in Group A receiving remedial teaching in reading twice weekly would make greater progress in reading attainment than boys in Group B helped only once weekly, was not supported at the end of the initial seven months experimental period. The mean gains of these two groups did not differ significantly, although Group A boys attended almost three times as many remedial sessions as those in Group B.

The second possibility, that at the end of the initial treatment period the groups that had been given remedial teaching in reading might have significantly higher reading attainments than the controls on both the Burt test and the Daniels and Diack test, was not confirmed. However, an initial spurt in progress of the groups receiving remedial teaching (found by many other researchers) was indicated in the differing rates of increase in scores between the groups on the Burt test.

The continuation of remedial help might have maintained the different rates of increase in reading attainment found in the three groups, thus producing significant differences favouring the treated groups in time. Other work by Cashdan, Pumfrey and Lunzer (1967), and by Lytton (1967) and Morris (1966) has shown that the continuation of remedial help in reading brings continuing improvement.

It seemed possible that a differential practice effect favouring the boys' scores on the Burt test might be found. This has been suggested by other researchers, including Curr and Gourlay (1960). But comparison of the three groups' scores on the Burt test and on the Daniels and Diack test at

A. Cashdan and P. D. Pumfrey

the end of the initial seven months of remedial treatment lends no support to this hypothesis.

The differential practice effect was also not found when the Neale Analysis provided a measure of comprehension which could be compared with the Burt test scores for the three groups.

The hypothesis that twenty-two months after the initial two-term period significant differences in reading ability would be found between the groups was also not supported. Thus, the findings agree with the somewhat depressing evidence produced by both Collins (1961) and Lovell (1966), although it may not be reasonable to expect short-term improvements in children's attainments to be maintained if the children are returned to the initial situation. The need for continuing compensatory education for children who fail to acquire reading at the junior level must again be emphasized (see Morris 1966).

We also investigated whether, on followup, any significant differences in attitude to reading would be found between the groups. None in fact were, although the groups' mean attitude scores were towards the favourable end of the continuum. Attitude to reading is probably less easily improved than reading attainment, at any rate with poor readers in the junior school (Dunham 1960). It must also be noted that the attitude scale used in this investigation was of a relatively coarse grading and to some extent its purpose must have been visible to the children to whom it was administered. Georgiades (1968) suggests an alternative technique which may have considerable promise in the measurement of attitude to reading.

Conclusion

The remedial teaching of reading to retarded junior school boys in two experimental groups did not improve reading attainment or attitude to reading when the groups were compared with a control group. The 'natural' improvement of the control group, which seems at first sight to be largely maturational, may be misleading. Very often, one suspects, the 'untreated' children get indirect help in the form of advice to their teachers from the remedial service, relief of pressure if some of their classmates are being helped, and so on. These are suggestions rather than firmly established facts which may help to explain awkward results. A more likely general conclusion is that the kind of children we are concerned with require a far more continuous programme of remedial treatment as an integral part of their normal school activities if they are to enter secondary education as literate children.

References

CASHDAN, A., PUMFREY, P. D. and LUNZER, E. A. (1967) A survey of children receiving remedial teaching in reading *Bulletin of the British Psychological Society* 67, 17A

CHAZAN, M. (1967) The effects of remedial teaching in reading: a review of research *Remedial Education* 2, no. 1, 4–12

COLLINS, J. E. (1961) *The Effects of Remedial Education* London: Oliver and Boyd

CURR, W. and GOURLAY, N. (1960) The effect of practice on performance in scholastic tests *British Journal of Educational Psychology* 30, 155–67

DUNHAM, J. (1960) The effects of remedial education on young children's reading ability and attitudes to reading *British Journal of Educational Psychology* 30, 173–5

GEORGIADES, N. J. (1968) The testing of reading today in J. Downing and A. L. Brown (eds) *The Third International Reading Symposium* London: Cassell

KELLMER PRINGLE, M. L. (1962) The long-term effects of remedial education: a followup study *Vita Humana* 5, 10–33

*LOVELL, K. (1966) The etiology of reading failure in J. Downing (ed) *The First International Reading Symposium* Oxford 1964 London: Cassell

*LYTTON, H. (1967) Followup of an experiment in selection for remedial education *British Journal of Educational Psychology* 37, 1–9

*MORRIS, J. M. (1966) *Standards and Progress in Reading* Slough: National Foundation for Educational Research

WILLIAMS, G. M. (1965) A study of reading attitudes among nine year old children Diploma dissertation University of Manchester

4.13 Implications for services: a postscript to the surveys

M. RUTTER, J. TIZARD and K. WHITMORE

Institute of Psychiatry; Professor of Child Development, Institute of Education, University of London; Senior Medical Officer, Department of Education and Science

Reprinted from M. Rutter, J. Tizard and K. Whitmore (1970) *Education, Health and Behaviour* Longman, pp. 358–77

In this paper we will examine some of the implications of our findings for the provision of services. The determination of the nature and prevalence of handicap is only one step in the programme of research required for the rational and informed planning of services. Consequently, the findings of the present study in themselves do not provide an adequate basis upon which to plan a comprehensive service for the care of children. Nevertheless, the Isle of Wight surveys have given rise to some very striking findings which do have immediate and direct implications for services. In discussing these we will point to the role of research in tackling the further questions which arise from the surveys and which still require answers.

Research and the planning of services

The planning of services cannot wait upon the results of definitive research —there are urgent problems which require action now. Such action must be taken in the light of the best evidence which is currently available, even if this is not as adequate as one would wish. But the development of services must be planned in such a way that research is built in to the development in order that planners in the future can know which steps have been effective and which have not. In the absence of research we can only move forward blindly, able to profit neither from our mistakes nor from our successes. Research and planning need to go forward hand in hand so that the questions for research can arise from problems in service provision and the findings from research can be taken into account when planning further services. The Seebohm Report (1968) put it like this:

> We cannot emphasize too strongly the part which research must play in the creation and maintenance of an effective service. Social planning

is an illusion without adequate facts; and the adequacy of services mere speculation without evaluation. Nor is it sufficient for research to be done spasmodically however good it be. It must be a continuing process, accepted as a familiar and permanent feature of any department or agency concerned with social provision.

It is this ongoing role of research which we wish to outline in the following discussion.

The need for experiment in the planning of services

Because of the paucity of research into treatment methods, many of the measures which we will advocate in this chapter on the basis of our findings from the surveys are relatively untested. This means that most of our recommendations for services will be accompanied by a recommendation that the methods be introduced experimentally so that the results of the changed services can be evaluated. People sometimes feel uneasy about the ethics of such an approach, doubting whether it is justifiable to deprive children of services (even if of unproven value) merely to demonstrate their worth (or lack of worth). It is as well, therefore, to consider this issue at the beginning of the discussion.

The key fact is that because of the present shortage of services of all kinds, many children who would benefit from them are willy-nilly denied them. This is an unfortunate situation but it does have consequences which it would not otherwise be easy to secure. As some children will in any case be deprived of services because of the overall shortage, it is as well to make sure that the services are deployed in such a way that comparisons can be made to test the contribution which the services make.

If services are really adequate to meet all the needs or supposed needs of a population, it becomes unethical to withhold them from some sections of the population unless there are very serious doubts as to whether the services make a significant contribution to well-being. Where services are in short supply, the alternative to their planned utilization is unplanned attempts to deal with a series of crises. Furthermore, where services are being expanded—as is happening at the present time—opportunities exist for systematic study of deliberately varied forms of expansion, to see which appear to offer the greatest cost and welfare benefits. To establish new services on an experimental basis is much easier than to attempt to modify for experimental purposes long established services running on traditional lines (Tizard 1966).

Applicability of findings to areas other than the Isle of Wight

The question arose of whether our findings could be generalized to other parts of this country or to other parts of the world. It was concluded that, because the social conditions on the Isle of Wight are generally better than those existing in the poor areas of most big cities, it is unlikely that the rate of handicap elsewhere would be less than that which we found. Studies of reading in London schoolchildren and in city children in other countries have shown considerably higher rates of reading difficulties than on the island. Unfortunately no exact comparisons are possible owing to differences in method and in the definition of reading retardation. In addition, we have evidence that, at least as judged from questionnaire studies, the rate of emotional and behavioural difficulties in London children is also well above that in the Isle of Wight.

The extent and nature of the differences between areas are unknown and require further study. One of us (MR) is carrying out an investigation comparing the Isle of Wight and a London borough in terms of reading retardation and psychiatric disorder in ten year olds. By studying school, social and family conditions in the two areas it should be possible to determine not only *how* the two areas differ but also some of the reasons *why* they differ. Further crosscultural studies are needed before the extent of the variability in rate and in type of handicap is known.

Local surveys or national surveys?

The relative merits and demerits of local and national studies may also be mentioned here. Local studies (such as the Isle of Wight survey) have sometimes been criticized because they are not representative of the whole country. This is true but it is not always appreciated that the converse is also true. A national survey no more represents the Isle of Wight, London or the Lake District than surveys in these areas represent the national scene. Planning for the country as a whole cannot be based on national figures for the very same reason—that is, that different areas have different problems and different needs. It might also be added that it is no longer possible to consider one country in isolation from the rest of the world and in this context a survey of the United Kingdom is also a local survey.

National surveys can be very worthwhile. But in our view, for most purposes, more is to be gained by comparative studies of several areas, each of which is fairly homogeneous and which differs from other areas in important respects, than by large-scale national surveys. In this way the extent, nature and reasons for regional variation can be assessed. Differences between areas can be related to differences in conditions and to differences in service provision. Local surveys also have the advantage that children can be examined by a relatively small team of trained workers using standardized methods. This is more difficult to achieve in a national survey. However, it should be added that comparative studies depend for their strength on the use of comparable standardized methods and this has not often been achieved.

Applicability of findings to other ages

That the rate of handicap in other groups is unlikely to be much below that we found at nine to twelve years has already been mentioned. However, this is a judgment necessarily based on the weak evidence which is so far available and there is no adequate answer to the question of how far the findings at other ages will be different. Further, even if the rates are roughly the same at other ages, it is most unlikely from what we know of the development of children that the *types* of handicap will be the same.

To investigate this issue we have recently undertaken surveys of educational and psychiatric disorders in Isle of Wight children aged fourteen to fifteen, using methods similar to those described for the present surveys. Unfortunately, resources did not allow a comparable survey of physical disorders. We have also carried out a much more limited survey of intellectual difficulties in five year old children and a questionnaire survey of emotional and behavioural difficulties in the same age group. More intensive studies of young children are required.

Persistence of handicaps

Any planning of services for children needs to be based not only on the prevalence of handicaps (by severity and type) but also on the persistence of handicaps. We have seen that, by definition, the disorders studied had been present for at least one year and in most instances for very much longer than that. Thus the children with reading difficulties had had difficulties in learning to read from the time they started school, and most psychiatric disorders had begun over three years before we saw the children. Handicapping disorders which have lasted as long as that require treatment, whatever the persistence of disorders after nine to twelve years.

Nevertheless, the extent and the kind of services required will be influenced by what happens to the children's difficulties during the latter half of their school days. This requires further study. The twenty-eight month followup of the children with reading difficulties already mentioned showed that *all* the children continued to have difficulties and most of them fell even farther behind, the group as a whole making only ten months' progress during the twenty-eight month period. This finding clearly illustrates the seriousness of the problem of reading retardation and underlines the necessity of providing adequate treatment for these children. A further study of the same children up to the end of compulsory schooling has recently been completed. A similar followup study of the children with psychiatric disorders from 10–11 years to 14–15 years has also just been carried out. Again, resources did not allow a similar study of physical disorders and this needs to be done.

M. Rutter, J. Tizard and K. Whitmore

Educational retardation

Many children who needed special educational treatment were not receiving it. During the twenty-eight months after the survey, largely in the absence of special help, the children made very poor progress. To what extent these educational problems are remediable is uncertain but there seems little doubt that given adequate treatment rather better progress than this should be possible.

The main reason why the children were not receiving help was that none was available. There was no trained remedial teacher in any of the ordinary primary schools. Furthermore, progress classes had been established in only eight of the junior schools, so that the majority of the children attended schools which could not provide any expert help in remedial teaching. However, unlike the situation in many other authorities, there was an adequate provision of places at the special day school for educationally subnormal children.

The provision of special educational treatment, particularly in small authorities, presents great problems of staffing and finance. Few teachers have special training in this field and these tend to work in special schools where both salary and staffing ratios are better. Of the five Isle of Wight teachers who had taken relevant advanced courses, four were at the special school, one at a graded post in a secondary school. Some of the larger primary schools had staff and accommodation which permitted the provision of one progress class much smaller than the rest, in which children needing special help could spend varying periods. This was much more difficult to arrange in the small schools.

To a much smaller extent, the lack of special educational treatment was due to a failure to use available services. Thus, five children with intellectual retardation, eleven with specific reading retardation, and twenty with general reading backwardness (a total of twenty-three children when overlap is taken into account) attended schools which provided progress classes, yet the children were in ordinary classes. Placement policy in these classes differed from school to school; age, attainment, prognosis and behaviour were some of the factors taken into consideration. Probably many children derived benefit from the eight progress classes running in 1964, but their value for the backward and retarded children we are discussing did not extend to any great improvement in their reading attainment.

Provision for remedial teaching differed more widely in the secondary schools to which these children progressed. In most of them some form of streaming would aim at smaller classes and special attention for those achieving poorly in basic subjects. This has been ineffective in improving the reading standards of these very poor achievers.

The treatment of reading retardation
Without treatment the prognosis for children with reading retardation is poor, and most of these children were not getting any kind of remedial

treatment. For most children with reading difficulties, the treatment, whatever it is, is going to have to be provided in ordinary schools. The high rate of reading difficulties makes it impractical, even if it were desirable, to provide special schooling for such a large segment of the school population. In any case, there is general agreement that the 'unnecessary' segregation of handicapped children is neither good for them nor for those with whom they must associate (Plowden 1967). If a child is going to spend his later life in the society of normal people it is not good that he spend his school days only in the company of other handicapped children.

However, the ordinary school can cope adequately with the educational needs of nearly all children only if it is organized to do so. We have shown that 'progress' classes, whatever their other merits, do not always provide the answer for the child with reading difficulties. Some other solution must be sought. At present very few trained remedial teachers are available in the ordinary schools and it is important that their number be *greatly* increased—in both the primary and the secondary schools.

However, even if there were immediate plans to increase the number, there are likely to be limited remedial resources for some time to come, because of the shortage of suitably trained people. This raises the administrative question of how to make the best use of such limited resources. A pilot study to answer this question was carried out on the Isle of Wight.

As a result of the survey findings the local education authority appointed one remedial teacher. One teacher was not enough to help all the children with severe reading difficulties, even those in the age-group we studied, but this inadequacy had an advantage from the point of view of research. Since the remedial teacher could only see some of the children, the eight Island secondary schools were divided into four groups; in two schools the remedial teacher himself taught the reading retarded children in very small groups of three or four, in two other schools he advised the teachers of the reading retarded children, in two others the children were already in remedial streams where special attention was paid to their reading and in the remaining two schools no special attention was given to their disability (Yule and Rigley 1968). The four groups of children (aged thirteen years or so at the start of the experiment) were compared according to their progress over the course of one year. The rate of progress was slightly (but only slightly) better in the group taught personally by the remedial teacher and was worst in the group where teachers had been advised by the remedial teacher. In this particular group, using the teacher as an adviser did *not* pay off.

However, the results concern only one remedial teacher and children nearing the end of their secondary schooling; also there was no measure of teaching standards. It proved to be a useful preliminary study but further investigations are required. If these are to provide clearcut findings it is essential that they include an evaluation of teacher quality and efficiency (see below).

333

Some would not expect that intervention at this late stage would have any effect. If inadequate teacher training plays a part in the children's difficulties in learning to read (see below), then help given to primary school teachers might be more effective than help given to children later. To this end we undertook another study, this time with teachers of eight year old children, for whom we ran a short in-service training course (Yule and Rigley 1968). Places on the course were offered only to those teaching in schools in a selected area of the Island. The children in their classes were matched with other classes on the basis of reading scores at the start of the experiment. At the end of the year, the children of the in-service trained teachers were reading at a level nearly two months ahead of those in the control classes. Obviously the study needs to be replicated but the results suggest that in-service training may be of value in improving children's progress in reading during primary school.

How best to teach reading to children with severe problems in learning to read is a question with as yet no satisfactory answer. On the whole, studies have shown that a 'phonic' emphasis when starting to teach reading is generally better than an emphasis on 'look and say' methods (Chall 1967), but this does not take us much further. Many of the children we studied had been taught by phonic methods but still they had not learned to read. Work with the Initial Teaching Alphabet shows some promise but its value for children with specific reading retardation has still to be assessed.

It has been shown that reading retardation is associated with developmental problems in speech, language, perception and motor coordination. It may be that special account of these factors will have to be taken in devising methods of teaching reading suitable for this hard core of children with very severe difficulties. Furthermore, most of the children with reading retardation have very poor concentration and many have become severely discouraged and disheartened by their repeated failures in school. Thus, attention must be paid to methods of gaining and holding the children's interest. Motivational problems are often the first and most serious difficulty to be overcome. There has to be a concern with the specific *skills* of teaching as well as with the *methods* used. This requires investigations in which there are systematic analyses of teacher–child interaction. There is little point in comparing one global method with another unless the quality of teaching is also taken into account.

The role of the expert

The ordinary classroom teacher will be responsible for the education of most handicapped children. But just as in medicine the general practitioner requires to be able to turn for advice to a medical consultant, so also the classroom teacher should expect to be able to turn to educational consultants for advice about teaching methods. If their advice is to be both useful and acceptable, it is necessary that these consultants should be experienced in the practical issues of classroom teaching. There are a fair number of people in most local authorities who should be able to fill this role—educational psychologists, local education authority inspectors (who would be more correctly called advisers), headteachers and heads of departments or colleagues who have attended special courses.

How best to make use of the specialist knowledge available in many areas has received remarkably little study. There is a tradition in education of referral of children to a doctor or psychologist for diagnosis and therapy if there is thought to be something wrong with the child. The tradition of asking a specialist in to see whether something might be done to improve the teaching is less well established. To do so is thought to imply criticism of the teacher rather than of the teaching. Whether the autonomy of teachers helps children to be better educated—or teachers to be better teachers—may not always be clear. The plain fact is that we apply to teaching different canons from those we apply to medicine and to other professional disciplines. If this means that the inexperienced teacher cannot even seek advice without losing face, it is likely to be harmful.

Overlap between reading retardation and antisocial disorder
The very substantial overlap between reading retardation and antisocial disorder has several important service implications. In the first place, it means that many of the children requiring special educational help for their reading difficulties are also those whose behaviour presents many problems in the classroom. Poor concentration, restlessness, mischief-making and poor relationships with other children are likely to be prominent features. The antisocial disorder may require treatment at the clinic or elsewhere outside the school but recent studies have also suggested that modification of the classroom situation itself may have a most important part to play in treatment (Becker *et al* 1967, Carnine *et al* 1969). The work of many investigators has shown that much can be done directly by the classroom teacher, using differential social reinforcement (or rewards), to eliminate behaviour which interferes with learning.

For many years educationists, psychiatrists and others have argued over the most effective use of praise and punishment in obtaining the best from children, but until very recently there has been little systematic study of the issue. Observation of classes in ordinary and in special schools soon shows that there is a strong (and very understandable) tendency for teachers to concentrate attention on the troublesome children and let the quiet ones carry on working on their own. When the class troublemaker actually settles down at last to doing what he is supposed to be doing, it seems natural for the teacher to sigh with relief, leave him to it and turn attention to someone else. However, recent studies suggest that this is just what should *not* be done. For example, Becker and his associates have found that rules by themselves made little difference to how children behave. General praise was also relatively ineffective, frequent punishment was not helpful, and simply ignoring 'bad' behaviour actually increased its frequency. In contrast, the combination of *systematically* praising and paying attention when a child behaved appropriately *together* with ignoring 'bad' behaviour was highly effective. However, this procedure had to be directed specifically to the behaviour of each child if it was to work—there was surprisingly little vicarious effect. Furthermore, even *sometimes* paying attention to 'bad' behaviour might increase it. As is well established, intermittent reinforcement is more efficient than continuous reinforcement.

These studies are still at a very preliminary stage and certainly no 'golden rules' for controlling disturbed behaviour in the classroom have been established. Many difficulties and many inconsistencies have yet to be investigated. Nevertheless, already the approach offers a most useful addition to our techniques for helping children. Some of the findings can be applied already and many others warrant further research. The extension of some types of therapy from the clinic to the classroom is likely to be highly rewarding.

A second implication from the overlap between reading retardation and antisocial behaviour comes from the suggestion that delinquency may sometimes arise as a response to educational failure. This is still a hypothesis, but if substantiated it follows that the early and effective treatment of reading retardation might prevent *some* cases of delinquency. This provides yet another reason for making better provision than at present for the treatment of reading difficulties. It also suggests that remedial teaching for delinquents who are backward in reading might be a useful approach in treatment. However, as the effects of this are still untested, it is also most important that there should be further experimental studies comparing the effects of different methods of treatment in children with both antisocial disorder and severe reading difficulties.

To what extent can reading difficulties be prevented?
Our studies were concerned with reading difficulties in nine to ten year old children, and so far in this discussion we have largely noted ways in which the treatment of established reading retardation might be improved. However, the survey results also have important implications for possible methods of *preventing* reading retardation. These may conveniently be considered under two headings: the teacher and the child.

1   *The teacher*
In view of the size of the problem of 'handicap' in childhood it is evident that the problems of handicapped children should figure large in the training of teachers, both of primary and secondary school children. Here, of course, we refer not just to reading retardation but also to the many other types of handicaps a teacher is likely to encounter. Child development, the psychology of learning, personality development, health education—these subjects are all important for good teaching. But just as the medical student is required to learn not only anatomy and physiology but also how to diagnose and treat disease, so the teacher in training needs to

be taught not only child development and educational psychology but also how to recognize children with special needs and how to teach them. A good deal of criticism has been levelled of late against colleges of education for their presumed failure to pay sufficient attention to pedagogy and it has been found that a high proportion of primary school teachers consider that their training was inadequate (Plowden 1967). The facts on training are hard to come by. At all events the teacher in training needs to learn the technical skills of teaching. This applies equally to university graduates who at present are accorded qualified teacher status without any professional training. In addition experienced teachers, like experienced doctors, require time to attend refresher courses and should be expected to do so.

2 *The child*

Reading retardation was found to be associated with language and speech problems, poor motor coordination and a difficulty in differentiating right from left. These are developmental functions in that it should be possible to identify children with these difficulties long before nine or ten years (the age at which we saw the children). As there are reasons for supposing that these developmental disorders play a part in the *causation* of reading retardation, it is important to diagnose the disorders early in order to help the children and to possibly reduce later reading difficulties.

To do this requires that the routine medical examination of children, both before and after starting school, should concentrate more on the details of a child's developmental progress. Medical students, paediatricians, child psychiatrists, welfare clinic doctors and school doctors need to be taught in their training about language, motor and perceptual development and how to diagnose abnormalities in these functions. This is already happening in some centres but such training needs to become more widespread.

There is also a need to introduce into preschool and school examinations more standardized and reliable methods of developmental assessment. At present examinations are mainly concerned with the diagnosis of diseases of various bodily systems and the detection of vision and hearing defects. The detection of sensory defects is most important, but our studies have shown that much of the rest of the usual school medical examination is unreliable and of very dubious value. There should be a reappraisal of the examination, inserting appropriate developmental assessments, retaining what is valuable in the traditional medical examination and throwing out what has been found to be unsatisfactory.

Some steps in this direction have already been taken. For example, a Spastics Society Working Party (of which MR and JT are members) has suggested what brief screening examinations of preschool children should include (Egan *et al* 1969). Also, one of us (KW) in collaboration with Dr Martin Bax, has developed an examination scheme for five year old children which focuses on developmental problems. This is being tried out on the Isle of Wight in the routine school entry medical.

The reliability of developmental assessment as carried out during a brief screening examination needs to be examined. Also, the value of a developmental assessment in detecting children who later have difficulties in learning to read has still to be determined. The finding that children with reading retardation have been delayed in their language development tells us nothing about the proportion of children with a language delay who later have difficulties in learning to read. For this purpose a *longitudinal* study of young children with developmental abnormalities is required. Some progress in this respect has been made by Ingram and his colleagues with regard to language and speech disorders (Ingram 1963; Mason 1967). Other studies on the early identification of children with reading disabilities are in progress (de Hirsch and Jansky 1966, McLeod 1966, Haring and Ridgway 1967, Sapir and Wilson 1967). In our own studies we are following all 440 infants who first entered school on the Isle of Wight in the autumn term of 1967. All of these children were tested on a battery of visuo-motor and language tests and were given a neurological examination. By following these children to age seven years we shall find out how successful our school entry examination was in predicting which children later experience reading difficulties. This is a pilot study and more investigations of this kind are required.

We have discussed in previous chapters how the language and other developmental disorders associated with reading retardation may be caused by both biological and social factors. Children in large families are often handicapped in their language development and adverse social circumstances can have widespread deleterious effects on children's intellectual development and scholastic progress (Haywood 1967). As already noted, the worst kinds of social deprivation were scarcely represented on the Isle of Wight and a similar study in a major city would doubtless reveal greater social problems than we found. Also, the Isle of Wight contained very few children born abroad. Language problems may be considerable in immigrant children not only because for some English is a second language, but also because their use of English developed in a different culture so that the way in which English is used in school may constitute a communication problem for them. Language involves not only an accepted code of words but also conventions of linguistic usage and styles of expression. Bernstein (1965) has pointed to the educational implications of different codes of language used by individuals from different social backgrounds and these differences are likely to be even more marked in relation to English-speaking cultures outside the United Kingdom.

How best to help children from socially disadvantaged homes is not completely understood. However, it seems that if intervention is to be effective it must begin early. The handicaps of the child from an adverse social background are already well established by the time he starts school and services are required during the preschool period. Again, what form they should take is not certain and research in this area is much required. Some form of nursery school provision is needed for both the biologically handicapped and the socially handicapped children. To what extent their needs are similar or different is not yet known.

The literature on the effects of nursery school attendance on scholastic progress is contradictory and inconclusive (Swift 1964, Haywood 1967). Nevertheless, it appears that while nursery school programmes have little effect on the educational progress of children of good intelligence from privileged homes, they have generally had a significant effect on the subsequent school achievement of socially disadvantaged children, of below average intelligence, if, and only if, the programme was directly focused on the specific defects (especially language deficiencies) of the children and if tutoring, instruction or training was provided to remedy these defects (Haywood 1967, Weikart 1967). In primary schools, too, a structured approach is probably more effective with these children than a permissive programme (Haring and Phillips 1962). Specialized preschool programmes for intellectually retarded children (Kirk 1958) and for culturally deprived Negro children (Gray and Klaus 1965, 1966, Eisenberg 1967a, Klaus and Gray 1968) have also been shown, in well controlled studies, to have beneficial effects. These studies have suggested that the preschool programme for the socially disadvantaged child is likely to be more effective the more the child's family can be involved in the extension and development of the child's learning experience. The gains have sometimes been quite small and even in the best programmes the children have only very partially caught up intellectually. A brief period of enrichment at four years of age is no more likely to be still effective at seven years than a good diet taken only at four years would protect a child from malnutrition at seven years (Eisenberg 1967). To be effective, the educational help must be continued.

Although it is only too evident that much further research is needed into the question of preschool provision for children with different types of handicap, certain conclusions can be drawn. If the 'nursery' consists only of an adult 'minding' a number of children there will be no benefit. Free play and an opportunity to experiment are valuable but on their own they are of little use to socially disadvantaged (and probably to language or physically handicapped) children who have not yet learned how to profit from such opportunities. What is suitable for a child from a professional background is unlikely to be suitable for a child from an overcrowded slum. Nursery schools must make deliberate efforts to provide *specific* training which is appropriate in relation to the children's handicaps, whatever they are. Unless this is done the conventional nursery school is not likely to be of much help to the handicapped child.

Yet again the plea for more provision must be linked with the need for experiment and evaluation. Preschool provision is required for handicapped children, but the ideas on how this should be organized and what should be provided need further testing.

M. Rutter, J. Tizard and K. Whitmore

Intellectual retardation

The findings on intellectual retardation have both psychiatric and educational implications. The children with intellectual retardation were found in a variety of settings ranging from the ordinary school to the mental subnormality hospital. Although there were marked differences between the children with the most mild and the most severe retardation there was no clear dividing line between *qualitatively* different groups as implied by the present sharp legally imposed distinction (in this country) between 'educable' and 'ineducable' children. This distinction has little educational justification; there are no grounds for placing the *education* of the most handicapped children in medical hands (as happens at present) and this health–education barrier makes the transfer of children from one school or class to another more difficult than it should be. Furthermore, the exclusion of some intellectually retarded children from education is rightly resented by parents. It is hoped, therefore, that local authorities will have regard for the proposed change in legislation and for the desirability of informal procedures when considering the needs of all intellectually retarded children.

The range of services required for the most severely retarded children and their families will not be discussed here since we have little to add to what has already been written about them by Tizard and Grad (1961) and Tizard (1964, 1969). Many of the shortcomings of existing services have arisen out of their isolation from paediatric, child psychiatric, educational and other social services, and in planning for the future this is the chief problem to be faced.

The first step towards a solution of the educational problems of intellectually retarded children lies in making a single department responsible for the education of *all* children. This arrangement, in itself, will have no necessary benefit, but it should facilitate improvements in the quality of education provided for retarded children. However, intellectually retarded children have many problems other than educational ones. As the survey showed, chronic physical handicaps and psychiatric disorder were common accompaniments of intellectual retardation, and of all the handicapped groups this was the one with the greatest family problems. The implications of these findings are that both the paediatrician and the child psychiatrist must be adequately trained in the diagnosis and treatment of intellectual retardation. Equally, the mental subnormality specialist must be adequately trained in developmental paediatrics and child psychiatry. In the past, he has largely been concerned with the care of patients in long-stay hospitals. As far as children are concerned, the training of mental subnormality specialists ill-equips them for this task which might be better undertaken in many instances by individuals trained in child care rather than in medicine. Hostel provision will not remove the need for hospital care, but it could allow hospital doctors to focus their attention on the smaller number of children who specifically require their attention.

At present, many mental subnormality specialists have no out-patient clinics. This is a deplorable state of affairs. As far as mental subnormality services for children are concerned, the bulk of the work should be out-patient, so that the medical, psychiatric, educational and family problems of intellectually retarded children attending ordinary and special schools and junior training centres, and those looked after at home by their parents, can be adequately dealt with. The mental subnormality specialist who deals with children must be first and foremost a child psychiatrist or paediatrician with a special interest in developmental medicine, and his training should reflect this.

Psychiatric disorder

To what extent are psychiatric disorders being adequately dealt with?
Most of the children with psychiatric disorder in the present study were receiving no kind of treatment and most had not had any psychiatric evaluation, however brief. This is an unsatisfactory state of affairs: the disorders were chronic and handicapping and the children needed help. The provision of child psychiatric services in the country as a whole is most inadequate and a very considerable increase is needed. In order to remedy this situation, more senior posts in child psychiatry are required. This is already officially accepted and more posts are being created, although the number planned for the next few years will still fall far short of minimal requirements. However, it is not enough that posts be created, it is also necessary that people be trained to fill them. Again, the number of training posts is already being increased but this must be linked with an expansion of training programmes and a considerable improvement in their quality (see below).

The need for more child psychiatrists is paralleled by an equally great need for a better training of general practitioners in child psychiatry. Very few of the parents of the children with psychiatric disorder had consulted their family doctor, and very few perceived him as someone who could help with psychiatric problems in children. As things stand now, they were probably right in this assumption with respect to many general practitioners. Until a few years ago most medical students received no instruction in child psychiatry, and few doctors have attended postgraduate courses in the subject. In most medical schools, there has been some increase recently in the amount of child psychiatry taught to students, but the situation is still far from satisfactory. In only one undergraduate medical school in the country is there a full-time university appointment in child psychiatry. Yet if child psychiatry is to be taught adequately it is essential that there be well-trained individuals with the time and facilities to develop a proper teaching programme. If this is to be possible, university departments of psychiatry in the future will have to include some child psychiatrists.

The survey findings also carry implications for the way child psychiatric services are deployed. Children with chronic physical handicaps (especially those with neurological conditions) had a high rate of psychiatric disorder and children with intellectual and with educational retardation had an even higher rate of disorder. This means that child psychiatry services must have *effective* links with both paediatric services and with schools. It also bears out the need for children referred to child psychiatric units to have a physical examination which includes a screening of neurological functions. The high rate of mental disorder in the parents of children with psychiatric problems (Rutter 1966) also necessitates close links with adult psychiatric clinics. Exactly how these links are provided must depend on the situation in each locality—it is very doubtful whether any standard pattern should be imposed. However, in the past child psychiatrists have often had to work in isolated clinics and whatever solution is found the isolation must be remedied.

Traditionally, in this country there has been a distinction (in training and in function) between the clinical psychologist who works in hospital clinics and the educational psychologist who works in local education authority child guidance clinics. It is evident from the overlap between disorders that this distinction is a false one. If child psychologists are to be maximally effective they must have both clinical and educational skills and they must be able to function equally well in the hospital as in the school. The (artificial) division between local authority clinics and hospital clinics has retarded the development of child psychiatry. The hospital psychologist who has no experience of schools is operating with his right hand tied behind his back, because many of the children he sees will have educational difficulties. Similarly, the psychological assessment of children referred to psychiatric clinics by schools often requires skills which up to now have been the prerogative of the clinical psychologist. Some means must be found of providing a clinical *and* educational training for all psychologists who will work with children.

How should psychiatric disorders be treated?
There is a considerable range of psychiatric treatments which may be used with children. Among those which have been tested and for which there is some evidence of their efficacy are short-term psychotherapy, various kinds of drug treatment, desensitization programmes, operant training procedures and classroom modifications. Most of these treatments are still inadequately assessed and much further research into their use is required. Nevertheless, enough is known now for them to be used to some extent in a rational and systematic way. It is clear, for example, that different kinds of disorders require different types of treatment (Eisenberg *et al* 1965). This is almost self-evident, yet there has been a tendency in some clinics for a similar approach to be taken to all problems. That not all clinics are making the best use of the existing (if limited) knowledge on treatment is due in part to the geographical and professional isolation of many child psychiatric clinics. If the people working in clinics are to be expected to keep abreast of the latest developments in their subject (as they should be)

they must have ready access to a well-stocked library and they must have the stimulus of discussion with their colleagues. Refresher courses should be available and proper facilities provided so that people may attend them. These conditions are largely lacking in the majority of clinics and the situation must be improved.

Part of the present difficulties in psychiatric treatment stems from inefficient utilization of existing resources and existing knowledge but part also stems from the vast areas of ignorance which still exist concerning child psychiatric disorder and its treatment. For example, much remains to be discovered about the treatment of antisocial disorder, the use of special schools, the use of remedial educative techniques, the treatment of disturbed family relationships and the use of new methods such as family therapy. There is deplorably little research in child psychiatry in this country (or in others). This is not surprising in that child psychiatrists have not been trained in research methods and furthermore there are very few positions open to anyone who wishes to make a career in research. There is a great need for the development of university departments (or units) of child psychiatry, both to develop research and also to develop training programmes.

In most places training in child psychiatry has tended to be rather haphazard and unsystematic. Things are improving but there is considerable room for further improvement. Psychiatric training must include both academic and clinical aspects of the subject (Royal Commission on Medical Education 1968). Child psychiatry is a developing subject and the trainee must be able to evaluate new developments, new findings and new theories as they present themselves. Learning must not stop on appointment to a consultant post, and an essential part of postgraduate training is to help the trainee learn how to learn. Facilities for undertaking research should be available and training in research methods should be provided by university departments (Rutter 1969). Recommendations have been made as to what an adequate training in child psychiatry should include (Royal Medicopsychological Association 1968), but there is a long way to go before these recommendations are implemented satisfactorily.

Who should treat children with psychiatric disorder?
The size of the psychiatric problem and the present shortage of psychiatrists means that, of necessity, most children with psychiatric disorder will need to be treated by people other than psychiatrists. Quite apart from the necessity of this, there are reasons for believing that even given unlimited resources this would still be the best approach for many children. If all doctors were better trained in child psychiatry as medical students, many of the problems could quite appropriately be dealt with by general practitioners or by paediatricians. The school doctor, if appropriately trained, might also have a major role to play. As already suggested, teachers could be helped to deal with many kinds of disturbed behaviour and the psychologist, too, has a crucial role to play. Emotional and

behaviour problems in children are often associated with social disturbances in the family, and social workers (both in the clinics and in the community) have an important part to play in treatment. Many more children than at present should be able to attend a psychiatric clinic so that their problems can be adequately evaluated, but often the role of the psychiatrist and the psychologist will be to advise others on treatment rather than to treat the child himself.

The identification of children with psychiatric disorder
The surveys showed that for every child with psychiatric disorder who was seeing a psychiatrist, there were many more who were not attending clinics. On the whole, those attending clinics had fairly severe disorders and although there were other children not attending clinics who had disorders of similar severity, it seemed that psychiatric services were being employed for a group of children who needed them. There is not, therefore, an immediate urgency to institute new methods of identifying children with psychiatric disorder—such a screening of the general population would only further overload already overloaded clinics. Nevertheless, the utilization of psychiatric services for the children who most need them is a serious concern. As services expand, efficient and standardized techniques for identifying children with psychiatric disorder should be introduced. As we have shown, this will need to be done both through the schools and through the parents.

Physical disorders

The treatment of children with physical disorder
We found that children with chronic or recurrent physical handicaps had an increased risk of both educational retardation and psychiatric disorder. Furthermore, many of the children had problems at home and presented difficulties to their parents. This means that the treatment of chronic medical conditions cannot be considered in isolation from the development of the child as a whole. Since the problem of severe infectious diseases in childhood has greatly diminished (following improvements in social conditions and the introduction of antibiotics), paediatric practice has come to be increasingly concerned with emotional and behavioural disorders and with *chronic* physical handicaps. This has obvious implications for paediatric training and paediatric practice (which we will not discuss further), but it also has implications for the organization of services. The finding that one in seven of children with a chronic physical handicap has a psychiatric disorder, and vice versa, suggests that there is a need for paediatricians and child psychiatrists to work closely together. This applies to children with epilepsy and other neurological disorders. In this context, too, it is important that the neurologist who deals with children should be aware of the emotional and educational development. The educational problems associated with physical handicap suggest the need for effective

344

links between the paediatric consultant and the school health service. One way of providing this is through the provision of joint appointments. Prompted by the survey findings, the Isle of Wight now has a consultant paediatrician who gives part of his time to the authority and a clinical paediatric assistant who is employed jointly by the Regional Hospital Board and by the local authority (as a medical officer). Such arrangements have, of course, been used previously by other authorities but in many, if not most, authorities the paediatric–school links leave much to be desired. In the long run the boundaries between hospital and local authority child health services must disappear; it is not without reason that university departments of child health are so called.

If teachers are to be expected to deal with chronically handicapped children in the ordinary schools (as they are and should be), they must be informed about the nature of the handicaps and the needs of the children. All too often this does not happen. For example, in a study of deaf children who had been transferred to ordinary schools, it was found that many of the teachers had little or no knowledge of the handicaps imposed by impaired hearing and their consequent effects upon speech and language development and upon communication and social growth (Ministry of Education 1963). Very few had received any guidance or help in the handling of deaf children and it was to be expected (as was found) that many of the deaf children therefore experienced considerable difficulties in adjusting to the transfer. Doubtless a similar situation applies to children with many other types of handicap, perhaps especially epilepsy.

That multiple handicaps are so common also suggests that the facilities for the assessment of physically handicapped children should be arranged to facilitate a multidisciplinary approach both to the initial assessment and also to the continuing treatment, care and education of the child. For some kinds of severe or unusual handicap, it may be essential to have regional assessment centres where consultants of different disciplines work together as a team. Such an arrangement may also carry advantages for other handicaps but the appropriate professional links and interdisciplinary coordination can also be developed informally given an appreciation of the need.

Special schools

The surveys showed a very considerable overlap between different handicaps. This finding has implications for the organization of special schools and special classes.

All countries with compulsory education recognize that some children are too handicapped to be educated in ordinary classes. In this country the Department of Education and Science recognizes ten categories of handicapped pupils for whom special educational treatment may be required (blind, partially sighted, deaf, partially hearing etc).

In addition, special schools are today being established for children with cerebral palsy, spina bifida, childhood autism, children with learning problems, dyslexics, delinquents and numerous others. As general education has become less specialized, especially during the early years of schooling, special education is becoming more specialized. Unfortunately, the more specialized the school, the larger must be the population from which it draws its pupils. Some of the more uncommon conditions (e.g. blindness) that are considered to make attendance at a special school necessary for the child, do not occur frequently enough in many areas to justify the expense of a small school or even group; in some of the smaller authorities this is even the case with relatively common handicaps. Consequently, the child either receives no special education or is placed residentially, sometimes hundreds of miles from his home.

How specialized must special education be? How exclusive must special schools be in the selection of children for admission? In our view, much of the small amount of special education in ordinary schools is not special enough, and this we have discussed; in the special schools, we think it is often too special in the sense that it is too exclusive.

For some of the children at present in special schools, particularly those with milder handicaps, it may be that just as effective education could be provided in ordinary schools if there were equally favourable conditions (in terms of small classes, skilled teachers etc). The best experimental studies of the value of the special class for slow learning children have produced equivocal results (Goldstein 1967). Special class children have been shown to make better progress than children in ordinary classes only in very limited respects and in many respects no differences could be found between the groups. Nevertheless, it is clear that for many handicapped children some kind of special educational provision will have to be made. The issues are the extent to which the special provision can be provided in ordinary schools and the extent to which different special schools or classes are needed for each different type of handicap.

Separation from ordinary school may be held to be organizationally necessary because of the difficulty of providing different regimes under the same roof. But the regimes of some types of special school differ little from those in the ordinary school; others, of course, differ very considerably. Separation may be administratively expedient in allowing the concentration in one school of children who need to be taught by methods that only specialist teachers can apply, or with the aid of equipment that would be too costly or bulky or sophisticated to supply to several ordinary schools. This might be the case with schools for deaf or cerebral palsied children, and possibly for the blind. It is convenient for the child if it allows him to receive both medical treatment and special teaching in one place, and thus to save valuable time for his education; this applies particularly to some physically handicapped children requiring physiotherapy. Separation is very likely to be a positive educational advantage to the child if it allows him to be in a small class and to receive more individual attention both in class and outside the classroom, in the smaller school community.

However, many of these features of a special school can be provided one way or another in ordinary schools if it is thought desirable to do so.

The same considerations apply to segregation within the special school system. It is administratively convenient to concentrate specialist teachers and equipment in one special school rather than several, and it is easier for one teacher to take a group of children together rather than each individually. However, once the numbers of children with the same disability require duplication of classes and equipment the convenience of having all the children in one special school becomes less, unless very specialized equipment or teaching is required, as for instance with deaf or cerebral palsied senior pupils taking domestic science or metalwork. Even then, the presence of such specialized equipment need not prevent the use of the classroom by children with other disabilities.

The main issues regarding segregation centre round the presumed need of children with certain disabilities to have specific teaching, treatment and school environment. And here it seems to us that the argument in favour of segregation according to handicap rests upon two assumptions which in general we find unproven.

The first assumption is that handicapped children with the same disorder or belonging to a single category of handicap have more in common with each other than with other handicapped children as regards their teaching, treatment and regime requirements. This may be so for deaf, for blind and for autistic children with respect to teaching requirements; and it may be so for children with haemophilia or spina bifida for treatment purposes; it may also be so for some maladjusted children with respect to the kind of regime they need. But it is not by any means so for these handicapped children in all three respects, nor necessarily for all other handicapped children in any respect. Nor should it be forgotten that whilst it is unusual for special schools to accept only those children who may be designated according to one category of handicapped pupils, in fact many of the children have another handicap; thus, schools for the educationally subnormal, delicate, physically handicapped and epileptic all have children with quite heterogeneous disorders. Our own survey provides numerical evidence of the overlap of handicaps.

The second assumption is that common educational treatment or regime needs are most beneficially provided by putting the children in an environment where they mix only with children with similar disorders. The rationale behind this is that the special school in question is providing very special education or treatment—so special, in fact, that it is too costly in personnel and money for the expertise to be dissipated. This may be true for some of the disorders with very special needs but it probably is not true for most.

Furthermore, this is only one side of the coin. The other side is the total well-being and development of the child. The more special the school the more uncommon and sheltered the environment. In addition, the more special the school the more likely it is to be residential. For some children

347

this is likely to be an advantage but for most the separation from home may carry grave disadvantages. Apart from any feelings of rejection a child may experience, it is likely to mean that the children lose their local friends so that friendships become increasingly restricted to children with similar handicaps. This is unlikely to be beneficial if the child is going to have to hold his own in the outside world when he leaves school.

The issues in relation to the provision of special schools are many and complicated. To discuss them fully would take us far from the findings of the Isle of Wight surveys. In addition, many of the facts needed in order to make rational decisions about the provision are not yet available. The point we wish to make is simply this. The degree of overlap between disorders is such that for the multiply handicapped child who is likely to require special schooling it is often a matter of arbitrary judgment whether he is classified, for example, as ESN, maladjusted, epileptic or dyslexic. The categorizing of children according to their presumed major handicap has now become restrictive in planning special education. Furthermore, the provision of schools for just one type of handicap has meant that perforce many of the schools have had to be residential (because of numbers) whether or not it was in the children's interest for them to be so.

It is suggested that special schooling be reconsidered from the point of view of the actual needs of handicapped children. Decisions should be taken as to what kind of special educational treatment is required, what kind of medical treatment, what kind of school regime and whether residential or day provision is preferable. By looking at these features it will be found that for certain children an exclusive special school may be required but for many others there will be advantages in the provision of a less exclusive school which takes children with several different kinds of handicap. The needs of yet other children may be best met by modifications to the arrangements in ordinary school. If special schools were to become less exclusive in their admissions, a small local education authority would have no difficulty in providing day special education for the majority of its young handicapped children.

Help for the child's family

All surveys, including this one, have shown that the families of handicapped children have a considerable burden to bear. In part this stems from the difficulties posed in the upbringing of a handicapped child and in the family adjustments which have to be made, and in part from worry and uncertainty about what caused the condition, whether the parents were to blame and what steps should be taken to help the child. In both respects many parents feel (quite rightly) that they do not receive the help they need. Time needs to be spent in explaining the nature of a child's condition, what to expect as he grows up, how the handicap will affect the child and his family and what kind of improvement or progress is possible. Parents need to be helped to work out ways of dealing with the day to day problems imposed by a handicapped child—such as how to cope with tantrums, how much a cerebral palsied child should be encouraged to do things without assistance and whether parents should try to teach the child at home. Of course, quite often no precise answers to these questions can be given, but this in no way diminishes the need for them to be as well informed as the situation allows. Advice and support are at least as necessary when there is no specific treatment as when there is. This is a continuing need which cannot be met by a single definitive statement, however comprehensive. The nature of a child's handicap changes as he gets older and parents should be helped to deal with each new issue as it arises rather than wait for a crisis to occur before seeking help.

These considerations apply with equal force to the child with intellectual or educational retardation and to the child with a psychiatric disorder, as to the child with a physical handicap. Severe intellectual retardation constitutes one of the most disabling of all handicaps and advice and support are particularly important for the parents of these children. Psychiatric disorder in the child can severely disrupt family relationships (as well as being responsive to disturbances in the home) and, as the survey showed, a high proportion of antisocial children also had severe educational difficulties. Parents need to be advised on how to obtain the most suitable schooling for their child, what alternatives are open to them and to whom they should go for further advice. Practical help may be needed with transport (to hospital or to a special school), with housing, financial matters, holiday arrangements and a host of other items of this kind. Parents frequently do not know what is available or how to obtain such services; the doctor, social worker or other adviser will need to help the parents with this.

Knowledge about services

It is not enough to provide services, it is also necessary to make sure the services reach those people who most need them. The better educated sections of the community tend to be better informed on how to obtain services, yet often it is the underprivileged groups who most need them.

There is no one answer to this problem; several different measures need to be taken. One solution is to make sure that there are adequate procedures for the identification of handicapped children. The surveys have shown that for every handicapped child under care or treatment there were several more who were receiving no help at all. In part this occurred because the existence of these children was not known to the clinics or to the authorities. Efficient screening methods may need to be introduced as a routine procedure. The ways in which this might be done have been mentioned in relation to the individual surveys. The timing of the introduction of screening methods also needs to be considered. There are problems in doing this when the existing services are already heavily overloaded.

A second need is for publicity about handicaps and about the services available for handicapped children. An informed public is better able to obtain the services it needs and, at least as important, to take steps to ensure that the proper services are provided where they are required. Parents' organizations have an important part to play in this, by advising and helping individuals, by providing information and by acting as a 'ginger group' to press for better service provision.

Lastly, it is important that professionals are fully aware of what other professionals and other groups have to offer. The paediatrician and psychiatrist need to be well informed in educational and social services and the teacher needs to know what the clinic, hospital and local authority services can do. Only in this way can the broader aspects of handicaps be adequately treated.

Conclusions

Inevitably, our work has raised more questions than it has provided answers. We hope that it has at least clarified some problems and has indicated in which directions research and service provision might develop. In the words of Binet and Simon (1914):

> May it also prove a guide—imperfect, no doubt, but still useful—for the organization of some of the social inquiries conducted in a strictly scientific spirit, which are becoming more and more necessary for the proper management of public affairs. . . . The essential thing to is understand that . . . methods of scientific precision must be introduced into all educational work, to carry everywhere good sense and light.

References

BECKER, W. C., MADSEN, C. H., ARNOLD, C. R. and THOMAS, D. R. (1967) The contingent use of teacher attention and praise in reducing classroom behaviour problems *Journal of Special Education* 1, 287–307

BERNSTEIN, B. (1965) A sociolinguistic approach to social learning in J. Gould (ed) *Penguin Survey of the Social Sciences* Harmondsworth: Penguin

BINET, A. and SIMON, T. (1914) *Mentally Defective Children* trans. W. B. Drummond London: Arnold

CARNINE, E., BECKER, W. C., THOMAS, D. R., POE, M. and PLAGER, E. (1969) The effects of direct and 'vicarious' reinforcement on the behaviour of problem boys in an elementary classroom

*CHALL, J. (1967) *Learning to Read: The Great Debate* New York: McGraw-Hill

*DE HIRSCH, K. and JANSKY, J. (1966) Early prediction of reading, writing and spelling ability *British Journal of Disorders of Communication* 1, 99–108

Implications for services

EDUCATION, MINISTRY OF (1963) *A Report on a Survey of Deaf Children who have been Transferred from Special Schools or Units to Ordinary Schools* London: HMSO
EGAN, D., ILLINGWORTH, R. S. and MACKEITH, R. C. (1969) (eds) *Developmental Screening: 0–5 years* London: Spastics International Medical Publications in association with Heinemann Medical Books
EISENBERG, L. (1967) Clinical considerations in the psychiatric evaluation of intelligence in J. Zubin and G. A. Jervis (eds) *Psychopathology of Mental Development* New York: Grune and Stratton
EISENBERG, L., CONNERS, K. and SHARPE, L. (1965) A controlled study of the differential application of out-patient psychiatric treatment for children *Japanese Journal of Child Psychiatry* 6, 125–32
GOLDSTEIN, H. (1967) The efficacy of special classes and regular classes in the education of educable mentally retarded children in J. Zubin and G. A. Jervis (eds) *Psychopathology of Mental Development* New York: Grune and Stratton
*GRAY, S. W. and KLAUS, R. A. (1965) An experimental preschool programme for culturally deprived children *Child Development* 36, 887–98
GRAY, S. W. and KLAUS, R. A. (1966) *Deprivation, Development and Diffusion* DARCEE Papers and Reports, vol. 1, no. 1
HARING, N. G. and PHILLIPS, E. L. (1962) *Educating Emotionally Disturbed Children* New York: McGraw-Hill
HARING, N. G. and RIDGWAY, R. W. (1967) Early identification of children with learning disabilities *Exceptional Children* 33, 387–95
HAYWOOD, C. (1967) Experimental factors in intellectual development: the concept of dynamic intelligence in J. Zubin and G. A. Jervis (eds) *Psychopathology of Mental Development* New York: Grune and Stratton
INGRAM, T. T. S. (1963) The association of speech retardation and educational difficulties *Proceedings of the Royal Society of Medicine* 56, 199–203
KIRK, S. A. (1958) *Early Education of the Mentally Retarded: An Experimental Study* Illinois: University of Illinois Press
KLAUS, R. A. and GRAY, S. W. (1968) The early training project for disadvantaged children: a report after five years *Monograph of the Society for Research into Child Development* 33, no. 4
MCLEOD, J. (1966) Prediction of childhood dyslexia *Slow Learning Child* 12, 143–54
MASON, A. W. (1967) Specific (developmental) dyslexia *Developmental Medicine and Child Neurology* 9, 183–90
PLOWDEN REPORT (1967) *Children and Their Primary Schools* Report of the Central Advisory Council for Education 1966 London: HMSO
ROYAL COMMISSION ON MEDICAL EDUCATION (1965–8) Report London: HMSO
ROYAL MEDICO PSYCHOLOGICAL ASSOCIATION (1968) The training of child psychiatrists. A memorandum prepared by a subcommittee of the child psychiatry section *British Journal of Psychiatry* 114, 115–17

351

RUTTER, M. (1969) The place of child psychiatry in postgraduate training in general psychiatry Working Paper RMPA/ASME Conference on Postgraduate Education: The Training of Psychiatrists London, March 1969

SAPIR, S. G. and WILSON, B. (1967) A developmental scale to assist in the prevention of learning disability *Educational and Psychological Measurement* 27, 1061–8 (Paper 5.3 in this volume, p. 380.)

SEEBOHM REPORT (1968) *Report of the Committee on Local Authority and Allied Personal Social Services* London: HMSO

SWIFT, J. W. (1964) Effects of early group experience: the nursery school and day nursery in M. L. Hoffman, and L. W. Hoffman (eds) *Review of Child Development Research* New York: Russell Sage Foundation

TIZARD, J. (1964) *Community Services for the Mentally Handicapped* London: Oxford University Press

TIZARD, J. (1966) The experimental approach to the treatment and upbringing of handicapped children *Developmental Medicine and Child Neurology* 8, 310–21

TIZARD, J. (1969) The role of social institutions in the causation, prevention and alleviation of mental retardation Proceedings of the Peabody NIMH Conference on sociocultural aspects of mental retardation, 10–12th June, 1968

TIZARD, J. and GRAD, J. C. (1961) *The mentally handicapped and their families* Maudsley Monograph no. 7 London: Oxford University Press

WEIKART, D. P. (1967) *Preschool Intervention* Ann Arbor, Michigan: Campus

YULE, W. and RIGLEY, L. (1968) A four-year followup of severely backward readers into adolescence in M. Clark and S. Maxwell (eds) *Reading: Influences on Progress* Edinburgh: United Kingdom Reading Association

5 Prevention

Introduction

Prevention involves breaking into a chain of cause and effect in such a way as to stop an effect developing at all or to reverse a trend which has begun to appear.

In the introduction to section 4 the point was made that many of the circumstances which seemed likely to be contributing to reading failure did not admit of any ready or direct cure. When we come to consider preventive measures on the other hand we think in a different time scale and in terms of a process that may be so gradual that its complete effects will not be seen in any one generation of school children.

Some long-term preventive measures have been adumbrated in earlier discussions and are therefore not represented again. Papers in this section cover roughly three areas of thought. First, there is emphasis on the need for the teacher to adapt the learning situation to the disadvantaged child and to think out what kind of experience will best compensate, if this is possible, for what has been lacking in his preschool years. Second, some attention is given to the early detection of the child who is 'at risk' and to the importance of fostering reading readiness instead of waiting for it to appear. Third, there is discussion of reading readiness, the value of becoming more aware of the child's learning problems—of what he is trying to do when he makes his early attempts at reading—and of the importance of making reading material more comprehensible, in linguistic terms, to those children who may be insufficiently familiar with much of the idiom and sentence structure of written stories.

Some of these measures will take effect more quickly than others, and they obviously do not provide a complete solution to the many problems outlined in the earlier parts of this book. Part of the answer undoubtedly lies in effecting an improvement in the quality of children's early lives and part in expanding the ancillary services and improving school conditions in general. But equally part of the answer lies in having an informed body of teachers in the primary school—teachers who are alert to the first signs that a child needs extra help and who are able to call on a wide repertoire of resources to meet his need.

5.1 Learning in the disadvantaged

CYNTHIA P. DEUTSCH
Professor of Psychology, School of Education,
New York University

Reprinted from M. Deutsch *et al* (1967) (eds) *The Disadvantaged Child*
Basic Books, pp. 147–62

In some respects, a title such as *Learning in the disadvantaged* is reminiscent of the *Honeybunch* series of children's books: the differing titles such as *Honeybunch in the country* and *Honeybunch in New York* served only to identify locales in which the saccharine little girl had the same experiences with the same kinds of people. Honeybunch herself always exhibited the same reactions and never changed. Similarly, in the title suggested for this paper, 'learning' could be regarded as a stable given, while the samples or populations or topics could be referred to as variable factors, having no intrinsic influence on the process itself. Thus, the particular social category of the learner is quite irrelevant to understanding and discussion of the process. There is historical precedent for considering learning in this way, in that it has been extensively studied in simple situations, such as maze running, with the aim of abstracting principles to be applied to other organisms, situations and levels of complexity. In other words, learning can be seen as a property of the organism—or, more accurately, of its nervous system—and a property which can be reduced to neurophysiological essentials. So a title such as *Learning in the disadvantaged*, like *Honeybunch in the country*, could be simply a device for altering minimally the arena of discussion rather than designating a particular content.

However, learning can be viewed in a manner which includes particular attributes of the learner, the context, and the content of the material to be learned. Despite the fact that the s–o–r paradigm offered a basis for such an emphasis, the experimental psychologists who specialized in learning theory twenty and thirty years ago eschewed it; as a result the findings from the multitude of learning studies yielded very little of relevance to human learning in a realistic social context. A variable such as the meaningfulness of what was being learned, in fact, was something

Cynthia P. Deutsch

that got in the way, so nonsense syllables were the content of choice for many experiments. The learning curves derived from such material find little application in the study of school learning, or in evaluating the differences in learning among differing populations.

With the current emphasis on education, and on the search for more effective teaching methods, learning theory has found its way through the maze and into the classroom. This process has brought about a focus on the learner and his specific characteristics—and in that context, a title such as *Learning in the disadvantaged* takes on a rather specific meaning. It is in this sense that this paper has been prepared. It includes, therefore, some discussion of the characteristics of the disadvantaged with respect to some of the skills underlying learning, and some treatment of the stimulus organization consistent with the learner's characteristics and the stimuli represented by the materials to be learned.

There are different kinds of learning and different kinds of disadvantage. For the population referred to in this paper, 'disadvantaged' is only the latest in a series of euphemisms, which have included 'slum dwellers' and just plain 'poor people'. These last two terms are concretely descriptive of the economic situation of these people, but by using the term 'disadvantaged' the intention is also to convey a categorization involving social or psychological variables. Since disadvantage exists only in a relative sense, the term needs somewhat further explication. For purposes of this discussion, the designation is used relative to the demands of the school and, later, the job market: the population being referred to are disadvantaged with respect to what is demanded for educational attainment and occupational mobility and advancement. The conditions of life at home for the children in this population are not continuous with the milieu of the school, and do not prepare them well for the demands placed on them by the school and by the broader society.

There are three major assumptions upon which the discussion which follows will be based:

1 The social milieu in which the child grows up is highly influential in determining the kind and degree of his experience. This is rather obvious on the macroscopic level: the slum child has a different milieu and therefore a different set of experiences from the middle class child. However, in current studies at the Institute for Developmental Studies (IDS), we are finding this true on a more microscopic level as well. An instrument known as the deprivation index, when applied to households of ostensibly the same socioeconomic status (SES) level, yields differences between families in social experience such as trips away from the neighbourhood, interaction between parent and child, organization of the home and of the family schedule, and the like. These differences are also found to be associated with scores on verbal and IQ measures given to the children.
2 The ease of acquisition of new knowledge and skills—learning—is based in large part on the prior experience and knowledge of the organism.

Ample documentation for this position is to be found in Hunt's (1961) *Intelligence and Experience*, which includes much work from many sources. 3 The nature of the stimulus—its organization, speed and manner of presentation, and the like—is influential in acquiring new knowledge. The relationship established between the experiential background of the organism and the nature of stimulus presentation is what Hunt refers to as the 'match'.

The discussion which follows concerns verbal, perceptual and attention characteristics of children who come from disadvantaged circumstances, and how these characteristics are related to their learning.

Let us begin with the verbal area. A large cross-sectional language study done at IDS has indicated that children from disadvantaged backgrounds enter school with a somewhat different language system than do middle class children. These differences obtain particularly in the grammatical structure of the language used, and in language used to relate one thing to another, as contrasted with the more simple descriptive uses. These differential language findings are consistent with the reports of Bernstein (1961, 1962) and with data reported by Jensen (1963). In general, the language used by the disadvantaged children may be described as simpler in syntax and less rich in descriptive terms and modifiers than is the language of the middle class child.

These differences come about apparently because the homes from which the children come are far less verbal than the average middle class home. Verbal interaction between parent and child tends to be in brief sentences and commands rather than in extensive interchange, and a great deal of communication in the very low-income home is gestural. Labelling objects and actions in the environment is not emphasized. There are few if any books or magazines in the home, and the child gets little exposure to the printed word as a source of information or of communication.

These differences in linguistic background between the disadvantaged and the more privileged home are too well known to belabour further here. The point to be made about them is that the verbal and linguistic experience of the child influences his learning. Not only does the child who has an impoverished verbal background have a more restricted vocabulary and especially, as indicated earlier, a narrower and simpler syntax for purposes of communicating with others, but in all probability he has what Jensen (1965) calls a 'higher threshold' for verbal mediation. Thus the child, as a result of his experiential background, is less able to solve problems by verbal mediation than would be true of the child with greater language experience. The potential importance of this background for learning cannot be overestimated, in view of the fact that the problems whose solutions are facilitated by verbal mediation are not limited to verbal problems, or even to problems verbally stated. In many so-called nonverbal tasks, verbalization plays an integral role, and many nonverbal problems are solved with the use of verbal mediation. Jensen (1965) points out the crucial role of verbal mediation in the solution to the problems posed by the Raven Progressive Matrices. Other examples may be found in such a test as the WISC. The picture completion subtest, for example, presents the subject with a series of pictures in which something is missing. This is of course a visual stimulus—but the response called for is a verbal one: a label. Another example would be the object assembly subtest on the same scale. There is considerable evidence to show that having labels for unfamiliar objects facilitates learning about them. Therefore, in tasks such as those in the object assembly, it may well be that the child who thinks in verbal terms—and is therefore more likely to label the incomplete object as he is working with it—will perform better even on such highly spatial tasks.

The exact nature of the verbal skills which underlie verbal mediational processes is still obscure. Whether simple exposure to a highly verbal environment lowers the threshold for the use of verbal mediation or whether what is important is extensive practice with verbal-type problems is not really known yet. While it will take extensive longitudinal studies on large samples to make such a determination, a promising tool has been formulated in the last several years: the Illinois Test of Psycholinguistic Abilities (ITPA). The test is a diagnostic test in the sense that what emerges for each subject is a profile of scores along several linguistic dimensions, such as auditory decoding, visual-motor association, vocal encoding and the like. In this way, as with any constructed scale, the components of a given overall score can be analysed in terms of patterning of strengths and weaknesses.

In an effort to learn more about the linguistic organization and growth of young children, especially those from disadvantaged backgrounds, we have been applying this test to the children in our preschool enrichment groups and to a control group. The preliminary results are that the experimental group performs at a higher level on the test than does the control, but that the subtest patterning of the two groups is almost identical. Apparently, the language experiences which the experimental group had during the enrichment year raised their overall level, but did not alter the patterning of language skills. Our same two groups of children were also tested on the Kendler (1963) concept-formation paradigm, but there was no significant difference between the experimental group and the controls in the number of subjects who could be designated 'mediators' according to Kendler's system. Further investigation and retesting, it is hoped, will determine if further language training does alter the ITPA pattern, and if such patterning can be predictive of mediational behaviour on the reversal shift technique. The level of performance of the experimental group on the ITPA was below the average, though on some subtests the difference was not significant; so it may also be that the overall ITPA score could predict mediation. If so, the implication would be that a language-enriched curriculum could foster the growth of verbal mediational processes in disadvantaged children, even without giving them any specific training in the use of verbal mediation.

Language was selected as one of the three areas of emphasis in this paper because it is obviously crucial to reading and to other academic performance. In the cross-sectional study previously referred to, one finding was that there were greater differences between the lower class and middle class children at the fifth grade level than at the first grade. While the data do not come from a longitudinal study, it still seems warranted to note that the disadvantaged children seem to become more disadvantaged, at least in the language area, as they go through school. What this fact indicates about the effects of the school on development is, for the moment, irrelevant. The point is that ground can be lost, relative to the development of the more privileged group. To the extent that language influences other learning, this developmental decline can be especially serious.

In evaluating possible remedies for poor progress in language development, cautious optimism seems the appropriate attitude. The ITPA results quoted above, as well as the test–retest gain of experimental enrichment groups on the Peabody Picture Vocabulary Test, indicate that such scores can increase following an experimental compensatory education programme. It is not yet known if such an increase will be maintained over long periods of time, with or without a continuing enrichment programme, or if language growth carries as a necessary corollary the growth in learning skills per se. As indicated above, one aspect of this question is being addressed in the ITPA study. Our longitudinal study—carrying the same groups of children through a special curriculum from the nursery year through the third grade, and continuing extensive evaluation of them through the sixth grade—will also yield some information on this question when completed.

In the meantime, Bernstein's work, the work of Bereiter and his group, that of Gray and her group, the Baltimore language study, and others, as well as our findings, are all contributing information and hypotheses in the area on language enrichment, an area which seems to be quite universally recognized as critical in the learning—and the teaching—of disadvantaged children.

In the perceptual area, where there is somewhat less widespread interest and work at the present, a greater emphasis is justified. Historically, theorists and researchers in this area have been concerned with the mechanisms of perception, and the influence that the organization of the stimulus field—particularly the visual field—exercises on what is perceived. The work on social influences on perception (with the exception of the well-known early study by Bruner and Goodman (1947) and a few scattered cross-cultural studies) has been concerned almost exclusively with the short-term influences of particular experimentally imposed or manipulated experiences. Unlike language, which is so obviously determined by social experience, perception has traditionally been regarded

Cynthia P. Deutsch

as a function quite independent of one's overall social milieu, an assumption which is open to serious question.

The fundamental contradiction to the assumption would be based on the proposition that experience and practice are influential in perceptual development. This does not seem so untenable when one considers the visual-deprivation experiments as examples, and it is certainly not unreasonable to view deprivation as a continuum. When so viewed, it becomes logical to assume that deprivation of varying degrees can be associated with perceptual disabilities of varying degrees. For example, as shown in the studies reported by von Senden (1932), people deprived of visual-form experience for varying periods of time will show varying degrees of impairment in form discrimination. Might it not be true also that people deprived *in varying degrees* of visual-form experience would show lesser, and perhaps more subtle, deficiency in form discrimination?

Slum homes provide few toys or other playthings for a child; neither are there picture books. Further, there is usually a paucity of household objects. Might it not be that such restrictions in the visual field inhibit the development of form perception? How can a child learn to differentiate the forms of a square and a triangle if the differences are not explicitly pointed out to him, even if his visual sensory apparatus is intact? What is the role of familiarity in accurate perception? Is it possible that new forms will be more easily differentiated if their components are more familiar, or if the child has a wider range of familiar forms against which to compare the novel? Fantz's work (1965) indicates that preference develops in accord with early exposure. Why shouldn't accuracy and ease of discrimination similarly relate to experience?

These questions have no definite answers at the present time. Posing them in this way places perceptual discrimination in a developmental and social context which is open to intensive experimentation, and, hopefully, removes the issue from the now sterile 'nativism–empiricism' controversy.

The suggested questions for investigation have related to visual perception primarily, but the inference should not be drawn that they are applicable only to vision. For further explication, let me briefly mention the hypothesis about auditory discrimination: that the noisy background and the weak signal conditions under which slum children live predispose them to learn early to tune out auditory stimuli. Both the signal-to-noise ratio itself and the inattention which it promotes operate to reduce the amount of auditory discrimination experience to which the child is exposed, and this eventuates in his later poorer performance on auditory discrimination tasks. While we do not as yet have sufficient data either to confirm or disconfirm this hypothesis definitively, so far our investigations in the area have supported the assumptions.

It is pertinent here to mention some recent specific analyses of auditory discrimination data which relate both to perceptual and to linguistic development. One of the primary tests used to evaluate auditory discrimination is the Wepman (1958). Item analysis of Wepman protocols done by my colleagues has shown that the most frequent items missed are those pairs which differ in the final phoneme, and that whenever in our samples groups of children with learning disabilities are compared with control groups, there are significant differences in final-phoneme discrimination whether or not the differences in initial-phoneme discrimination are significant. It seems fairly certain that the differences in performance by placement of phoneme are real ones. The implications for grammar and syntax are obvious, since most grammatical inflections in English are carried at the end of the word. There are also conceptual implications, in that accurate definition of number and tense can be very important in both stating and solving problems. Here it is relevant to note that, in the ITPA study, the subtest patterns show for both the experimental and the control groups the poorest performance in those which involve auditory stimuli and call for knowledge of grammar and of function. Perhaps even more interesting is the fact that these are also the two subtests on which the experimental group is farthest above the control group. Unfortunately, data on the Wepman for these groups are not yet analysed.

That discrimination can be successfully taught to young children can be implied from the experimental-control group differences in the ITPA data. Whether it can be trained in older children, especially those who already show considerable deficiency, is less clear. A study recently concluded at the Institute involved the testing and training of auditory discrimination in a group of third grade reading retardates. The purpose of the study was to determine if training in auditory discrimination would enable retarded readers (who, we have found, are deficient in this skill compared to average or good readers) better to profit from reading instruction. Four groups were defined: one which received regular auditory discrimination training and also remedial reading, one which received only auditory training, one which received only remedial reading and a control group which received neither. The second two groups also had a play period (during which the activities were neither auditory nor book or reading related) in order to equalize the time spent with the tutor. A battery of eleven auditory discrimination tests was administered before, immediately after and twice more at spaced intervals after, the training period, which was one school semester's length for each group. The special work given the children was in addition to their regular schoolwork. Overall analyses indicate no differential auditory discrimination improvement for those children who had specific auditory training. The more microscopic analyses are still underway, and it is not yet known whether some differential performance or patterning of performance will be defined.

Attentional processes are, in essential respects, a part of both perceptual and linguistic development, and are being considered separately here only for convenience. It is obvious that experience will mean little unless the input channels are sufficiently open and attuned to the stimuli being presented. Both the state of the organism and the organization of the stimuli and the field in which they are presented influence attention. The state of the organism can be considered to include both the neural state and the motivational state. While the former may not be too directly influenced by the social environment (though the possibility of a somewhat indirect influence must not be negated), certainly the latter is; and here the social environment quite directly influences the selection of stimuli which are perceived.

The educators of the thirties were quick to point out that if children lose interest they do not attend and therefore do not learn. Therefore, much effort was expended to attract the children's attention. Unfortunately, almost all of this effort was directed towards making the stimuli compelling. Virtually no care was taken to ensure the kinds of experience that would influence the motivational state of the child. A child who feels lost in school because demands and materials are unfamiliar and discontinuous with what he previously experienced at home will not attend properly to the stimuli presented. A child who has not previously been exposed to as much as ten minutes of uninterrupted speech will have great difficulty in listening all the way through so long a statement. Furthermore, a child who has not previously learned to respond to rather elaborate spoken directions will not be able even to attend to, let alone follow, all the directions. Such difficulties have strong negative effects on motivation and as a result negatively affect the child's attentiveness and therefore his learning. Once the attentiveness has been, as it were, tuned out on the inside, it is difficult to reinstate it, no matter how attractively and seemingly effective attention has been engineered by organization of the stimulus field. Further, the stimulus organization, to be effective, must relate to the child's background of experience.

Very early a child learns to be selective in what he perceives: this is a prime necessity, inasmuch as one is always assailed by many more stimuli than it is possible to respond to. Hierarchies of attentional and response systems are established, apparently on a neural as well as an experiential level, related to sensory modality preference and efficiency as well as to the 'compellingness' of individual stimuli. A stimulus-field organization, to be effective in channelling a child's attention to the aspects most relevant to the learning task, should be consistent with a child's already learned hierarchies. What these are for different children at different ages are far from clear, and many experimenters and teachers have found a child relating to what was conceived of as a nonessential part of the stimulus material. It is probable that a child's background yields not only particular amounts and kinds of stimuli, but also some *channelling* of his attention to particular aspects of the stimuli present. Here it may well be that the middle class background gives a child not only a great amount and variability of stimuli, but also an attentional channelling which is consistent with his response to aspects of stimuli which are most relevant for his school performance.

Apart from these built-in hierarchies and proclivities, however, one must address the question of the manner in which attention is engineered by stimulus-field manipulation, and how often the original purpose is overwhelmingly defeated. The best example is the modern primer. Because colour attracts attention, it is used quite lavishly. Because children like pictures—or are thought to like pictures—they are included multitudinously. But by these measures, the children's attention is of course attracted to the coloured pictures rather than to the print, which is the stimulus to be learned. The child is confronted with the task of attending to a relatively small black and white stimulus in the face of a strong, competing, large coloured one. It is good to note that some of the new experimental reading series have abandoned this format, whether or not for conscious reasons of better visual and attentional coordination. Another example of self-defeating stimulus organization may be found in many elementary school classrooms. The rooms are often a riot of colour: posters all over the walls, pictures the entire length of the room etc—all distractions from the teacher's voice and from whatever content is placed on the blackboard or the bulletin board, or in the pupil's notebook in front of him. These comments do not reflect support for a movement back to the austere, dull and undecorated classroom, but simply for a movement towards a judicious use of attention-getting aids. A stimulus analysis of the classroom and the learning materials presented would yield considerable information about the objects to which attention is really being called. Then, a redesigning of the placement of the stimuli and of the stimuli themselves should enable the creation of attractive classrooms and materials without the danger of engineering the child's attention to the nonessential stimuli.

With regard to other correlates of attention, I would like to cite a series of studies at the Institute involving the use of our modification of the Continuous Performance Test. Our version uses coloured dots, inasmuch as the subjects for whom it was adapted were young children and retarded readers. Briefly, the task is a vigilance one, which involves attending continuously to a series of stimuli and pressing a button when the one previously designated as correct is presented. The visual form of our test uses a memory drum, on which coloured dots are presented at the rate of one per second. Each dot appears in the aperture for 0.6 second, and there is 0.4 second between stimuli. This is subjectively rather a rapid rate, and it is necessary to pay close attention in order not to miss a stimulus. Subjects are told to press the button every time the red dot appears. An auditory analogue uses the naming of the colours in the same order and at the same rate, with the same stimulus—red—being the correct one. In all our studies using this device, the clinical-type sample has always done more poorly than its control group. For example, retarded readers perform more poorly than good readers. The original scoring of the technique involved a simple tabulation of incorrect and correct presses, and missed presses (i.e. when the correct stimulus appeared and the button was not depressed). However, more recently we have connected the device to an electronic clock, so it is possible to record the elapsed time between stimulus presentation and button press. When these results are analysed, what is found is that many of the responses labelled incorrect by the old scoring method are really simply late responses to the correct stimulus. That is the retarded readers, for instance, are responding correctly to the stimuli, but their responses are made too late to be recorded as correct. (They occur too soon to be real responses to the stimulus following the correct one, so it is obvious that they are slow but correct.) Since the Rosvold, Mirsky and colleagues (1956) studies with the CPT indicate that the test is sensitive to central changes in arousal or attention, it seems most reasonable to view the children with learning disabilities as having faulty or slow attentional processes.

Recent drug studies by Kornetsky and his colleagues (1964) indicate that there are differential effects of various substances, depending on whether the timing of a task like the CPT is experimenter- or subject-controlled. While the drug studies as drug studies are irrelevant for this discussion, the fact that the two types of stimulus presentation control can be differentiated is highly relevant—and relevant to understanding the role of attention in performance.

Even before the implications of all these CPT findings for children's learning have been investigated experimentally, their relevance for the classroom seems obvious. What is needed is a well-engineered stimulus field and a speed of presentation adjusted to the children's actual rate of response. This latter may be harder to accomplish than it looks. Some classroom observational data collected by some of my colleagues show that, without being at all aware of it, many if not most teachers tend to give less response time to the child whom they see as a poorer student than they give to the child who they are more sure knows the answer. This practice results in less time being given to the child who in reality takes longer to respond than is given to the child who actually needs less time. This kind of teacher behaviour also influences directly the number of success experiences of the slower responding child, and also influences his performance indirectly, by conveying subtly that the teacher does not expect him to know the answer. For the children are aware of the differential time allotment and of its implications even though the teachers in the sample are not.

What are the implications for 'learning in the disadvantaged' from these brief discussions of the verbal, perceptual and attentional processes? Many of the studies referred to drew samples from lower class and middle class groups in order to make direct comparisons between them. Other data, gathered for other purposes, also yielded information on such comparisons. For example, in the studies of retarded versus normal readers, we are dealing with populations which are biased on SES lines. That is, the prevalence of reading retardation is much higher (estimates range from four to ten times higher) in disadvantaged groups than in middle class groups. Hence, whatever characteristics are found in retarded readers will be found in a larger proportion of disadvantaged children than in middle class children.

The burden of the data and hypotheses presented is that disadvantaged children suffer in the three areas mentioned, and that these areas represent crucial underlying skills in school learning. Further, the implication is that these children are deficient in these skills as a result of the deficits they experience in their home backgrounds. Data are adduced to show that skills in these areas can improve, though there is not yet concrete evidence to indicate that such improvement will result in overall academic or conceptual improvement. There are no data to the contrary; it is simply that the whole approach to the specific areas is too new to have permitted as yet the gathering of definitive data.

Another fairly clear point is that children from more privileged backgrounds are superior in most of these skills, and that groups of such children show a lower rate of reading and other learning disabilities. Therefore, it does seem reasonable to conclude that improvement in these skills could result in better progress in school learning, and a lower rate of learning disabilities.

Evidence may be adduced from the fact that many of the disadvantaged children who have difficulty with school learning learn many other things most adequately, when their experiential background is appropriate for such learning. For example, large numbers of five year old children are quite capable caretakers for their infant and toddler siblings. These children can be quite independent in personal care from a very early age, dressing themselves and then helping younger siblings to dress at ages when middle class children do not do so. More examples could be cited, but the point is made: these children do not show the same disabilities in learning when the behaviour called for is consistent with their experience. Perhaps this is an instance in which the old concept of cultural relativism is appropriate. The middle class children learn well those tasks which are consistent with their training and experiences, and so do the lower class slum children. The problem is that it is the school-type learning which is related to the values of the broader society—and to the later job needs of the children—and this is the type for which the middle class child's background best equips him. The implication is, therefore, that it is not the learning ability per se of the slum child which is deficient, but only his background of experiences. It is on this basis that compensatory education programmes have been established by us at the IDS and by various other groups around the country. As both our measuring instruments and our curricula are sharpened, the answers to many of the questions posed in this paper should be forthcoming.

Two words of caution are in order before concluding. One is that despite the cultural-relativism hypothesis put forward above, it must be recognized that the deficiencies which seem to exist in the slum child have to do in part with cognitive and concept-formation behaviour, and these are skills which underlie many problem-solving abilities, even in nonverbal areas. If, as is hypothesized, it is impoverishment of experience which negatively affects the development of these skills, then that impoverishment is associated with a debilitation at the centre of the growth of basic learning skills, and not with more superficial, and presumably more easily compensated, skills.

The second word of caution applies especially to the area of training and curriculum. It is highly likely that experience alone is not enough to enable the disadvantaged child to overcome the poverty of his background. That is, what is probably necessary is experience that is engineered, labelled, verbalized and repeated in such a way that it is made relevant both to the child's previous experience and to his later activities. In other words, a trip to the zoo will not in itself make up the child's lack of previous trips, acquaintance with animals, with the use of transportation to get there and the like. What is necessary is the organizing of the trip in such a way that it reinforces knowledge the child already has, and imparts specific labels and procedures that he can make use of in the future. For example, a trip to the zoo can contribute to an understanding of the concepts 'larger' and 'smaller' by making obvious for the child the sizes of the various animals and comparing one to the other in the words of the concept: the elephant is *larger* than the monkey; the ostrich is *smaller* than the horse. Simply taking the child to the zoo and expecting him to acquire this concept himself is unrealistic.

That this is true can be seen in unplanned real-life examples as well as in pedagogical theorizing and evaluation of enrichment curriculum experiences. I recently had occasion to meet a number of children of migrant workers. These children are disadvantaged not only by their impoverished home backgrounds, but by their irregular school attendance as a result of the family's travel from one crop harvest to another. But the children, in contrast to city slum children, are not disadvantaged by a geographical narrowness: by the age of ten, those to whom I spoke had travelled thousands of miles, usually in cars or small trucks. When some of the children from city slums who have never been more than ten blocks in any direction from their homes show little concept of distance, geography or mileage, it is easy to attribute their deficit to simple lack of experience. But when migrant children show the same type of deficit, it becomes apparent that experience alone is not enough. The migrant children, who were interviewed informally and with no sampling procedure, had a very poor concept of distance and time. These children gave for the width of the continent estimates which varied from ten to one hundred miles, even though they themselves had travelled from Oregon to Texas and back several times, with a trip or two from Texas to Florida in between. It seems clear that their deficient knowledge and unrealistic estimates were due to the lack of any attempt to specify and make meaningful their extensive geographical experience. Apparently, a child can travel thousands of miles, but if the time, the mileage and the geography are not pointed out to him in some meaningful manner, little specific learning about distance is gained.

Curricula which simply present a cafeteria of experience, and experiences which do not include some direction, cannot be expected to succeed—or to accomplish much—in ameliorating the school learning disabilities manifested by the disadvantaged child. Therefore, the evaluation of the specific skills and deficits of children from varying backgrounds should continue, and the attempt should be made to devise curricula and experiences which will be consistent with the current skills of the child and which will be effectively directed towards his growth in the areas of deficit.

References

BERNSTEIN, B. (1961) Social structure, language and learning *Educational Research* 3, 163–76

BERNSTEIN, B. (1962) Social class, linguistic codes and grammatical elements *Language and Speech* 5, 4, 221–40

*BRUNER, J. S. and GOODMAN, C. C. (1947) Value and need as organizing factors in perception *Journal of Abnormal Social Psychology* 42, 33–44

FANTZ, R. L. (1965) The origins of form perception in P. H. Mussen, J. J. Conger and J. Kagan (eds) *Readings in Child Development and Personality* New York: Harper

*HUNT, J. McV. (1961) *Intelligence and Experience* New York: Ronald

JENSEN, A. R. (1963) Learning in the preschool years *Journal of Nursery Education* 18, 2, 133–8

JENSEN, A. R. (1965) Verbal mediation and educational potential Unpublished manuscript

KENDLER, TRACY S. (1963) Development of mediating responses in children in S. C. Wright and J. Kagan (eds) Basic cognitive processes in children *Monograph of Social Research in Child Development* 28, 33–48

KORNETSKY, C. and ORZACK, MARESSA HECHT (1964) A research note on some of the critical factors on the dissimilar effects of chlorpromazine and secobarbital on the digit symbol substitution and continuous performance tests *Psychopharmacologia* 6, 79–86

ROSVOLD, H. E., MIRSKY, A. F., SARASON, E., BRANSOME, E. D., Jr and BECK, L. H. (1956) A continuous performance test of brain damage *Journal of Consultative Psychology* 20, 343, 350

SENDEN, M. VON (1932) *Raum- und Gestaltauffassung bei operierten Blindgeborener vor und nach der Operation* Leipzig: Barth cited by D. O. Hebb (1949) *The organization of behaviour* New York: Wiley

*WEPMAN, J. (1958) *Manual of directions: Auditory Discrimination Test* Chicago: Author

5.2 Reading failure: its causes and prevention

A. E. TANSLEY
Staff Inspector for Special Education,
City of Birmingham Education Authority

Reprinted from A. E. Tansley (1967) *Reading and Remedial Reading* Routledge and Kegan Paul, pp. 60–80

Despite the improvement in reading standards in recent years there are still many children who find reading difficult and who leave school with attainments too low for reading to be a useful and pleasurable activity. These failing children have great difficulty in developing healthy attitudes towards themselves and others; they either isolate themselves from social contacts and become withdrawn and depressed or, in order to compensate for feelings of inadequacy, become aggressive, uncooperative, unreliable, pleasure-seeking and perhaps delinquent. It is well known that the incidence of reading backwardness is much higher in delinquents than in the population as a whole. Whatever the causal relationships, teachers who work with delinquents and emotionally disturbed children know that dramatic improvements in behaviour often occur with improvements in reading. The causes of failure may be difficult to determine, the relationship between causes and symptoms may be obscure, but the results of failure are usually obvious. Without success in reading, educational progress in general will be retarded. Teachers must therefore be cognizant at all times of their obligation to prevent reading backwardness if possible, and to treat it with all the skill and understanding they can muster when it arises.

What can be done to prevent reading failure?

Failure in reading is due to a variety of causes which are always interrelated and interdependent. The failure may be due to a combination of inherited, congenital, physical, emotional or environmental factors, but the relationship between them is never easy to determine, particularly in children who have been failing for a long time. With them the original causes often become overlaid by acquired symptoms. Thus failure may be ascribed to poor intellectual endowment, e.g. as indicated by a low IQ; however, we have already stressed that a low IQ is no certain indication of poor biological inheritance. There is, of course, abundant evidence in research to confirm that a poor biological inheritance is generally worsened by any physical or sensory handicap, emotional disturbance or deprived environment. Again, failure may be due to organic causes—mild cerebral dysfunction is likely to result in psychomotor disability, perceptual disturbance, aphasias, attentional defects, personality deviations and environmental difficulties due to consequent mismanagement and lack of understanding. In such cases, it is often impossible to determine to what extent the failure to read is due to the brain damage per se or to the psychological and environmental *sequelae* of it. Yet again, failure may be due to emotional disturbance caused by too hasty an introduction to reading by over-ambitious parents or teachers; here the child may set up defences against learning to read, display psychosomatic conditions, show deterioration in intelligence test scores and become progressively more difficult to motivate.

It is thus often difficult to isolate causes and to differentiate between causes, effects and symptoms. Teachers working in a normal school setting may therefore feel that much time would be wasted in attempting to diagnose causes before they begin to take remedial steps. In any case, few teachers are at present sufficiently well trained to attempt a comprehensive diagnosis let alone relate scientific treatment to it. Consequently they approach the problem empirically and often achieve surprisingly good results. However, their methods usually constitute nothing more than intensive systematic coaching using well-tried methods and reading schemes, such as those mentioned earlier. Much of what is described as remedial work is nothing more than this. Of course this coaching is valuable and doubtless prevents much ultimate backwardness.

These teachers should realize, however, that in many cases the treatment they give is what may be described as *peripheral* rather than *fundamental* or *basic*. They might find it helpful to think in terms of two types of backwardness: pseudo or conditioned backwardness due to environmental and psychogenic factors, and real backwardness caused by etiological factors such as brain injury, sensory deficiencies, markedly inferior intelligence, mental disorder or other pathological conditions.

These two types or classes of backwardness cannot, of course, be differentiated absolutely nor can their degree be reliably measured except in terms of chronological age. However, the concept of pseudo-backwardness is a useful one in that treatment becomes primarily concerned with manipulating the environment to organize success and good motivation. A detailed diagnosis of backwardness may in such cases be unnecessary because success may result from systematic coaching based on good teacher–child relationship. However, some measure of *present* intellectual status is generally desirable in order to avoid overoptimism. One danger inherent in making an assessment of intelligence is that a mental age may be used to set the upper limit of reading attainment or to assess readiness. There is now sufficient research evidence, and our own experience over the past fifteen years supports this, to raise serious doubts about the predictive value of mental ages as indicators of optimum levels of attainment, particularly in reading, and especially in relation to children with severe reading disability. The variation of abilities within the individual, which are masked by any global assessment or measure such as an IQ, can also often upset any prediction of success or failure. For example, a child with a low IQ may well possess abilities which make good levels of reading quite possible. This is often seen in some educationally subnormal children who find mechanical reading quite easy.

When intensive coaching fails to produce results the teacher may be faced with true or real backwardness which is more intractable. A thorough, comprehensive diagnosis then becomes essential. Nevertheless, there is now mounting evidence that even this backwardness can be limited in severity by early diagnosis and scientific, systematic, related remedial treatment. The degree of backwardness and its exacerbation by faulty or delayed treatment can be progressively reduced.

The above discussion indicates that every effort should be made, particularly in the earlier stages of children's education, to prevent backwardness and reduce its many serious effects. This effort should be based on the following considerations.

1 *Poor linguistic backgrounds*
Attempts must be made to ameliorate the disadvantages of language deprivation resulting from poor linguistic backgrounds. Special attention must be given to providing stimulating experiences of a broad and varied character. Thus in the case of immigrant children, no real progress in reading is likely to be made until they have become conversant with our language and culture. A reading readiness programme for them must include many explorations of the environment and ample opportunities for talk and discussion. Without these, the books we use can be rather meaningless, and reading may be good mechanically but poor in comprehension. These children need also play experiences with the materials used by children in our culture so that they have the same opportunities for the adequate development of those sensori-motor skills, constructive abilities and perceptual and conceptual processes needed for learning in our educational system. We have met coloured children whose language development was so poor that they were quite unable to pin concepts to words they were able to read mechanically.

Of course, many British children suffer under similar handicaps; indeed, it is often difficult for teachers from middle class backgrounds to appreciate how little communication exists in the homes of some deprived children. The 'average' child of six should have a spoken vocabulary of 6,000–7,000 words; many backward children of six have spoken vocabularies of 1,000–2,000 words or less. They therefore have great difficulty in understanding the language they hear from other children and teachers, and if they are able to read, are unable to comprehend and to have rich concepts. They are still further handicapped because they have even less awareness of the meaning and use of words which are vital in the development of relational thinking, e.g. prepositions, adverbs and adjectives. They therefore find it difficult to make abstractions from and generalizations about their environment. *They are unable to learn how to learn.*

Many backward children have had little contact with books, periodicals, magazines or newspapers. The school must therefore remedy the deficiency by surrounding the child with these media of communication. Looking at well-illustrated books will do much to stimulate a desire to communicate, to become curious and interested in things, and to seek and exchange information and ideas.

2 *School organization*

Teachers must not only be made aware of the psychology of individual differences; they must also receive training in how to organize their teaching to tackle the educational problems created by these differences. It seems that few colleges of education make any serious attempt to show students how to arrange their teaching so that they are capable of making some attempt at providing each child with an education suited to its age, ability and aptitude. There is, of course, some value in showing students how to prepare, plan and present a set lesson and, in the first place, such a lesson may have to be given to a whole class. A little experience of *class* teaching soon demonstrates to the sensitive teacher its inefficiency and inadequacy. Post-lesson tests will clearly indicate that the response of the children varies considerably and this obtains no matter what the age or intellectual status of the class may be. The good, well-trained teacher must therefore be capable of dividing her class into groups of convenient size, of carrying on several 'lessons' simultaneously, of remaining flexible in the methods and curriculum she uses, and of providing learning situations which are tailored to the psychological and educational needs of every child. This is perhaps asking too much of teachers, particularly at present when class sizes are much too large. However, it should be stressed in order to make teachers appreciate that *class* or *mass* teaching should be anathema to them.

The exponents of streaming will, of course, put forward the plea that they believe in streaming because it helps teachers to deal more adequately with a more limited range of individual difference. However, even in large schools where streaming might be expected to result in groups which are fairly homogeneous for learning purposes, a detailed look at the children will reveal a very wide range in learning ability, to say nothing of differences in personality, backgrounds, interests and emotional and social development. In the author's school which caters for educationally subnormal pupils who have been screened for low intelligence, a comprehensive survey has clearly shown that the population in it is as heterogeneous as that found in any group. The children have been examined medically, neurologically, psychologically and educationally, and family and case histories have been completed for each child. The data obtained have shown that each child is different and presents a 'unique' individual educational experiment. We are certain that a similar result would be found for any group of children irrespective of age, class or school. For example, an analysis of children in an A stream in a large grammar school would yield similar results and indicate the inefficiency of much of the subject-centred teaching that prevails.

To prevent backwardness, therefore, schools must be prepared to examine not only their methods but also their organization. Since the main attack on prevention of reading failure must be made in the primary school, let us briefly examine what changes might be tried. Some schools have already made changes and are engaged in exciting experiments.

First, we should think about using more flexible systems of grouping children. The class system is often applied very rigidly and a child, once placed in a class, tends to remain in it for far too long. An organization based on cross-classification or 'setting' for various subjects or groups of subjects might be tried. This system can be very flexible and allow children to move across 'sets' as the speed and depth of their learning change. Again, some schools have experimented with so-called family groupings. In this, children may be grouped in 'families' which cover the whole or part of the age range of the primary school and ignore attainments and intelligence ratings. This has obvious social benefits but it could also lead to improvements in attainments, particularly if it were supplemented by cross-classification, and special groupings for remedial work.

The evidence for and against streaming is not yet sufficient to lead to reliable conclusions. Statements have been made that unstreaming reduces the incidence of backwardness without detriment to brighter children. My own school is unstreamed and the evidence suggests:

1 There has been no deterioration in the attainment gains made by brighter children in basic subjects.
2 The failing children, and particular older ones, have gained in confidence and social status and in most cases have been helped by their more successful friends.
3 Children with acute learning difficulties have been more strongly motivated to accept and benefit from remedial help.
4 Teachers have had to individualize treatment. They have therefore gained knowledge and experience in handling a wider range of learning problems and their teaching has become more systematic and inspiring.
5 With the desegregation of the slowest learners all teachers have become more aware of the needs of these children and have made greater efforts on their behalf.
6 Children with marked reading disability have needed extra help.

All primary schools should have at least one teacher who has been thoroughly trained in the diagnosis and treatment of reading disability. Large schools should have a remedial department to give special, systematic help to poor readers either within their own class or grouping, or in specially arranged reading classes. For extremely difficult cases of reading failure, the remedial teaching staff should be helped and guided by the school psychological service working *in the school* and playing its part not only in diagnosis but also in treatment. The present arrangement whereby children are sent out of schools to a clinic is usually inefficient for the following reasons:

1 Much of the time spent on intelligence testing and diagnosing is wasted because it is not followed up by appropriate, related education in schools.
2 Educational psychologists are not always capable of interpreting their test results to indicate what form of treatment should be given. For instance, it is of little use to apply an intelligence test without suggesting what the result means in terms of teaching. Simply to inform a teacher that a child's IQ is so and so, that he has a poor memory for visual or auditory material, is suffering from mild 'brain injury' which interferes with perception and attention, or merely to supply a catalogue of item responses on the test, is of no use to most teachers. We should surely expect more assistance from educational psychologists than this. Of course, they cannot be expected to do much actual teaching. They must, however, be sufficiently experienced and knowledgeable to suggest to ordinary teachers what changes or modifications in method and approach might be made or what new techniques might be tried.
3 Many teachers are sceptical about or openly dissatisfied with the service provided at present.

When efforts to help slow readers in the primary school's normal organization have failed, and particularly when marked failure is generalized to all basic subjects, special classes should be organized for them where possible. These classes should be for about fifteen children and should be taken by good, specially trained teachers. Conditions in such classes should be on a par with those in special schools. The segregation of such children should be as limited as possible—they should combine with other children for as many activities as they are able to profit by. If the need is too great for one special class to meet, and if more than one class is impossible to organize, then priority should be given to the younger children, say, the seven and eight year olds.

The primary school in its efforts to prevent backwardness in reading must organize its teaching so that it truly educates the *whole child*. An atomistic approach based on the teaching of individual subjects fitted into a rigid, timetabled programme will not achieve the total, well-integrated, orderly development of each child. In respect of reading, for instance, the development of reading skills depends upon what happens in all lessons—physical education, art and crafts, music and number, as well as in reading or language lessons per se. A successful start to reading cannot be made until a certain level of psychoneurological maturity has been reached. The child must have certain visual and auditory perceptual skills, motor and psycholinguistic abilities before he becomes capable of perceiving, organizing and interpreting the symbols and sounds involved in the reading process. A total, integrated approach is therefore necessary in which the teacher uses *all* her teaching as a contribution to developmental reading.

Backwardness is perhaps as much a social problem as it is an educational one. Somehow or other the primary school, and indeed all schools, must be involved in the sociological aspects of education. Attempts must be made to enlist parental cooperation, to change those influences in a child's background which militate against his educational progress. The size of the problem is so frightening that teachers often feel that they are impotent to do anything about it. Nevertheless, some schools make valiant attempts chiefly through such things as open days and parent–teacher associations. More often than not, however, these fail to attract the parents of backward children. It then becomes necessary for the school to take itself to the children's homes and parents. Some teachers of slow learners do visit the children's homes, but teachers should not be expected to become part-time social workers in addition to their professional work.

Realistic attempts to prevent backwardness must involve social workers and health visitors working as members of the school staff or, failing this, in much closer cooperation with schools than exists at present. This would almost certainly lead to the arousing and sustaining of the parents' interest in the school's work and its efforts to educate children as individuals. It is well known that backward children are often not interested in school. They come from homes where education is viewed as being of little importance and in which strong antagonisms exist towards schools and teachers. Children from such homes are thus likely to find school irksome and to have difficulty in understanding the importance of learning. They lack determination and persistence and are difficult to motivate.

Many teachers can cite examples to demonstrate the great improvements that can accrue from attempts to change parental attitudes and to obtain their cooperation. In my own school we have had surprising gains in reading attainments and personality when, as a result of the joint efforts of teachers and our social worker, parents have become enthusiastic about the school and anxious to cooperate fully with it in helping their children.

3   *Identifying the problem*

The early identification of potential reading difficulty is, of course, an important factor in prevention. It is a tragic, yet not an infrequent occurrence, to encounter children whose reading backwardness has not been dealt with by the time they reach the postprimary stage in their education. Of course, reading difficulty will have been noted by teachers before this, but only by the child's failure to respond to teaching and his consequent lack of achievement. Prevention of reading failure, however, depends on an early identification of the *reasons* why a child is failing to respond to the school's reading programme. These reasons are never particularly easy to isolate even by a highly trained and skilled diagnostician. The author proposes to list some of the signs and conditions which may indicate to *a class teacher* that difficulty in reading is likely to arise.

The following suggestions are intended as a guide to teachers of younger children to help them more readily identify children to whom reading may be difficult. They might also, in some cases, be suggestive of preventive methods.

1 *Estimate the child's level of intelligence*
This cannot be done by using group intelligence tests which depend upon reading. Nonverbal or more accurately nonreading group tests such as the Otis Primary or Sleight Nonverbal tests may be used, but too much reliance must not be placed on any IQ or mental age arrived at for giving a definite indication of intellectual readiness for reading. Perhaps the best guide is to assess the child's language level in relation to his peers by noting the size of his spoken vocabulary, the facility with which he communicates, the length and complexity of sentences he uses, and his ability to respond to commands and requests and to interpret stories. If test results and an assessment of language development indicate a poor intellectual level, then it is usually wiser to defer formal instruction in reading and concentrate on developing readiness, particularly in the language area.

2 *Estimate the level of the child's neurological and perceptual development*
Such an estimation will be new to most teachers. However, there is now mounting evidence that these aspects of growth are of significant importance in the acquisition of reading skills.

Of course, teachers cannot be expected to be neurologists, but they can observe signs which indicate neurological immaturity or abnormality. The following are some of the things to look for in assessing a child's readiness:

1 Do his movements appear to be awkward, jerky and uncontrolled?
2 Is there evidence of difficulty in eye-muscle control?
3 Does he find it difficult to balance on either foot?
4 Does he appear to be lacking in rhythm, e.g. in walking, marching, running, skipping, singing?
5 Does he have difficulty in using a pencil or paint brush?
6 Can he draw the following forms as well as the majority of his peers?

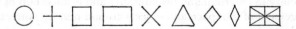

In assessing the quality of these drawings, teachers should remember that it is the accuracy of form perception which is important. Children with motor difficulties which, for instance, interfere with the fine manipulation of a pencil point may not *draw* the figures well but their drawings may still indicate good ideas of form.

We have now studied the drawings of over a thousand children, the majority of whom were in the age range four to eight years. The remainder were older children who were experiencing considerable difficulty in learning to read. Teachers from all over the country sent drawings to the author and gave each child's chronological age and reading age on the Burt and Schonell Graded Word Tests. It appeared that, except in some older children who through practice and sophistication could draw the figures, a child was unlikely to make successful progress in reading if his form perception of any of the figures was poor. What constitutes poor form perception is at present somewhat subjective (as is the case, for instance, in the Binet-type tests where examples are given as a guide). We are working on an analysis of the drawings in an attempt to arrive at an objective assessment or scoring system. All we can claim at present is that the quality of the form perception indicated by the drawings does appear to be a very useful guide to reading readiness if a visual approach is to be used. For a child who is unable to read, if the drawings indicate good form perception then some other causes of failure should be sought; for example, the child may have auditory, emotional or attentional difficulties, or he may have been taught by wrong methods. On the evidence of the drawings, reports have been written for teachers giving indications of readiness and/or possible reasons for reading failure. Many have written to say how very useful the reports were in helping to improve teaching either by giving more emphasis to a readiness programme or by changing the methods used.

7   Does cerebral dominance appear to have been established? This is particularly important when looking at older children because dominance ought to have been established by 6–7 years. Children before this age may be more or less ambidextrous and show reversals in writing letters and words or drawing figures and shapes. They may also show rotational difficulties when copying figures and shapes—these rotations may be complete inversions such as writing 'u' for 'n' or turning figures through ninety degrees, e.g. 8 may be reproduced as ∞. Lack of cerebral dominance will also reveal itself in the child having difficulty in right–left orientation. The child is not certain of the left and right side of his body; he is unable to indicate his left hand, right ear, left foot etc with absolute certainty. If parts of his body are touched, he has confusion in distinguishing his own *laterality* (i.e. internalized right–left discrimination). He may also have difficulty in externalizing his laterality and is uncertain of the right–left arrangement of the space and objects around him (i.e. directionality is uncertain).

Poor laterality and directionality may be shown by a child's poor representation of his body image and concept when drawing a man. He may also have difficulty in crossing his own mid-line when drawing, e.g.

when drawing a circle he may draw one half first (usually the left) and add the other half separately; he has difficulty in completing the drawing of the circle in one continuous movement. If these difficulties persist after the age of 6–7 years, reading difficulty may exist.

8   In most children the left cerebral hemisphere becomes dominant (at birth the two hemispheres probably have an equal potential for dominance). This is perhaps due to the fact that those parts of the human brain concerned with language are usually found in the left hemisphere. Thus, since most of our actions are mediated by language, the left hemisphere assumes dominance because more nerve fibres are involved in it. We need not go into brain function in any greater detail here except to point out that there does appear to be a definite relationship between the development of higher language functions and the establishment of cerebral dominance. Neurological immaturity and abnormality may therefore manifest itself in poor language development, speech defects and difficulties in language reception and expression.

Extreme forms of language difficulty may be due to aphasic conditions: receptive aphasia when the child has difficulty in decoding language symbols although the receptor organs are healthy; expressive aphasia in which the child can receive language stimuli and deal with them internally but cannot express the end result in words and/or writing although the motor aspects of expression may be intact. Such cases are fortunately rare, but mild aphasia or dysphasia may be more prevalent in young children than we imagine, at least until the psycholinguistic processes have reached maturity.

The psychoneurological aspects of reading will be dealt with more fully later, but the above list of symptoms of neurological disturbance give some indication of what class teachers may look for. They also suggest that teachers should organize activities which will help to hasten the orderly organization of the child's neurological processes. Physical education should include activities and exercises:

a   to give the child a greater awareness of his own body—its structure, symmetry and balance
b   to develop laterality and directionality
c   to develop rhythmic abilities, good posture and graceful movements.

Art and craft lessons should provide training in form appreciation and reproduction, and in visual rhythms, and give opportunities for the development of tactile abilities. In my own school, we actually train children to appreciate and accurately produce the shapes given above. We think that this training improves visual learning and helps the child to get meaning out of visual perception. The child draws round templates of the shapes in various sizes, he feels the shapes while they are hidden from view and classifies them. He *talks* about them, draws them freehand, and uses them in constructing pictures and patterns.

As we shall see later, it may be advantageous to encourage unilateral dominance once it becomes clear that the child has begun to show a preference for one side or the other. The importance of this is still the subject of much debate and more work of an experimental nature is required before firm acceptance is possible. It is still impossible to say, for instance, whether *mixed dominance* (a lack of clear preference for one side in all activities—handedness, footedness, eyedness) or *cross-laterality* are important causes of poor reading. However, many children with severe reading disability and language difficulties do show clear evidence of mixed dominance. It might be advisable to strengthen the child's preferred side—particularly hand and foot—until unequivocal preference has been established. Once this has been done the child may later develop ambidexterity without detracting from reading progress. Training in the correction of reversals must certainly be undertaken whether the child is right- or left-handed.

3 *Make sure that the child's visual acuity and hearing are within normal limits*
If they appear to be deficient, take the necessary steps for diagnosis and treatment to be effected.

4 *Ascertain whether there is a familial incidence of reading difficulty as evidenced in the retarded development of those abilities and skills involved in learning to read*
There is no evidence that this is inherited, but congenital and other factors may be involved—complications during gestation, difficult births, abnormal parent–children relationships—predispositions towards certain illnesses such as meningitis, high fever, recurrent bronchitis and other respiratory diseases, nervous conditions, epilepsy. If the child is known to have intelligent parents and is very markedly the 'odd man out' in an otherwise normal family, suspect some pathological condition and expect emotional complications. Children whose development appears to have been influenced by these factors may be beyond the help of a teacher working in a class situation. They usually constitute severe behaviour problems in any case. However, much can be done if expectancy levels are lowered and a more intensive application of the readiness programme already outlined is used.

5 *Observe and anticipate difficulties as progress in reading is being made*
We have stressed the developmental nature of reading and outlined the way in which we believe this development takes place in the majority of children. The results achieved in the author's school suggest strongly that the general thesis upon which the developmental reading programme is based is acceptable. There are, of course, some children who because of variations or anomalies in growth and development, require modifications to the programme. For instance, because of the individual differences we have noted, some children may need a phonic approach more or less from the beginning. Their auditory perception seems stronger than visual, and they are therefore able to use an analytical approach much earlier. There are those who respond to a visual method very quickly and, often because they are more intelligent or strongly motivated, appear to cope

with phonic analysis without the need of an organized phonic programme. Thus, several bright children using our early readers have progressed so dramatically in all aspects of reading development that at seven they have reading ages of between ten and twelve years. Perhaps it is likely that they would have been excellent readers no matter what scheme had been used.

In identifying reading problems class teachers should therefore be watchful of each child's progress and be prepared to be diagnosing and treating any difficulties which hinder the orderly, continuing acquisition of reading skills. This does not mean that they have to use published diagnostic tests. The observant teacher can discern difficulties in the course of her teaching. She does not need tests to discover that a child suffers from reversals, directional confusions, has difficulties in blending or comprehension, reads individual words rather than phrases and so on. These things are obvious to her. When she finds them, treatment based on the suggestions already given should follow immediately. If these fail, then she should use an appropriate remedial method from those described later in this book, if this is possible in her teaching situation. If failure persists, she should then seek expert advice and not be afraid to admit that she and the child need additional help and guidance.

Teachers may now be better aware of the many abilities involved in learning to read and the widely differing rates at which they develop not only in different children but also within the individual child. Early identification of difficulties and variations in development is thus of very great importance in designing efforts to reduce backwardness.

5.3 A developmental scale to assist in the prevention of learning disability

SELMA G. SAPIR and BERNICE WILSON

Scarsdale Public Schools; Teachers College,
Columbia University, New York

Reprinted from *Educational and Psychological Measurement* (1967) 27, pp. 1061–8

This research is part of a pilot study which hypothesized that children with problems in perceptual-motor, bodily schema and/or language development can be identified by kindergarten age and then trained in areas of deficit. The Sapir Developmental Scale C (Sapir 1966) was used to identify children with developmental lags at the kindergarten age.

Levels of development have been considered good predictors of intellectual and academic growth (Gesell 1925). Emphasis has been placed on perceptual-motor functioning (Silver and Hagin 1965), visual perception (Frostig 1965), bodily schema (Kephart 1960), language development (Deutsch 1964) and sensory integration (Birch and Lefford 1963), and their relationship to reading and intelligence.

The following hypotheses will be tested:

1 developmental differences can be identified at the kindergarten level
2 they tend to persist in first grade
3 developmental performance, as measured by the Sapir Developmental Scale C (Sapir 1966), can predict academic performance at the end of first grade.

Subjects

The subjects were 54 children, 36 girls and 18 boys, aged 5 years 1 month to 6 years 2 months at the time of testing. The children were the total kindergarten population of a suburban primary public school in a high socioeconomic community.

Instrument

The Developmental Scale was constructed to reflect differences in developmental patterns of kindergarten children in three major areas: (i) perceptual-motor skills; (ii) bodily schema; and (iii) language development. Perceptual tests consist of visual discrimination, visual memory, auditory discrimination, auditory memory, and visual-motor skills. Tests of bodily schema include (i) directionality-laterality, (ii) body image and (iii) visual-motor spatial relationships. Language development includes tests of concepts of orientation to the environment and vocabulary.

The following items make up the Sapir Developmental Scale C:

1 Visual discrimination
a Child asked to match 4 forms on a card with 6 forms on it.
b Child asked to determine likenesses and differences in pairs of words shown.
c Child asked to find embedded triangles in complex designs.

2 Visual memory
a Forms shown for 5 seconds, then removed. Child told to identify form from 6 forms.
b Forms shown for 5 seconds. Child asked to reproduce from memory.

3 Auditory discrimination
a Child asked to determine likenesses and differences in pairs of words.

4 Auditory memory
a Child asked to repeat series of numbers heard.
b Child asked to repeat backwards series of numbers heard.
c Child asked to repeat tapping rhythms.

5 Visual motor
a Copy square, triangle and diamond.
b Draw two horizontal parallel lines 13 mm apart.
c Draw circle and cut it out with scissors.

6 Directionality/laterality
a Right–left directionality: eyes open and eyes closed.
b Laterality with record of eyedness, handedness and footedness.

7 Orientation to environment
a Child asked to answer questions about the relationships of size, time, movement in the environment.

8 Visual-motor spatial relationships
a Child asked to copy designs developed by White and Phillips (1964).

9 Body image
a Draw-a-person test.
b Child asked to identify parts of body.

10 Vocabulary
a   Child asked to define the first ten words of the Stanford–Binet Vocabulary subtest. Child's definitions are analysed by level of usage.

Procedure

The Sapir Developmental Scale C was individually administered in January of the kindergarten year and data were recorded on standardized forms. Designs and words were standardized on 223 × 280 mm oak tags, written with a black magic marker pen. Thirteen millimetre square blocks were used for counting. The 12 White and Phillips (1964) designs, approximately 223 × 223 mm each, were on the blackboard for the child to copy. The examiner, sitting beside the child, explained that there were games to play and asked the child to sit at a desk next to the examiner just over half a metre away, facing the blackboard.

In the autumn of first grade, approximately nine months later, the Marianne Frostig Test of Visual Perception was administered to the same population. One month later the New York State Reading Readiness Test was given. Subtests are as follows: word meaning, listening, matching, alphabet, numbers and copying.

One year after the administration of the Developmental Scale, an independent neurological survey was conducted in the public school by a leading paediatric neurologist. The children were seen individually in the school setting by the neurologist and they were rated neurologically on a 1–10 scale, 5 designated as borderline.

The Stanford Achievement Test, Primary I Form W with subtests; word meaning, paragraph meaning, vocabulary, spelling, word study and arithmetic, was administered to this population in June at the completion of the first grade programme.

Results

Norms were established in terms of scores at the seventieth percentile, and eighteen children placed below this percentile were judged with this scale to be developmentally deficient. These eighteen children scored below 61 on the scale (range 0–95) and revealed deficits in at least two of the three areas: bodily schema, perceptual-motor function or language development. The range of scores in the total first grade population was 39–84 with 'normal' population mean score 69.06, and standard deviation 8.41. For the 'deficit' population, the mean score was 50.0, and the standard deviation was 9.03. For a t of 7.66, p was less than .001. Thus the difference between means of the two groups was significant beyond the .001 level.

Thirteen of the children in this first grade population were diagnosed by Dr Arnold Gold, paediatric neurologist of the Neurological Institute to have 'minimal cerebral dysfunction'. These thirteen children were among the eighteen children which the scale designated 'deficit'. None of the 'normal' children was so rated by the neurologist. Because two of the 'deficit' children were ill, only sixteen of the eighteen were seen by the neurologist. Thus 81.25 per cent ($p < .001$) of the 'deficit' children seen were diagnosed by Dr Gold to have 'minimal cerebral dysfunction'. The subtests of the Sapir Developmental Scale were able to differentiate children with 'minimal cerebral dysfunction' from 'normal' children beyond the .001 level of significance.

Table 1 shows a comparison of the 'normal' and 'deficit' population with the developmental scale, the New York State Reading Readiness Test, and the Marianne Frostig Test of Visual Perception. The last two tests were administered eight months after the children had been so diagnosed with the Sapir Developmental Scale. This again validated the findings of the Developmental Scale. All tests showed significant differences between populations beyond the .01 level.

TABLE 1   *Comparisons of performance for 36 'normal' and 18 'deficit' children*

Test	'Normal'		'Deficit'			
	Mean	SD	Mean	SD	t	p
Sapir Developmental Scale	69.06	8.41	50.00	9.03	7.66	$<.01$
Sapir Perceptual-Motor	30.92	2.57	24.22	4.73	6.76	$<.01$
Sapir Bodily Schema	24.75	6.92	14.22	5.94	5.52	$<.01$
Sapir Language	13.39	1.27	11.56	1.92	4.20	$<.01$
N.Y. State Readiness	77.72	7.90	62.72	7.73	6.62	$<.01$
Marianne Frostig Test of Visual Perception	107.58	12.33	94.39	12.83	3.66	$<.01$

Correlations between the Sapir Developmental Scale and the New York State Reading Readiness Tests and its subtests, and the Marianne Frostig Test of Visual Perception and its subtests, administered eight months after the Developmental Scale, are shown in Table 2. The Developmental Scale and all its subsections correlate significantly beyond the .01 level with the total New York State Reading Readiness score ($r = .66, p < .001$) and its subtests; Matching ($r = .63, p < .001$), Alphabet ($r = .53, p < .001$), and Copying ($r = .57, p < .001$). These are the subtests that Gates and Bond (1958) have listed as most significantly related to reading. The lack of correlation between the language section of the Developmental Scale and the New York Reading Readiness Test is very puzzling. Further study is required.

Correlations of the Developmental Scale with the Marianne Frostig Test of Visual Perception show more variability. The total test scores correlate significantly ($r = .45, p < .001$), but subtests Form Constancy and Position in Space do not ($r = .27; r = .16$).

TABLE 2   *Correlations between Sapir Developmental Scale and New York State Readiness and Marianne Frostig Test of Visual Perception with 54 children*

	Total Sapir Scale	Perceptual-Motor Sapir Scale	Bodily Schema Sapir Scale	Language Sapir Scale
	r	r	r	r
NY State Readiness	.66***	.66***	.53***	.44**
Word Meaning	.22	.24	.15	.23
Listening	.27*	.25	.21	.30*
Matching	.63***	.51***	.60***	.36**
Alphabet	.53***	.48***	.48***	.27*
Numbers	.03	.16	.07	.10
Copying	.57***	.55***	.50***	.26
Marianne Frostig Test of Visual Perception	.45***	.31*	.47***	.14
Eye–hand	.46***	.38**	.45***	.16
Figure–Ground	.45***	.34*	.45***	.21
Form Constancy	.27*	.16	.30*	.04
Position in Space	.16	.08	.20	—.002
Spatial Relationships	.49***	.35*	.49***	.23

$*p = <.05$
$**p = <.01$
$***p = <.001$

TABLE 3   *Correlations between scores on Sapir Scale and Stanford Achievement Test N = 54 children*

Test	Total Sapir Scale	Perceptual-Motor Sapir Scale	Bodily Schema Sapir Scale	Language Sapir Scale
	r	r	r	r
Stanford Achievement (Form A)	.64***	.68***	.47***	.50***
Word Reading	.47***	.50***	.34*	.40**
Paragraph Meaning	.65***	.68***	.50***	.44***
Vocabulary	.30*	.32*	.19	.42**
Spelling	.71***	.76***	.55***	.46***
Word Study	.51***	.53***	.42**	.27
Arithmetic	.52***	.58***	.36**	.50***

$*p = <.05$
$**p = <.01$
$***p = <.001$

The Sapir Developmental Scale and its Perceptual-Motor section correlate significantly beyond the .01 level with all the subtests except Vocabulary of the Stanford Achievement Test administered at the end of first grade, seventeen months after the administration of the Developmental Scale. Table 3 shows that the Bodily Schema section of the Developmental Scale correlates with all but the Vocabulary subtest of the Stanford Achievement Test beyond the .02 level. The Language section of the Scale correlates significantly beyond the .01 level with all subtests but Word Study of the Stanford Achievement Test.

Two test–retest reliability studies were completed. The first study was within a two week interval with eleven kindergarten children in Queens Public School No. 201, New York City and a reliability coefficient of .92 was obtained. The second was with this population with a nine month interval (Sapir 1966) and the Pearson test–retest correlation coefficient was .84.

Discussion

The study has shown that with this population developmental differences were identified at the kindergarten level, persisted in the first grade and correlated significantly with the academic performance seventeen months later. The Developmental Scale is now being used with a larger population, and the results will be studied to see whether the scores continue to correlate with academic achievement.

It must be emphasized that the Sapir Developmental Scale C is a survey instrument to be used with a total kindergarten population. With it, children can be selected for specialized training. One of its major assets is that it is a short test, taking at most thirty minutes to administer. It can eventually be used by kindergarten teachers carefully trained. In a very general way, the instrument can highlight areas of deficiency in a child and can indicate the strength or weaknesses of sensory modalities. It is hoped that with such an instrument children could be selected for 'transition' (De Hirsch, Jansky and Langford 1966) or 'maturity' (Swedish Royal Board of Education 1964) classes to prevent later academic failure.

References

Birch, H. G. and Lefford, A. (1963) Intersensory development in children *Monograph of Social Research in Child Development* 28
*De Hirsch, Katrina, Jansky, J. and Langford, W. S. (1966) *The Prediction of Reading, Spelling and Writing Disabilities in Children* Report to Health Research Council of City of New York
Deutsch, M. (1964) Facilitating development in the preschool child *Merrill Palmer Quarterly* 10
Frostig, Marianne (1965) Introduction to the symposium on learning

S. G. Sapir and B. Wilson

difficulties American Psychological Association Meeting, Chicago, Illinois, September 1965

GATES, A. and BOND, G. (1958) Factors determining success and failure in beginning reading in C. W. Hunnicutt and W. J. Iverson (eds) *Research in the Three Rs* New York: Harper

GESELL, A. (1925) *The Mental Growth of the Preschool Child* New York: Macmillan

KEPHART, N. (1960) *The Slow Learner in the Classroom* Columbus, Ohio: Charles E. Merrill

SAPIR, SELMA (1966) Sex differences in perceptual-motor skills *Perceptual and Motor Skills* 22

SILVER, A. and HAGIN, ROSA (1965) Specific reading disability: teaching through stimulation of deficit perceptual areas Paper read at American Orthopsychology Association meeting in New York, March 1965

SWEDISH ROYAL BOARD OF EDUCATION (1965) Personal communication, Laroplan for Grundskolan, Stockholm

WHITE, MARY ALICE and PHILLIPS, MARION (1964) Psychophysiological prediction of test performance using group screening techniques Paper presented to American Orthopsychology Association meeting, Chicago, March 1964

5.4   What is reading readiness?

JOHN E. MERRITT
Professor of Educational Studies, Open University

Reprinted from *Where* (1970) 49, pp. 83–5

Many children are ready for reading well before five. It will be clear why some are not when we look at what 'reading readiness' means. It occurs as a result of the complementary processes of maturation and of learning: that is, natural growth and development on the one hand, and the effect of experience on the other. Thus children who are maturing slowly, who have a mental age lower than their chronological age, will be delayed in achieving reading readiness. The same holds for children whose range of early experience has, for any reason, been very restricted.

We can consider the reading process in terms of three levels of response. First, the child must recognize units—letters, or groups of letters—and associate these with sounds or with meanings. A boy does this when he recognizes the letters of his name, or can pick out the odd word in a picture book that is being read to him. These may be thought of as 'primary skills'.

Next, the child must be able to relate the sequences of printed words and symbols to the sequences which are familiar in his spoken language. Thus, a child who can read a number of separate words may be able to read these words fluently if they are put together in phrases or sentences, even if he is too young to understand the meaning. This ability to read fluently and with appropriate intonation is the area of 'intermediate skills'.

Of course, there is little point in getting a child to read material he cannot understand, even at the earliest stages. Even if the child is reading the words on the cornflakes packet he should be doing so for sheer enjoyment or to satisfy curiosity. Thus he can build the richer comprehension skills which he will need as an adult, when he must be able to evaluate the patterns of thought and respond imaginatively, or critically, or both. This is the area of 'higher order skills'—the skills which represent the whole point and purpose of reading. Each of these three levels of skill involves both maturational and learning factors.

J. E. Merritt

Recognizing letters

Only some two-thirds of the letters of the alphabet differ in shape from all other letters. The others differ in orientation. Thus, in the case of b–d–p–q, n–u and t–f, for example, the letters in each group differ from each other only because they are printed in reverse, or upside down, or both.

From four years onwards most children should have little difficulty in distinguishing letter-like shapes. One need only look at the remarkable facility with which so many identify minute differences in Matchbox toys to realize that they do not have a problem of inadequately developed vision or perceptual ability. If such children do not learn their letters this is a learning/teaching, not a maturation, problem.

Learning letters like b–d–p–q presents an additional and quite different problem. Here, we must realize that the preschool child has already learnt that objects *do not change* into something else when they are reversed or rotated. His teddy bear, his toy car and almost every other object in his everyday experience, retains or 'conserves' its identity regardless of its orientation—which way up it is. Children therefore learn that the orientation of an object does not affect its identity. This is known as a 'learning set', but it is totally inappropriate when a child is responding to letters. The habit of attending to 'form' rather than 'orientation' for recognition purposes, must be changed so that he attends to orientation as well as form. This is not easy. Indeed, even adults have difficulty in learning names assigned to shapes such as the following which differ only in orientation:

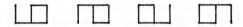

They can remember the names, and they can recognize the orientation but they have difficulty in saying which goes with which.

Not only do many children have difficulty in learning to distinguish b–d–p–q, and so on, they also muddle 'on' and 'no', 'won' and 'now', 'saw' and 'was' and so on, and for much the same reasons. This difficulty can persist with normal children until eight.

What can be done to help correct this? At a very early age children can practise 'sorting' a wide variety of materials. Construction toys of all kinds are useful—but even the sorting of materials for convenience of storage helps. When children can cope with this, they are ready for sorting and selecting pictures, as in 'snap' and 'pairs'.

Once children can sort out pictures they can progress to similar games using shapes instead of pictures—simple outline objects like trains and cars are probably better than abstract shapes like triangles and circles to begin with. If suitable games are not to hand they can be made up from pictures and symbols cut out of children's puzzle books.

Once children have got a 'learning set' to look carefully at shapes, very simple orientation problems can be presented. These too can be found in children's books of puzzles. For teaching children to respond to sequence, children's comics are quite useful. The pictures should be cut out and the children can sort them out from left to right in accordance with the story sequence. Unless it is a very obvious sequence the children should know the story first.

Orientation and sequences are not the only problem in recognizing letters: there is also the variety of letter forms. The forms of the 'same' letter A–*a*–a, for example, are more different from each other than the 'different' letters *a*–o–c. Similarly:

Ggg, Ttttt, Qqq, Yyyyy

This is like learning that the first 'letters' below are the 'same' but that the second 'letters' are all different letters:

ᴧ ⌊ L , ⌐ ⌐ ⌐

Since preschool children have all the perceptual equipment required for learning the 26 lower-case letters of the alphabet and the 19 or so differently shaped capital letters, there is no reason why they shouldn't start to do this at an early age. Most children can take letter variations in their stride once they are reading fluently, for reasons which will become clear when we consider the intermediate skills.

2   Letter–sound association

The first requirement is the ability to discriminate the speech sounds of the language. This presents no problem even to the less able preschool child, provided that he has adequate opportunities for listening to speech—and encouragement to express himself clearly. Lack of satisfactory language experience, rather than maturity, is the real problem with many children. *Any* child can be helped, however, by encouragement to pay particular attention to the sounds of speech—in learning nursery rhymes, say.

The next stage is the association of letters, or groups of letters, with sounds or words. This level of maturation is normally achieved by the preschool child. Even small babies seem to recognize pictures of familiar objects. Then when they begin to talk they soon learn to name them. Learning to respond vocally to letters or groups of letters requires precisely the same perceptual abilities and ability to associate sounds and symbols.

There is one big difference, of course. Children will be much more interested in acquiring speech, and even in naming illustrations of familiar objects, than they will be in learning to read. So some children will be poor at letter–sound association or whole-word recognition, because they are *poorly motivated* to attend to the significant features.

Intermediate skills

These are the skills required in associating the sequences which occur in the spoken language with the sequences signalled on the printed page. This is important in recognizing unfamiliar words, and in reading sentences never seen before. The printed form 'toughicionk' is readily pronounced 'tuffishunk' by most adults, because they are familiar with the sort of sequences of sounds which are common in English, as well as with the variety of possible spellings. A child who encounters an unfamiliar word is faced with a rather similar problem. If he can begin the word, for example, acci-, he knows immediately that only a limited number of sounds can follow. Only some of these make real words, and *dent* is perhaps the most probable ending. A child who has encountered a great number of words orally is thus able to cope with the problem. Without this ability he can read only those words he has been previously taught and which he has thoroughly learned. Given the inconsistency of English spelling, a child without this ability is very severely handicapped.

Anticipating sound sequences relies of course on the convention of scanning letters from left to right. This is not innate, and it does not develop automatically as a result of maturation. Certain languages, in fact, are written from right to left, or from top to bottom. One reason why children can have so much difficulty with this is simply that most reading schemes do not provide adequately for the development of left to right scanning. They may have only one or two words to a line, or else use a sentence which reads equally well from right to left: 'Look, Tom, look.' No teacher has time to supervise every child and to see that he attacks words from left to right, without missing any out. Children can therefore spend a long time steadily accumulating faulty reading habits.

Useful groundwork can be done in this respect by running a finger under words read aloud to a young child, for example. (Perhaps the best idea for helping children here was that of the mother who made her children their own 'books' from the start—on family, friends, holidays and outings—so that the children got accustomed to the 'front to back' and 'left to right' convention in books without any conscious effort being made. See *Where* 37. This practice can easily be adapted to school as well as home-based activities.)

Properly designed games can also be useful: perhaps on the same lines as ludo, but the counters should be moved from left to right along each line of squares, and from top to bottom, as in reading a page.

Now let us consider the development of the ability to read meaningful sentences. In the sentence 'Tom Harrison went to Helton by t . . . .' the adult will almost certainly respond with 'train' thus following the several language cues given in the sentence. There would have been little difficulty had the sentence been printed as 'T□m H□rris□n w□□t t□ Helt□n by t□□□□.

Clearly, reading depends almost as much on the reader's ability to anticipate sound sequences and word sequences as it does on what is actually presented. If language development is inadequate, then such anticipation is not possible.

Relating this language to the printed word is another matter. So many reading schemes are banal, and quite divorced from the child's speech, that it is scarcely surprising that young children do not respond. That is why some teachers use a 'language experience' approach to reading, writing out a child's *own* sentences. She will encourage the child to notice that the words are written down in the order in which they were spoken. If children have already developed some idea of the relationship between a single spoken word and a single written word, they will then 'see' their speech being translated into writing and more readily make the link.

Higher order skills

Reading may be thought of as 'thinking within the context of print'. So children have not really learned to read until they have developed the skill of critical and constructive reading. So far as preschoolers are concerned, however, this means helping children to acquire primary skills without interfering with intermediate or higher-order skills. Any encouragement of children to 'bark out' the names or sounds of letters can result in an impediment to fluent reading. Similarly, learning to recognize sets of isolated words, with no emphasis on meaning, can produce a 'learning set' to read without comprehension.

Some general points in helping children to achieve reading readiness:

1 Be careful not to interrupt if the child is engaged in the important business of amusing himself, or if he is 'tetchy'. If his eyes light up when he sees you, proceed.
2 Be a little bit wary of materials which resemble favourite board games —they may suffer from the comparison. On the other hand, if you can make your materials superior in some way—in a board game, for example, one can use magnets on a metal board, instead of plastic counters which tend to slide about—you may gain a bonus.
3 Occasional failure can act as a stimulant. It can also become an addition. Expectation of failure is an inducement to avoid the effort of trying. A steady success rate, however limited the rate of progress, provides the best possible basis for later learning.
4 If you feel anxious when a child does not 'catch on', don't persist.

J. E. Merritt

You have merely made a bigger jump in difficulty level than he can cope with at that time. Make the material easier or more attractive.

Specific suggestions

1 *Language*
Talk to young children, not at them or down to them. If you wish them to attend when you speak, be sure to listen carefully when *they* speak.

Tell children stories with and without the aid of a book. Pictures are important—but they must learn to accept the words on their own. Be sure to discuss the stories, following any points of interest the child raises —why people behaved as they did, alternative endings had they behaved otherwise and so on. This ensures that listening becomes an active process, not merely a form of passive titillation.

2 *Letters*
Play any game which causes the child to attend closely to the differences between letters. Example: Rummy using letter cards. The child either saves sets of the same letter (a a a) or alphabet 'runs' (e f g).

3 *Letter–sound association*
As above, but with pictures on the reverse side (e.g. apple, axe, anchor). The child should not be expressly taught that the letter 'stands for' the initial sound. But once he starts to talk about the relationship his questions can be answered.

4 *Whole-word recognition*
Play any game in which sets of words having the same initial letter are collected—one player saves cat, clock, cupboard, another collects dog, duck, dustbin. Thus the player must look at the first letter to decide if he wants the word. The child can play the games using the picture first, then proceed to word and picture, then word only, with pictures on the back as a check.

5 *Phrase reading*
Use any game in which a child must read words in a left–right sequence, for example, one in which the child must read the first word to decide if he wants a card, and then recognize the second word to decide where it goes. Example: each child has his own board, as in bingo.

one cat	two cats
one horse	two horses
one train	two trains
one bus	two buses

Matching cards with pictures on the reverse side, are placed in a pack and the players take alternately from the pack. The object is to cover each phrase with a matching card drawn from the pack.

These are a few of the methods that can be devised to encourage language development and to induce appropriate word-attack habits. For the development of intermediate and higher order skills perhaps the most important factor is the encouragement of curiosity—and the use of reasonable discussion to discover how best to achieve its satisfaction.

5.5 Children's comprehension of syntactic features found in some extension readers

JESSIE F. REID

Centre for Research in Educational Sciences, University of Edinburgh

Occasional Paper, Centre for Research in Educational Sciences, University of Edinburgh (1972)

In his introduction to *Sentence Structure and the Reading Process*, Schlesinger (1969) remarks on the dearth of experimental work on the influence of sentence structure on reading. He observes that readability studies have been aimed at providing helpful yardsticks to assess the difficulty of a given text, rather than at offering explanations of the ways in which syntax may interfere with or facilitate the reading of it. Further, he claims that sentence length is the only true syntactic variable to appear in readability formulae; and that this seriously limits their experimental usefulness.

The experimental work reported by Schlesinger (1969) is concerned with studying the dependence of features of reading performance such as eye–voice span, recall, reading rate and comprehension on some isolated and controlled syntactic variables. The failure to verify some of his experimental predictions leads him to question the 'syntactic decoding hypothesis' which states that syntactic decoding is not dependent on semantic factors. He postulates instead a model in which semantic and syntactic factors both operate and he suggests that sentences which as a result of their syntactic form contain a potential ambiguity may be particularly difficult to read.

The importance of syntax as a variable in early reading material is now quite widely recognized (Fries 1962, Strickland 1962, Lefevre 1963, Reid 1970). There is already some evidence that supplementary teaching methods emphasizing language structure can produce improvement in learning (Ruddell 1968), though the interaction between structural elements and phonological ones (i.e. the degree of consistency maintained in spelling patterns) appears to be significant. Moreover, several studies have shown that children learning to read try to make use of their implicit knowledge of the grammar (Merritt 1968, Clay 1969, Weber 1970). Merritt using approximations to English generated from a store of thirty common words, showed that the speed and accuracy of reading in eight year old children was directly related to the degree of approximation.

Clay analysed the reading errors of 100 beginners throughout their first year, and found a marked preponderance of 'syntactically correct' errors over 'phonically similar' errors. Weber, in a similar study, found that 90 per cent of errors were syntactically correct in terms of preceding context, and concluded that children 'bring their knowledge of grammatical structure to bear on their performance from the outset'.

It has also been shown recently, however, that although children over the age of five have mastered the basic grammar of the language there are still specific areas where their knowledge can be shown to be incomplete. Menyuk (1969) has traced some of the growth of syntactic understanding in groups of children between the ages of four and seven. More recently Carol Chomsky (1970) has shown experimentally how certain systematic misinterpretations of syntactic form occur in children between the ages of five and ten, and how these errors can be interpreted as mistakes in identifying the deep structure of the sentences involved. Such findings have important implications not only for the better understanding of all forms of language acquisition, including the acquisition of literacy, but also for the practical task of making literacy less difficult to achieve. By the time they are seven, many children have already left their basal reading scheme behind and are on 'extension readers'—texts aimed at presenting a wide variety of reading matter, mostly fictional narrative, but also some descriptive and informative writing. Many children, however, (as many as 50 per cent in some areas) fail to progress with these books. See, for instance, Kellmer Pringle (1967).

The hypothesis on which the present experiment is based is that certain syntactic features of the language in reading books and textbooks written for children of around seven to eight years of age make comprehension difficult, and that they do so by

1 making use of grammatical and stylistic features which do not occur at all, or occur relatively rarely in speech, and which many children have not learned to interpret
2 inviting misinterpretations of structure which the semantics of the sentence are sufficiently ambiguous to permit.

Under this hypothesis (as in Carol Chomsky's experiments) certain sentences found in these books will have predictable wrong interpretations. This experiment tests the effect, on choice of interpretation, of restructuring sentences in a form closer to spoken language, while retaining their semantic content.

Method

Materials

A search was made in some extension readers used with children aged from 7–8 years, and sentences were chosen which appeared to exhibit both of the features specified above. They were judged to be deviant from the speech forms used and heard by most 7–8 year olds, and to be potentially ambiguous in certain respects if complete account was not taken of the syntax. These sentences were taken as syntactic models for a set of nineteen experimental sentences. For each sentence, a question (one sentence had two questions—items 17 and 18) in binary choice form was constructed in which the alternative response to the correct one represented a specific predicted misinterpretation. For example, the sentence: 'If only David had known, the dog was quite tame.' was followed by the question: 'Did David know that the dog was tame?' (yes/no). The two correct answer positions (first or second) were randomly assigned to the 20 items, but in order to control for position preference, one half of the subjects was given the answer choices in reverse order to the other half. These 20 sentences with their accompanying questions constituted version A of the test.

Version B was constructed by rewriting each sentence so as to replace the syntactic feature judged to be confusing by a structure of a form more likely to be found in speech. For instance, the sentence quoted above was replaced by the sentence: 'The dog was quite tame, but David did not know that.' Each simplified statement was then followed by the same question as before, with an exact duplication of the order of choices and randomization of correct answer position. These 20 items constituted version B of the test.

The overall vocabulary load was kept low. In version B, unless the syntactic feature concerned was an inversion of some kind, all the restructurings required some vocabulary change, either by addition, subtraction or morphological variation, or a combination of these. The mean sentence length for version A was 9.6 words, and for version B, 10.0 words. In constructing version B, the following words were removed: anything, both, if, neither, nor, only and or. The following were added: are, at, be, her, it, that, when and which, so that a slight advantage in the total number of different words lay with version A. In addition, 'known' in version A was replaced by 'know'.

The alternative to the null hypothesis (of no difference between performance on the two versions) was that version B would be easier than version A. The level of α was set at .01.

Subjects
Six classes were selected from six local authority schools in a predominantly working class area in central Scotland. The mean age was 7 years 4 months, and over 93 per cent of the children were aged between 6 years 10 months and 7 years 9 months. They were in their third year of primary school.

Procedure
A briefing session was held with the class teachers who were to administer the test, and the local primary adviser and educational psychologist were

available for consultations. Within each class, the two versions of the test were distributed in class register order. The time allowance was generous, since it was important to give every child a chance to try every item. Practice items were given before the test proper.

Results

Eighty-seven scripts were obtained for each version of the test. The distribution of total scores for each version is given in Table 1 (possible total score = 20). The contrast in the form of the two distributions is marked. For version B, 50 per cent of the scores lie between 18 and 20, while for version A, only 12.6 per cent of scores reach this level. The observed difference between the medians (5.1 points of raw score) is very highly significant ($\chi^2 = 29.78$ for 1 d.f.; $p < .0005$). The prediction that version B would be easier than version A is therefore very substantially supported.

TABLE 1 *Distribution of raw scores on versions A and B of the reading test*

Interval	Version	
	A	B
18–20	10	43
15–17	15	19
12–14	24	7
9–11	26	14
6–8	12	4
	87	87

In order to see how individual items were contributing to this difference, an analysis of score differences was performed. Table 2 shows the percentage correct and the percentage difference between versions for each version of each item.

Two things are clear from Table 2:

1 The majority of the items were easier in version B by more than 10 per cent.
2 Of those which did not reach this level, all but one contributed something to the overall difference: so that altogether 19 out of the 20 items showed a positive (B—A) figure.

Discussion

It is clear that the changes made in producing version B constituted a major simplification of the reading task. It is also clear that this simpli-

Jessie F. Reid

TABLE 2 *Percentage correct on each version of each item and percentage difference*

Item	A%	B%	B−A%
*1	41.4	88.6	+47.2
2	82.8	93.2	+8.4
*3	43.7	80.5	+36.8
4	86.3	87.4	+1.1
*5	65.6	75.9	+10.3
6	78.2	86.3	+8.1
*7	39.1	64.4	+25.3
8	54.0	63.3	+9.3
9	80.5	78.2	−2.3
*10	63.3	79.4	+16.1
11	85.1	87.4	+2.3
*12	64.4	80.5	+16.1
*13	58.7	69.0	+10.3
14	82.8	86.3	+3.5
*15	64.4	80.5	+16.1
16	71.3	74.8	+3.5
*17	39.1	81.7	+42.6
*18	36.8	80.5	+43.7
*19	69.0	81.7	+12.7
*20	57.5	81.7	+24.2

* Items in which (B−A)% > 10.

fication cannot be attributed either to the removal of difficult lexical items, or to the provision of shorter sentences. Both of these are popularly regarded as major contributors to the difficulty of reading material, and both appear as variables in readability formulae. Here, however, the independent variable associated with difficulty is the syntax of the sentences.

The items contributing most to the overall difference (see Table 2) show a variety of syntactic features and will be looked at in some detail.

Item 1
A   The girl standing beside the lady had a blue dress.
B   The girl had a blue dress and she was standing beside the lady.
Qu.   Who had a blue dress? (The girl/the lady)

Item 1A contains a reduced clause separating the verb 'had' from its subject. It was interpreted by 59 per cent of subjects as though the extended version were: 'The girl was standing beside the lady and *the lady* had a blue dress.' The 1B version was clear to all but the poorest readers.

Items 17 and 18 (based on one sentence)

A   Mary's dress was neither new nor pretty.

B   Mary's dress was not new and it was not pretty.

Qu. Was Mary's dress new? (yes/no)

Qu. Was Mary's dress pretty? (yes/no)

These items, which came next to item 1 in order of (B—A) contrast, concerned the syntax and meaning of 'neither . . . nor'. More than 60 per cent of subjects did not interpret these as negatives but apparently ignored 'neither' and took 'nor' to be equivalent to 'and'.

Items 3 and 20

3A   Tom's mother was anything but pleased.

3B   Tom's mother was not pleased at all.

Qu. Was Tom's mother pleased? (yes/no)

20A If only David had known, the dog was quite tame.

20B The dog was quite tame, but David did not know that.

Qu. Did David know that the dog was tame? (yes/no)

Both these items contain, in version A, what might be termed idiomatic concealed negatives. Both convey negative meaning without any formal negative on the surface, but in ways accepted in adult speech and writing. Item 3A invited almost as much error as item 1A, and item 20A, though easier than item 3A, was markedly harder than 20B.

Item 7

A   The princess was both clever and beautiful.

B   The princess was clever and beautiful.

Qu. How many princesses? (one/two)

Version A contains 'both' as an intensifier preceding two adjectives. The sentence was interpreted wrongly by 60 per cent of subjects, but it is important to note that the difference (B—A), though round 25 per cent leaves 34 per cent of subjects who failed to deal with version B. So either they read 'princess' as a plural (i.e. as 'princes'), and accepted the singular verb, which is what many would use anyway, or else the presence of two adjectives ('clever and beautiful') even without 'both' caused them to choose a plural interpretation. The feature in this item needs further study.

Items 10, 12 and 19

10A The dog did not like the cat, who always took the best place by the fire.

10B The cat always took the best place by the fire, so the dog did not like her.

Qu. Who always took the best place? (the cat/the dog)

12A Tom walked in front of Dick and carried a flag.

12B Tom walked in front of Dick and Tom carried a flag.

Qu. Who carried the flag? (Tom/Dick)

19A Tom went back without his brother and was met by Mrs Brown.

399

Jessie F. Reid

19B   Tom was met by Mrs Brown when he went back without his brother.
Qu.   Whom did Mrs Brown meet? (Tom/Tom's brother)

These items form another interesting group, in that the A versions show the apparent confusion of two contrasting deep structures.

To interpret 'Tom walked in front of Dick and carried a flag' (12A) as meaning that Dick carried the flag, is to interpret 'and' as a relative pronoun, equivalent to 'who'; and to interpret 'who always took . . .' in item 10A as referring to the *dog* is to regard 'who' as equivalent to 'and'. Item 19A shows the same confusion as item 12A, '. . . and was met . . .' being apparently interpreted by some 42 per cent of subjects as a relative clause.

Items 13 and 15
15A   John was followed by David.
15B   David followed John.
Qu.   Who went first? (David/John)
13A   Under the big stone was a wooden box.
13B   A wooden box was under the big stone.
Qu.   Was the stone under the box? (yes/no)

These items concern the match/mismatch between the word order and the spatial positions of the referents. In 15A, the order of naming agrees with the sense of the statement, but that statement is passive. In 15B, the active form, David is mentioned first, but as having 'come' second. This confusion, however, is apparently less serious than that caused by the passive. A somewhat similar item is 13, in which the first mentioned object (in 13A) is not the one which is 'under'. In this item, there is a possibility that 'under the big stone was . . .' has been read as if it meant 'the big stone was under . . .'. The form of the question may also have been confusing, however, because the B version did not show as big a contrast as might have been expected. An unpublished study by Marshall (1965) used sets of items in which similar pairs of structures had to be matched to diagrams. He showed that the form used in 13B was much easier than that used in 13A, in that many subjects matched the A structure to a diagram showing the *opposite* state of affairs.

Items 2 and 5
2A   The dog was not only big but also wild.
2B   The dog was big and it was also wild.
Qu.   Was the dog big? (yes/no)
5A   The little swans, or cygnets, can swim very well.
5B   Cygnets are little swans, and they can swim very well.
Qu.   Cygnets are (little swans/big swans)?

These remaining two items with (B—A) per cent < 10 have nothing in common in their A versions except an idiomatic use of two very common words; in one case 'not' and in the other case 'or'. Item 2A contains the expression 'not only . . . but also'. In this expression 'not' is used to negate

400

'only wild', and not 'wild' itself. In other words, what is negated is not the attribute but its sole status. 2A obviously confused some of the poorer readers. In the remaining item, number 5, the A version uses 'or' to introduce the synonym 'cygnets' for 'little swans'. The hypothesis here was that subjects would interpret 'or' as a disjunctive, and conclude therefore that cygnets were not little swans. The relatively low success level even in 12B is notable, since 12B states 'cygnets are little swans'. The fact that the sentence began with an unknown, or at least an unexpected, word, may have been enough to confuse children who could otherwise have read the rest of the item.

Most of the remaining items resemble in type those already discussed, but show less contrast between versions. This would suggest that study is needed of groups of items with similar syntactic features but different semantic content.

These results have obvious implications both for the study of language acquisition and for the teaching of literacy. Most importantly, they indicate that the bridging of the initial gap between speech and its graphic representation is only one part of the problem. A study by Brandis and Henderson (1969), in which the authors look for connections between educability and indices of communication between mother and child, draws attention to what the authors call 'powerful forms of cultural discontinuity' existing between the homes of some children and the schools they attend. Among items which contribute to the measures of mother–child communication are 'mothers who read frequently to the child' and 'library membership of mother or child, or both'. The authors appear to see these activities merely as helping, in a fairly general way, to foster 'favourable educational orientation'. The present study suggests, however, that the lack of them can be viewed as a source of deficit of a much more specific kind than Brandis and Henderson envisage.

There is a dimension to the experience of having stories read aloud which goes beyond general familiarizing with the idea of books, and even with the notion of written language, of marks on paper that stand for words. It is that of becoming familiar with the linguistic forms in which stories are couched. Some of these forms are normal constituents of written as opposed to spoken language, and arises from the medium. Davies (1969) calls them in fact 'medium' features of register. Others are highly conventional almost stylized features, intended to produce dramatic tension and to highlight significant points in ways which are (a) important to children and (b) effective *when a text is read aloud*. They are what Davies (1969) calls 'stylistic' and 'function' features of register. A child's early familiarity with all these kinds of features can come only from hearing written language spoken aloud, and deprivation in this area will therefore constitute an educational barrier of some gravity.

But even for those who have not been so deprived, it is by no means certain that the level of comprehension achieved when listening will be transferred to the situation where they are reading alone and in silence.

Jessie F. Reid

The examples that have figured in the present study have made use of language patterns that will doubtless have been heard many times by some of the children in the sample. Yet the misinterpretations they have invited have not been confined to the poorest readers, but have also been found at a level where attainment as shown in the simpler version is reasonably good. It is true that the findings are from a test composed of unconnected sentences, where contextual help is limited. However, the possibility that the confusion would be lessened in a continuous narrative is not supported by Bormuth et al (1970), who have shown that serious deficits in the understanding of 'between-sentence syntactic structures' can be found in children as old as nine. Moreover, Reid (1958) found that children were unable to recognize, in an unfamiliar syntactic and semantic context, words they had previously read correctly. It is therefore possible that in this present study the unfamiliarity of the syntax was producing failure at a word recognition level as well.

The findings from this experiment indicate that the language used in reading books and textbooks for 7–8 year olds needs much systematic scrutiny and experimental study. They also argue for regarding the forms of written language in general, and those of the 'story telling register' in particular, as aspects which children have to be explicitly helped to understand and not just left to pick up in a haphazard fashion. In a wider context the study indicates an area of developmental psycholinguistics about which so far very little is known.

References

BORMUTH, J. R., CARR, JULIAN, MANNING, JOHN and PEARSON, DAVID (1970) Children's comprehension of between- and within-sentence syntactic structures *Journal of Educational Psychology* 61, 5

*BRANDIS, W. and HENDERSON, D. (1969) *Social Class, Language and Communication* London: Routledge and Kegan Paul

*CHOMSKY, C. (1970) *The Acquisition of Syntax in Children from 5 to 10* Cambridge, Massachusetts: MIT Press

*CLAY, M. (1969) Reading errors and self-correction behaviour *British Journal of Educational Psychology* 39, 47–56

DAVIES, A. (1969) The notion of register in *The State of Language* Birmingham Educational Review 22, 1

*FRIES, C. C. (1962) *Linguistics and Reading* New York: Holt, Rinehart and Winston

*KELLMER PRINGLE, M. L. (1967) *11,000 Seven Year Olds* London: Routledge and Kegan Paul

*LEFEVRE, C. (1963) *Linguistics and the Teaching of Reading* New York: McGraw-Hill

MARSHALL, C. D. D. (1965) A study of the effect of question form upon performance in a test of relational concepts Unpublished dissertation, Department of Psychology, University of Edinburgh

MENYUK, P. (1969) *Sentences Children Use* Cambridge, Massachusetts: MIT Press

MERRITT, J. E. (1968) Assessment of reading ability: a new range of diagnostic tests? *Reading* 2, 2

REID, J. F. (1958) A study of thirteen beginners in reading *Acta Psychologica* 15, 4

REID, J. F. (1970) Sentence structure in reading primers *Research in Education* no. 3

RUDDELL, R. B. (1967) Reading instruction in first grade with varying emphasis on the regularity of grapheme–phoneme correspondences and the relation of language structure to meaning—extended into second grade *The Reading Teacher* 20, 730–39

SCHLESINGER, I. (1969) *Sentence Structure and the Reading Process* The Hague: Mouton

*STRICKLAND, R. (1962) The language of elementary school children: its relationship to the language of reading textbooks and the quality of reading of selected children *Bulletin of the School of Education* 38, 4 Bloomington: University of Indiana

WEBER, R. M. (1970) A linguistic analysis of first-grade reading errors *Reading Research Quarterly* 5, 3

5.6 Implications of recent research for teaching techniques

GEOFFREY R. ROBERTS
Department of Education, University of Manchester

Reprinted from M. M. Clark and S. M. Maxwell (1968) (eds) *Reading: Influences on Progress* United Kingdom Reading Association, pp. 57–64

I think we have created difficulties and confusion in the past by searching for one simple method which would solve all the problems of teaching children to read—a sort of Aladdin's lamp with a simple mechanism that could be used with the minimum of thought and effort. The result has been that only in very recent years have a few people begun to accept the fact that this is an impossibility and that learning to read is a complex problem which can only be examined by splitting it up into component parts and then probing these restricted areas in depth.

Furthermore, there is a strong tendency amongst teachers to give information—'That word says . . .'—rather than to explain the process that has constituted that information—'That word says . . ., because . . .' or to engage the child in actively thinking out reasons—'What makes that word say . . .?' The learner needs to be helped to gain insight, otherwise blind acceptance can easily lead to confusion. Reid's (1966) work is striking and relevant here and I feel that much would be gained if we adopted her approach in seeking what the child understands, but at all stages of the learning process, not only at the beginning. We should be careful not to assume understanding where none exists.

These two features appear to me to have inhibited our approach to the examination of reading problems and to the methodology of teaching children to read. I hope to show in this paper the ways in which a few research workers are beginning to apply research techniques to the problems that face the teacher, but which the teacher cannot investigate amidst all the diversity of classroom activities.

Letter discrimination

If we accept that part of the reading process is decoding, then before a child can attach a composite sound to a new or unfamiliar word, he must be able to discriminate between the various letters, because these are the signs which show him how he should shape his mouth and control the flow of air. This does not necessarily entail knowledge of the sounds these letters represent. Muehl (1960) neatly demonstrated that during the pre-training period children used single letters for matching words. Hence, by that fact, they need to distinguish one letter from another.

Gibson *et al* (1962) showed that it is not merely a matter of immediate recognition of differences and that some letters can be differentiated more readily than others. That is, a child can *learn* to do this more easily with some letter shapes than with others. If this is so, then the need for more attention to perceptual training in letter discrimination at the pre-reading stage is underlined. Tansley (1967) makes various suggestions which can be adapted for most situations, and Gibson (1967) makes a significant deduction from recent research by Pick, that this training should be concerned with contrasting pairs of letters, for example C and O, rather than letter by letter. In this way, children would be forced to draw their own comparisons.

A point of procedure which faces the teacher of a reception class is whether or not to teach children the names of letters. There is some re-search (Durrell (1958), Olson (1963)) which demonstrates that both the name and the sound are necessary for the learner after, of course, he has learned to discriminate between letters. I should like to speculate about my reasons for thinking a knowledge of letter names is an advantage, not for word identification so much as for understanding word formation and for reference. Letter names are a much easier form of reference than the sound. For example, when in the later stages of differentiating between letters the teacher wishes to discuss two letters with the child, 'Show me *aitch*' is easier than 'Show me /h/.' Also, in dealing with words, a know-ledge of the names and their repetition, overtly or covertly, emphasizes the correspondence between the order of the letters and the order of the sounds. And I have the notion that it does this more effectively than any phonic method, because it is a clearer and more easily articulated form of labelling symbols (Roberts and Lunzer 1968).

Sound–spelling irregularities

The irregularities of English, although sensationally overemphasized by some, do cause confusion; but again the problem facing the teacher during the early stages is not quite so simple as would appear at first sight. It is not one which can be solved purely by logic, because there are two equally viable courses of action. The teacher can take the apparently logical course and keep to regular words only, as Bloomfield (1961) suggested. Then at a later stage she can introduce the irregularities in the corres-pondence between sound and spelling patterns. On the other hand, the teacher can begin with both regularities and irregularities, which un-doubtedly will make the task more difficult during the early stages of learning, but which may prove to be a better preparation for the later stages of learning to read.

The need to choose between the two is always present but it will become more obvious in the near future as more books, such as the Merrill Readers (Fries *et al* 1966) and the Bloomfield and Barnhart Scheme (1961), appear on the market. Fortunately, there is one piece of significant research by Levin (1963). His results suggest that it is better to introduce the irregularities during the early stages, because although this may create initial difficulties, it does create in the mind of the child an expectation of irregularities, which will make it easier to learn new letter–sound correspondences. There is in effect a developing and cumulative process, in which each stage is made easier by having mastered the difficulties of the previous stage. And surely a set for flexibility and searching behaviour is what we wish to create in the child's mind.

Harlow's (1949) theories about a 'set' to learn different material more readily and Levin's results suggest strongly that it is probably better to begin with a mixture.

There is one further point. Whilst it is advantageous to create this expectation of irregularity of correspondence between grapheme and phoneme, this need not impinge upon another aspect of early reading instruction, which aims to show the child that there is much that is regular in our written code (Fowler 1964). For this purpose it seems obvious that regular words would be used exclusively on those occasions when the teacher was dealing with regularity of correspondence.

Cross-modal transfer and verbal labelling

Birch and Belmont (1964, 1965) demonstrated that amongst poor readers there is the difficulty of integrating what is seen with the sounds that should be attached to these symbols. That is, the difficulty lies in a particular process rather than in the direct application of known matter and as such it is one remove away from learning to read: it is learning to learn to read, or, in other words, the difficulty lies in understanding the nature of the task.

It is obvious that the practice of engaging the children in writing will have great significance as a means of stressing, in a manipulative manner, the link between the order of print and the speech sounds represented by that print. Awareness of this would lead the teacher to take every opportunity of drawing attention verbally to the link between sound and print.

Blank and Bridger (1966) took up the experiments of Birch and Belmont, agreed that there was a problem of intramodal transfer, but they went on to explain that the deficiency was that of attaching verbal labels to the stimuli. This may be a crucial factor, for as Langman (1960) pointed out, good readers have the 'ability to direct attention to the significant visual and auditory stimuli in word recognition situations, while at the same time they resist the distraction of other less relevant stimuli in the same modes'. They also have flexibility: the ability to reject, replace and to shift responses. Hence, it may well pay dividends to the teacher, when teaching a child to recognize a word, if she were not to stick specifically and rigidly to that word but preferably to work through and round the word, introducing contrasting words and following all manners of clues and trails, even if they have to be rejected and other clues taken up. This more flexible treatment of the process of word identification would act as a model upon which the child could base his procedure of word attack on future occasions.

Blending and the critical units of language

'Looking at and around words' in the last section leads to my next point. There is substantial evidence to show that a reader does not engage in sequential processing letter by letter. Dodge (1906) showed that perception only occurs during fixations; Cattell (1885), Newman (1966) and Kolers (1963) demonstrated the possibility of reading words at high tachistoscopic rates. Furthermore, Chall et al (1963) demonstrated how important it is to be able to blend letters; yet we know how difficult this can be for the beginner. Jeffrey and Samuels (1967), examining the effects of letter and word methods upon initial learning and upon transfer of learning to new words, found the superiority of the letter method and thought it contingent upon the phonic blend training that all the children received.

Thus, the crucial significance of Gibson's (1962) work on the critical units of language becomes evident. Very briefly, she sees the grapheme–phoneme cluster, in which each letter bears a specific relationship with the other letters, as the basic unity of language. Thus the *o* in *boat* and *bomb* is not to be seen as a hopeless irregularity, but rather as an instance of a particular letter in a specific relationship with other letters. In other words, learning to read is, in part, gaining familiarity with groups of letters with an invariant pronunciation when placed in juxtaposition with other letters and clusters.

These findings of Gibson et al (1962, 1963, 1964) fit into Miller's (1956) theory that 'chunks' are made from 'bits' of information in order that the mind is able to carry greater quantities of information.

Therefore, it seems to me that after the initial introduction of the child to three-letter words, the emphasis of teaching should be reorientated away from individual letters towards clusters, blends and digraphs, such as *tr* and *sh*, in the first instance and gradually the span should be increased to three, four and more letter strings, so that towards the end of the 'decoding part of the programme' the child's span will reach words and even phrases in many instances. It is ludicrous to find children at approximately the book 3 level of reading still going through a word such as *slightly* letter by letter–sound. At that stage they should be able to split the word into clusters—*sl/ight/ly.*

Geoffrey R. Roberts

Learning; familiarization; language

There are a few small carefully controlled experiments which have been designed to answer clearly defined and restricted problems concerned with the ways in which children learn to read.

Whenever we leave the preparatory stages of learning to read and begin specific instruction in decoding written symbols, we are faced with the central problem of how many letters/words to introduce at a time and whether the words should be similar in letter components or should they be as different as possible. Look-and-say enthusiasts favour wide differences, whereas Daniels and Diack advocate fine distinctions.

This is of course a very complex problem, but some small progress has been made towards a solution by a few recent experiments. Samuels and Jeffrey (1966) and Jeffrey and Samuels (1967) examined the problem of learning words and then transferring this knowledge to new words. Their reports are rather complicated but the experiments are neat. They indicate quite strongly that the words we train our children on have important repercussions during the next stage of word identification. For example, they suggest that if we select words which are highly similar, the child will become accustomed to make fine discriminations—and he can only do this by looking at *all* the letters—whereas if we select words quite dissimilar from one another, the child when he comes to identify new words will be more likely to attempt this by looking at less than the total number of letters. Incidentally, this is one of the less desirable consequences of look-and-say.

The significance of these experiments is that they suggest an answer to the very common problem of children, in the middle stages of learning to read, who will persist in recognizing words by reduced cues when there are no other constraints, semantic or syntactic, to enable cued guessing. For example *then* for *there*, *the table* for *the tablet*. These experiments strongly emphasize the fact that it is the teacher's task to prevent this by so arranging the words used in the training sessions that the child is forced to consider every letter in the word. This will establish a set for fine distinctions between words. The *Royal Road Readers*, Book I; parts 1 and 2, attempt to do this.

Familiarization is another aspect of learning which has been applied to reading skill. What it amounts to is that the child should be familiar with some at least of the basic factors in any new learning or problem-solving situation. Muehl (1960) showed the positive effects of previous training on words of similar construction in learning to read new words.

Samuels (1966), Strickland (1962), Ruddell (1965) and Lefevre (1964) all apply this notion to the context of children's readers, and they stress the fact that it should closely resemble the language patterns of the children themselves, so that confusion is avoided and the flow of ideas is unimpeded. Bernstein (1961) has demonstrated the existence of two types of language which each child possesses in varying degrees: the elaborated code of formal language, as represented in books and formal relation-ships, and the restricted code used for intimate personal communication, as in the language of play and intimate relationships. In addition to this, Postman and Conger (1954) make the point that usage of words, as op-posed to merely seeing them in print, plays an important part in speed of recognition. Hence the need for a rigorous programme of speech develop-ment alongside the reading programme in order that the child may use words and, equally important, develop through new relationships a famili-arity with the elaborate code which he will have to interpret in his reading books. Furthermore, this should be matched wherever possible with the selection of reading books which bear a closer affinity with the language facility of the child.

Indeed, one wonders whether we do not apply the wrong procedure when we begin too soon to ask children in the early stages of reading to look at print and then supply a verbal interpretation of the symbols: would it not be better to ensure that the child knows the verbal context *before* he looks at the print? The horse is then put before the cart and doing so will ensure that the child is at least familiar with, if not practised in, the language patterns of the text.

The content of basic reading books

The research of Miller and Isard (1963) shows that it is the semantic and syntactic constraints in a sentence that makes it intelligible and memorable. '*The boy spoke a triangle* is grammatical, but semantically anomalous.' We can take this further. The writer has noticed amongst a small group of five year olds an ability to read with greater fluency from their school basic reader than from parallel books in other series in the home, even when there has been preparatory work on the words but not the language structure in the home books. The apparently obvious conclusion is that the difficulty lies in the interpretation of the meaning or structure of the language.

From this a problem emerges. Is it advisable during the early and critical stages of learning to read—books 1 to 4 level—to restrict a child to one set of basic readers and their accompanying supplementary books in order to avoid semantic and/or syntactic confusion or should several sets of reading books be used in order to induce a set for diversity? If the latter course is accepted, then steps should be taken to introduce the child to the variations, rather than wait until he stumbles upon them.

Another problem concerns the use of pictures in reading primers. Every-one loves to look at an interesting picture, but the fundamental question is whether the pictures function as distracting stimuli. Samuels (1967) demonstrates that they do divert attention and give incorrect cues and, furthermore, he demonstrates that in the case of poor readers pictures of the type used in primers impede learning. In the case of the more skilled readers, the pictures made no significant difference. This experiment should not be used as an argument against having books with beautiful pictures; it does, however, indicate that the actual book on which the child is practising during the early stages may not be the appropriate place for pictures.

There are many other things that could be said about the paucity of content in most of the widely used primers in the United Kingdom. We are all aware of the mutilation of the English language that takes place in the laborious and tedious pursuit of a 'controlled' vocabulary. However, that could form another paper in itself.

Reflection–impulsivity

Finally, a new field of investigation has been opened by Kagan (1965, 1966), who distributes human beings along a reflection–impulsivity dimension. He contends that the impulsive child who does not pause to consider the alternative hypotheses in a word identification or recognition situation is less accurate in word recognition than the reflective child who does actively consider the alternative answers.

This is a very interesting proposition for it suggests that a considerable proportion of children may benefit from specific training in reflection. For example, when he impulsively reacts to a word, the teacher might indicate to the child the alternatives which could be considered. Indeed, we may ask ourselves whether in emphasizing rapid responses to words and stressing the desirability of quicker reading, we are not discouraging the very children who are doing what should be expected of them, that is, considering all the reasonable alternatives to the problem.

Conclusion

A survey of research on reading illustrates how little research work there is into the more fundamental aspects of learning to read. However, it is hoped that the work referred to in this paper indicates the advent of a more hopeful era of research.

To summarize the implications of this research, I think we should give more thought to the preparatory period—the period of letter discrimination, word and sound awareness where look-and-say has a proper part to play, and the introduction to the skill of listening. Secondly, the attitudes which we foster to the performance of the various skills will crucially affect the way in which a child attacks a word: whether he looks for alternative hypotheses and is prepared to reject and replace initial decisions. Thirdly, we should proceed from Gibson's work to look for ways of teaching children to develop and process their awareness and use of the critical units of language, so that it is not left entirely to the child to find his own ways of 'building up words'. And perhaps above all we should pay more attention to the development of the language of children and to the adaptation of both books and teaching to meet the needs of all children.

References

BERNSTEIN, B. (1961) Social structure, language and learning *Educational Research* 3, 163–76

BIRCH, H. G. and BELMONT, L. (1964) Auditory–visual integration in normal and retarded readers *American Journal of Orthopsychiatry* 34, 852–61

BIRCH, H. G. and BELMONT, L. (1965) Auditory–visual integration, intelligence and reading ability in school children *Perceptual-Motor Skills* 20, 295–305

BLANK, M. and BRIDGER, W. H. (1966) Deficiencies in verbal labelling in retarded readers *American Journal of Orthopsychiatry* 36, 840–47

BLOOMFIELD, L. (1961) Teaching children to read in L. Bloomfield and C. L. Barnhart *Let's Read: A Linguistic Approach* Detroit: Wayne State University Press

BLOOMFIELD, L. and BARNHART, C. L. (1961) *Let's Read: A Linguistic Approach* Detroit: Wayne State University Press

CATTELL, J. McK. (1885) The inertia of the eye and brain *Brain* 8, 295–312

*CHALL, J., ROSWELL, F. G. and BLUMENTHAL, S. H. (1963) Auditory blending ability: a factor in success in beginning reading *The Reading Teacher* November

DANIELS, J. C. and DIACK, H. (1960) *Royal Road Readers* London: Chatto and Windus

DODGE, R. (1906) Recent studies in the correlation of eye movement and visual perception *Psychological Bulletin* 3, 85–92

DURRELL, D. *et al* (1958) Success in first grade reading *Journal of Education* 140, 1–48

FOWLER, W. (1964) Structural dimensions of the learning process in early reading *Child Development* 35, 1093–1104

FRIES, C. C., WILSON, R. G. and RUDOLPH, M. K. (1966) *The Merrill Linguistic Readers* Columbus: Merrill Books

*GIBSON, E. J., GIBSON, J. J., PICK, A. D. and OSSER, H. (1962) A developmental study of the discrimination of letter-like forms *Journal of Comparative Physiology and Psychology* 55, 897–906

GIBSON, E. J., PICK, A., OSSER, H. and HAMMOND, M. (1962) The role of grapheme–phoneme correspondence in the perception of words *American Journal of Psychology* 75, 554–70

GIBSON, E. J., OSSER, H. and PICK, A. (1963) A study of the development of grapheme–phoneme correspondences *Journal of Verbal Learning and Verbal Behaviour* 2, 142–6

GIBSON, E. J., BISHOP, C. H., SCHIFF, W. and SMITH, J. (1964) *Journal of Experimental Psychology* 67, 173

GIBSON, E. J. (1967) Learning to read in N. S. Endler, L. R. Boultes and H. Osser (eds) *Contemporary Issues in Developmental Psychology* London: Holt, Rinehart and Winston

Geoffrey R. Roberts

HARLOW, H. F. (1949) The formation of learning sets *Psychological Review* 56, 51–65

JEFFREY, W. E. and SAMUELS, S. J. (1967) Effect of method of reading training on initial learning and transfer *Journal of Verbal Learning and Verbal Behaviour* 6, 354–8

*KAGAN, J. (1965) Reflection—impulsivity and reading ability *Child Development* 36, 609–29

KAGAN, J. (1966) Developmental studies in reflection and analysis in J. H. Kidd and A. H. Rivoire (eds) *Perceptual Development in Children* London: University of London Press

KOLERS, P. A. and KATZMAN, M. T (1963) Paper presented before the Psychonomic Society, August 1963

LANGMAN, M. P. (1960) The reading process: a descriptive, interdisciplinary approach *Genetic Psychology Monograph* 62, 3–40

*LEFEVRE, C. A. (1964) *Linguistics and the Teaching of Reading* New York: McGraw-Hill

LEVIN, H., BAUN, E. and BOSTWICK, S. (1963) in E. J. Gibson, H. Osser, W. Schiff and J. Smith *A Basic Research Programme on Reading* Project 639 Office of Education, Department of Health, Education and Welfare USA

LEVIN, H. and WATSON, J. (1963) in E. J. Gibson, H. Osser, W. Schiff and J. Smith *A Basic Research Programme on Reading* Project 639 Office of Education, Department of Health, Education and Welfare, USA

MILLER, G. A. (1956) The magical number seven, plus or minus two: some limits on our capacity for processing information *Psychological Review* 63, 81–97

MILLER, G. A. and ISARD, S. (1963) Some perceptual consequences of linguistic rules *Journal of Verbal Learning and Verbal Behaviour* 2, 217–28

MUEHL, S. (1960) The effects of visual discrimination pretraining on learning to read a vocabulary list in kindergarten children *Journal of Educational Psychology* 51, 217–21

NEWMAN, E. (1966) Speed of reading when the span of letters is restricted *American Journal of Psychology* 79, 272–7

OLSON, A. (1963) Phonics and success in beginning reading *Journal of Developmental Reading* 6, 256–60

POSTMAN, L. and CONGER, B. (1954) Verbal habits and the visual recognition of words *Science* 119, 671–3

REID, J. F. (1966) Learning to think about reading *Educational Research* 9, 56–62

*ROBERTS, G. R. and LUNZER, E. A. (1968) Reading and learning to read in E. A. Lunzer and J. F. Morris *Development in Learning Volume 2* London: Staples Press

RUDDELL, R. B. (1965) The effect of oral and written patterns of language structure on reading comprehension *The Reading Teacher* 1, 270–75

SAMUELS, S. J. (1966) Effect of experimentally learned word associations on the acquisition of reading responses *Journal of Educational Psychology* 57, 159–63

SAMUELS, S. J. (1967) Attentional process in reading: the effect of pictures on the acquisition of reading responses *Journal of Educational Psychology* 58, 337–42

SAMUELS, S. J. and JEFFREY, W. E. (1966) Discriminability of words and letter cues used in learning to read *Journal of Educational Psychology* 57, 337–40

*STRICKLAND, R. G. (1962) The language of elementary school children: its relationship to the language of reading textbooks and the quality of reading of selected children *Bulletin of the School of Education* 38, 4 Bloomington: Indiana University

TANSLEY, A. E. (1967) *Reading and Remedial Reading* London: Routledge and Kegan Paul

Bibliography

ABLEWHITE, R. C. (1967) *The Slow Reader* London: Heinemann
BRITTON, J. N. (1970) *Language and Learning* London: Allen Lane Penguin Press
BUTCHER, H. J. (1970) *Human Intelligence: Its Nature and Assessment* London: Methuen
DECHANT, E. (1971) (ed) *The Detection and Correction of Reading Difficulties* New York: Appleton-Century-Crofts
DOWNING, J. A. and THACKRAY, D. V. (1971) *Reading Readiness* London: University of London Press
GAHAGAN, D. M. and GAHAGAN, G. A. (1970) *Talk Reform: Explorations in language for infant school children* London: Routledge
HARRIS, A. J. (1961) *How to Increase Reading Ability* New York: Longman
HOGGART, R. (1957) *The Uses of Literacy* London: Chatto and Windus; Penguin 1968
HOLT, J. (1964) *How Children Fail* London: Pitman; Penguin 1969
LEE, W. R. (1957) *Spelling Irregularity and Reading Difficulty in English* Slough: National Foundation for Educational Research
KIRK, S. A. (1966) *Diagnosis and Remediation of Psycholinguistic Disabilities* Urbana: University of Illinois Press
LERNER, J. W. (1971) *Children with Learning Disabilities: Theories, Diagnosis and Teaching Strategies* Boston: Houghton Mifflin
MILES, T. R. (1970) *On Helping the Dyslexic Child* London: Methuen
NATCHEZ, G. (1968) *Children with Reading Problems* New York: Basic Books
RAVENETTE, A. T. (1968) *Dimensions of Reading Difficulties* Oxford: Pergamon
RAWSON, M. B. (1968) *Developmental Language Disability* Baltimore: Johns Hopkins Press
SPACHE, G. D. (1969) *Reading Disability and Perception* Newark, Delaware: International Reading Association
STRANG, R. (1969) *Diagnostic Teaching of Reading* New York: McGraw Hill